The Ultimate Guide to Clean, Cleaner, and Cleanest Foods

EAT CLEAN, STAY LEAN

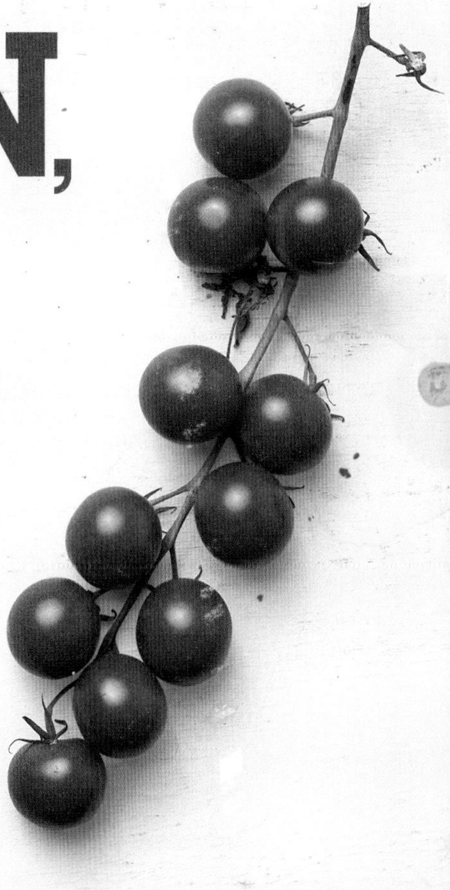

The editors of
Prevention
with Wendy Bazilian, DrPh, RD

RODALE

This book is intended as a reference volume only, not as a medical manual. The information given here is designed to help you make informed decisions about your health. It is not intended as a substitute for any treatment that may have been prescribed by your doctor. If you suspect that you have a medical problem, we urge you to seek competent medical help.

Mention of specific companies, organizations, or authorities in this book does not imply endorsement by the author or publisher, nor does mention of specific companies, organizations, or authorities imply that they endorse this book, its author, or the publisher.

Internet addresses and telephone numbers given in this book were accurate at the time it went to press.

Rodale books may be purchased for business or promotional use or for special sales.
For information, please write to:
Special Markets Department, Rodale Inc., 733 Third Avenue, New York, NY 10017.

Prevention is a registered trademark of Rodale Inc.

Printed in the United States of America
Rodale Inc. makes every effort to use acid-free ♾, recycled paper ♲.

Art direction and book design by Amy C. King
Photographs by Mitch Mandel/Rodale Images except "not clean" image on page 56 © Corbis
Food styling recipes: Khalil Hymore
Food styling categories: Chelsea Zimmer
Food styling cover: Chris Barsch
Prop styling recipes: Kira Corbin

Library of Congress Cataloging-in-Publication Data is on file with the publisher.
ISBN-13: 978-1-62336-528-8

Distributed to the trade by Macmillan

2 4 6 8 10 9 7 5 3 1 paperback

RODALE.

We inspire and enable people to improve their lives and the world around them.
rodalebooks.com

*To anyone who eats clean,
has tried to eat clean,
or has even once thought about
eating clean.
You inspire and motivate us.*

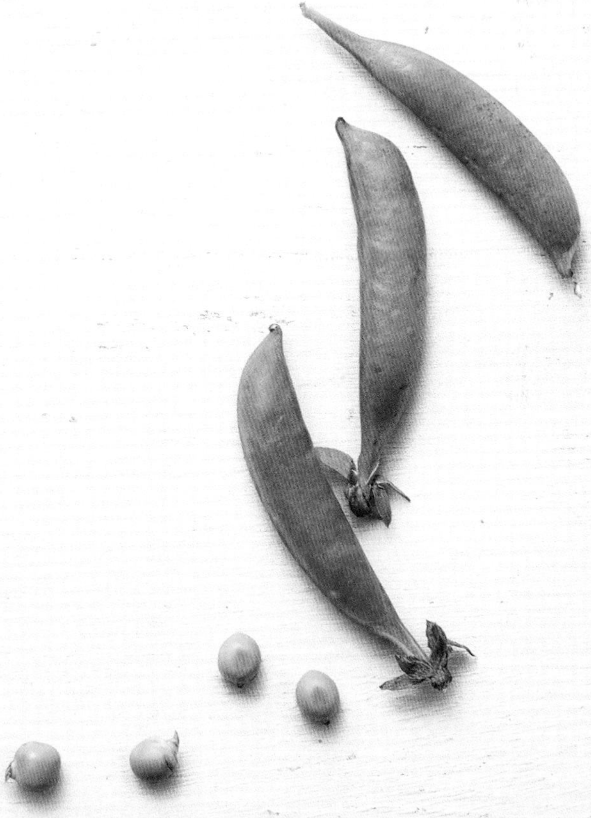

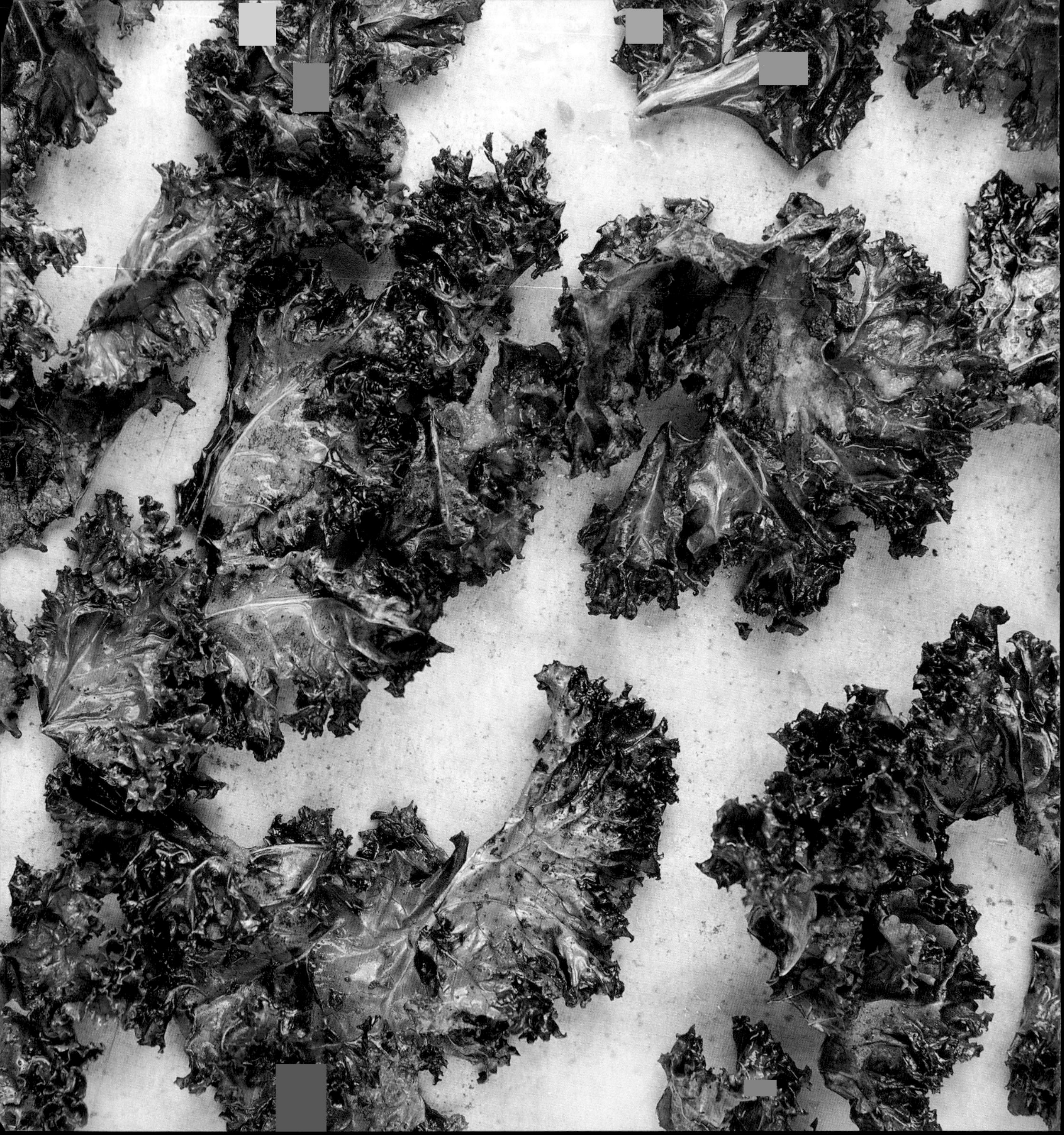

CONTENTS

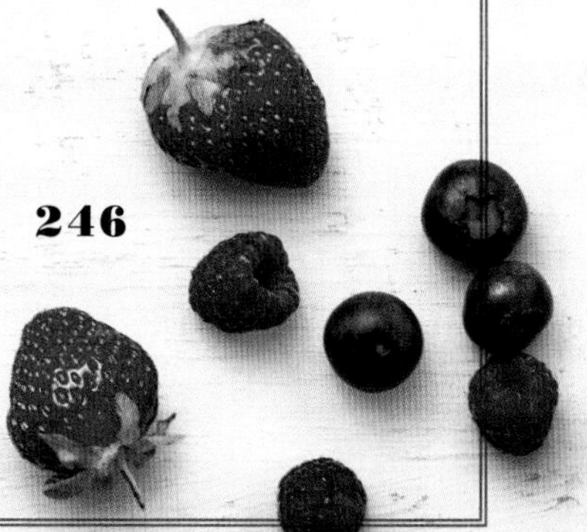

The single best investment you can make daily for your health is to *eat well*. Eating well is about eating quality foods, in delicious combinations, on a regular basis, giving you energy to run on, mental clarity to make those 1,001 daily decisions, and a glow that reflects your inner beauty and overall health. As a doctor of public health, a registered dietitian, and a certified exercise physiologist, I constantly evaluate scientific research on health so that I can help people come up with solid, practical food and fitness solutions for the real world we live in. With my clients, we talk about food a lot, from the freshest produce to the most overprocessed, packaged stuff. And we look at food labels. But my favorite foods are those without a label: The cleanest foods you can eat are real foods themselves—whole, fresh foods that haven't been highly processed, refined, and poured into big boxes, crinkly bags, or shiny wrappers. Research shows that these whole, foods are the best at creating, restoring, and preserving the healthiest bodies.

Real whole foods come first, but what about convenience? Packaged foods made up of more than one ingredient make life easier, for sure—and, fortunately, there are plenty of clean options out there—you just need to know how to find them. The pages ahead will help you navigate the *bazilians* of choices in the places you like to shop so that you can learn to distinguish those clean nutritional superstars from the imposters. It's really pretty simple—and fun—once you get the hang of it. The best part is that you will feel and see the rewards quickly as you journey toward an energized, vital, and leaner you.

At the end of the day, the pleasure from eating flavorful food feels so good! And ultimately, while being healthy itself is a compelling goal, you know you probably won't stick with a plan if it doesn't also taste delicious. Great news: Clean foods, prepared creatively like the recipes you'll find inside, will tantalize your taste buds, too.

Enjoy each step—and bite—of your clean-eating journey!

Wendy Bazilian, DrPH, RD

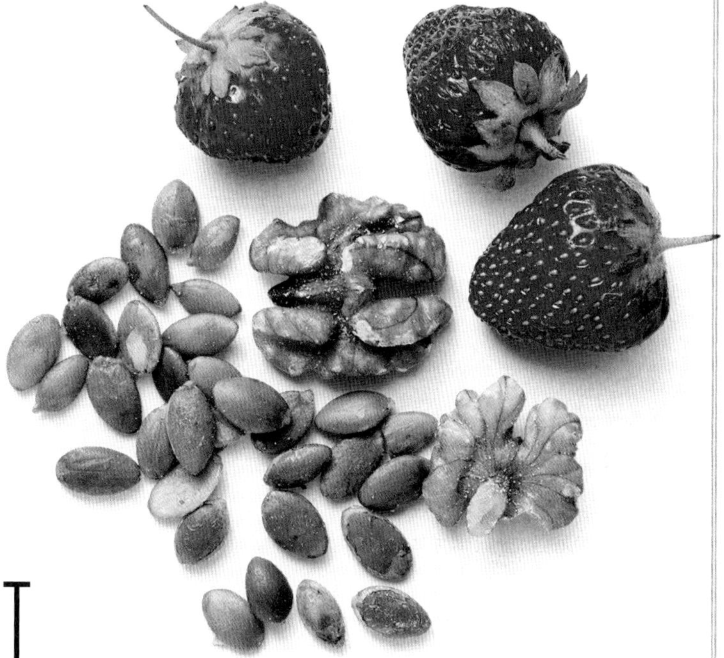

WHAT IS CLEAN EATING?

You've undoubtedly seen it on magazine covers and heard it rolling out of the mouths of celebrities, athletes, nutritionists, maybe even some of your friends. But what the heck does "clean eating" really mean? If you're confused, you're not alone. In today's world, we're all bombarded with so much information about different diets, new food studies, and food-packaging labels that seem to promise big but hidden health benefits—gluten-free, sugar-free, Paleo-friendly, low-fat, high-fiber, all-natural, organic, grass-fed, the list goes on—that it's hard to know what to put in your mouth on a daily basis, let alone what to buy for the week.

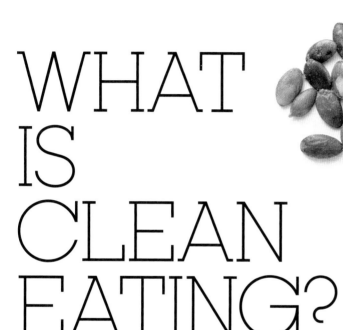

THE WHOLE STORY

Throughout this book, you'll hear a lot about "whole foods." They're at the core of the clean-eating lifestyle, but what are they, exactly? Whole foods are foods like fresh fruits, vegetables, unprocessed meats and fish, and unrefined grains—unadulterated foods that are straight from the earth and nature. They are pure, untouched, and full of the nutrients your body needs to thrive. By definition, whole foods have not been refined in any way and nothing's been added to them, so they do not contain any added sugar, salt, fat, preservatives, or chemicals.

On the opposite end of the spectrum, processed foods are far from natural—they result when whole foods are manipulated into other products, and they usually bear little resemblance to their original, natural state. Many processed foods contain artificial ingredients and often lack nutrients and contain excess or added sugar, fat, or salt. Unfortunately, many of the snack foods, prepared meals, and drinks we reach for today are highly processed to last longer on store shelves. If a food is in a package, chances are it's been processed in some way.

But unlike traditional and fad diets, eating clean isn't just shopping for one food label or eating a specific way, where you give up gluten or dairy, or start slashing calories, carbs, or sodium. "Eating clean" has nearly replaced "eating healthy" in how we talk about food. And the reason so many people are talking about it is that it's simple to do, not a fad, and best of all—it makes you feel *and* look great.

So what is clean eating? While the term means different things to different people, the root of it all is the effort to consume as many whole foods as possible that have undergone as little processing as possible—foods that look and taste like they came fresh out of the ground or from a tree, a farm, the ocean, or even someone's kitchen, not like they are fresh off the conveyor belt of a factory. Eating clean means choosing foods that don't have a ton of (or any) added chemicals like pesticides, herbicides, preservatives, or artificial sweeteners, flavors, and colors. For many, eating clean also means trying to eat organic and local whenever possible.

A diet rich in unprocessed whole foods automatically increases your intake of vitamins, nutrients, minerals, and phytochemicals, and decreases unhealthy fats, added sugar, excess sodium, chemicals, pesticides, and preservatives. In short, clean eating is a simple and delicious way to stay lean, healthy, and feeling great.

But clean eating isn't just about health and weight loss—it's about enjoying more of the foods you eat every day. Clean eating opens your diet up to a delicious and fresher array of flavors and textures. You'll start to crave garden-picked fruits and vegetables, hearty whole grains, savory beans, crunchy seeds and nuts, filling cuts of lean meat, and just-off-the-boat seafood. You'll feel fuller and more satisfied eating clean, which means you'll naturally want to avoid all the fried foods, sugary treats, and processed junk found in the Standard American Diet (SAD, for short). We know all this because while the idea of clean eating has grown in popularity lately, the practice is hardly new: Before Western society turned toward eating more and more processed foods, most of our ancestors ate clean without even trying or thinking about it—and they were naturally thinner, had lower incidence of chronic disease, and likely had more energy as a result.

The purpose of this book is to show you the many benefits of eating delicious, nutrient-rich foods, not only for your health and waistline, but also for your taste buds—and energy levels, sleep quality, skin, hair, and overall mood. Best of all, choosing whole and minimally processed foods in the supermarket, at restaurants, and when you're traveling or out with friends and family is easy—and rewarding—when you know what to look for, and *Eat Clean, Stay Lean* makes it easy by showing you which common foods to reach for at stores, restaurants, and even in your own home: Consider it your shopping and everywhere dining guidebook. You'll learn how a diet of whole foods benefits your body, controls your appetite, triggers weight loss, and contributes to better overall well-being. You'll understand how "foods" with mile-long ingredient lists and toxic additives are closer to a science experiment than a culinary creation, and affect your body in ways nature never intended. You'll learn that nutrients added to processed foods won't cancel out all the crap, and don't even come close to matching the power and quality of naturally packaged vitamins, minerals, and antioxidants in whole foods. You'll understand why going organic is important, and you'll see how mindful eating and an active lifestyle perfectly round out a diet of clean foods.

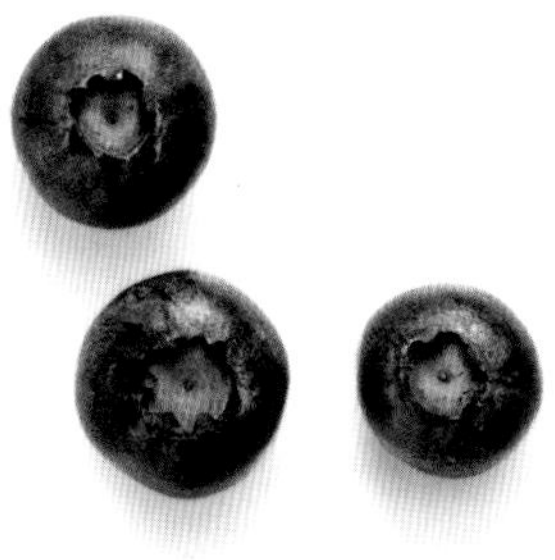

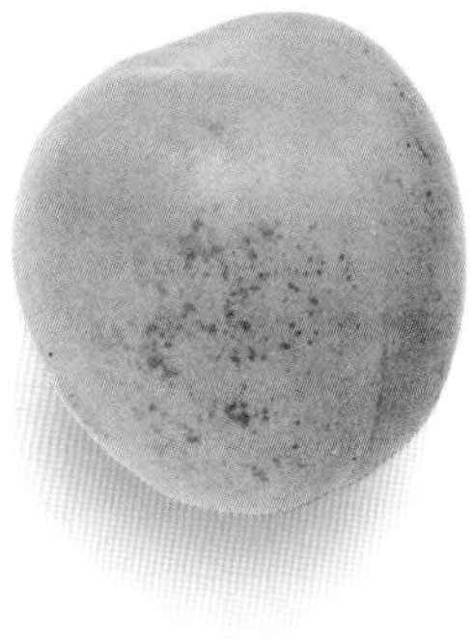

 INTRODUCTION

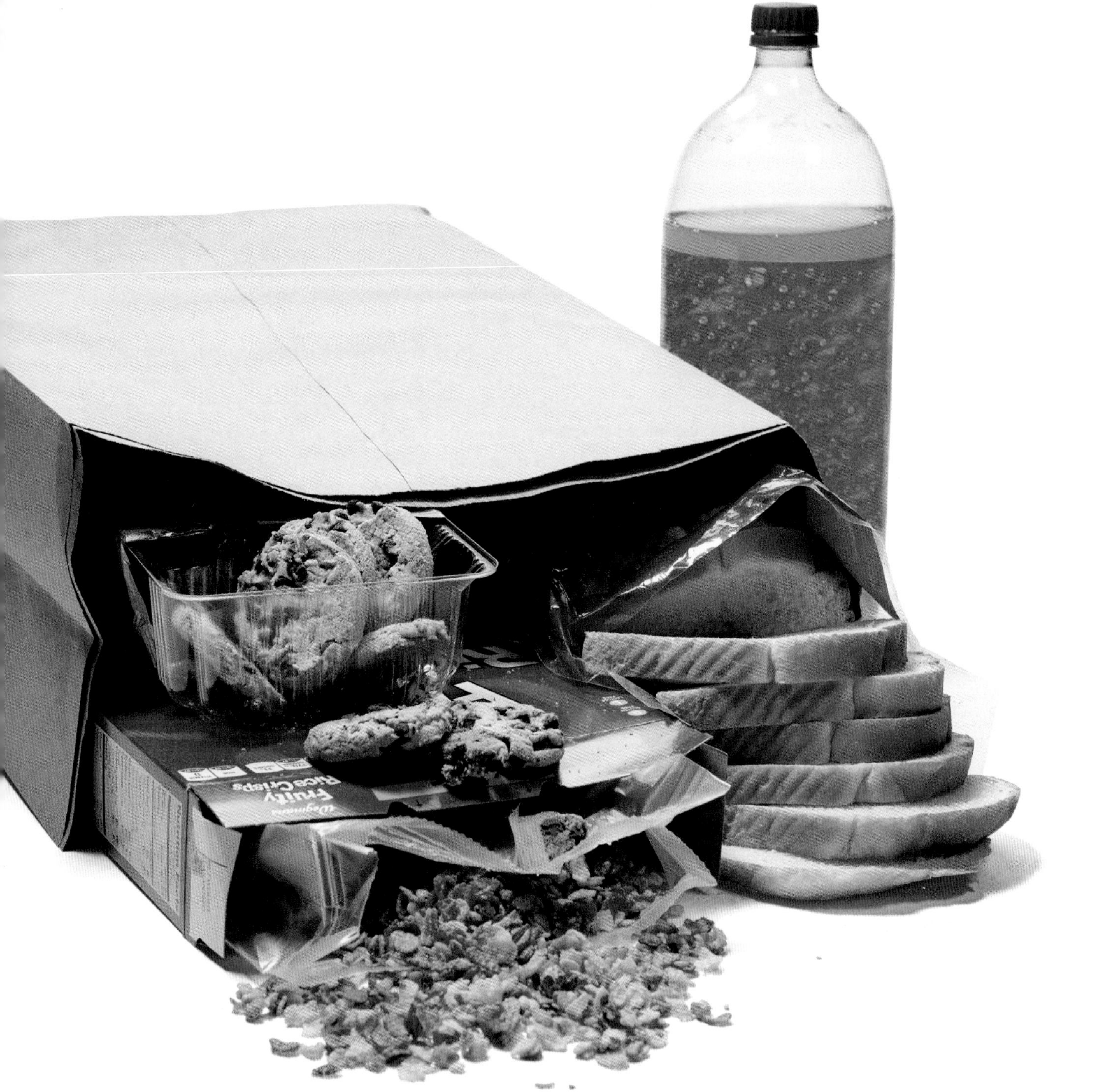
Wegmans
Fruity
Rice Crisps

PART 1

The Ultimate Diet for Health and Weight Loss

Are you ready? You're about to learn some not-so-savory things about much of the food sold on grocery store shelves. For starters, it's making you fat and sick. The good news: We've got your back, and a bunch of solutions to keep you slim and healthy. Here, we'll help you understand just what makes a clean food clean and how to avoid the marketing hype of processed junk in disguise—nope, not all those promising labels are actually worth paying attention to. (High-fiber? Pass!) Plus, we'll provide loads of practical tips to make clean eating easier, even if you don't have the time or money to spend your days whipping up organic meals from scratch. We think—nah, we know—you're ready. Let's get started!

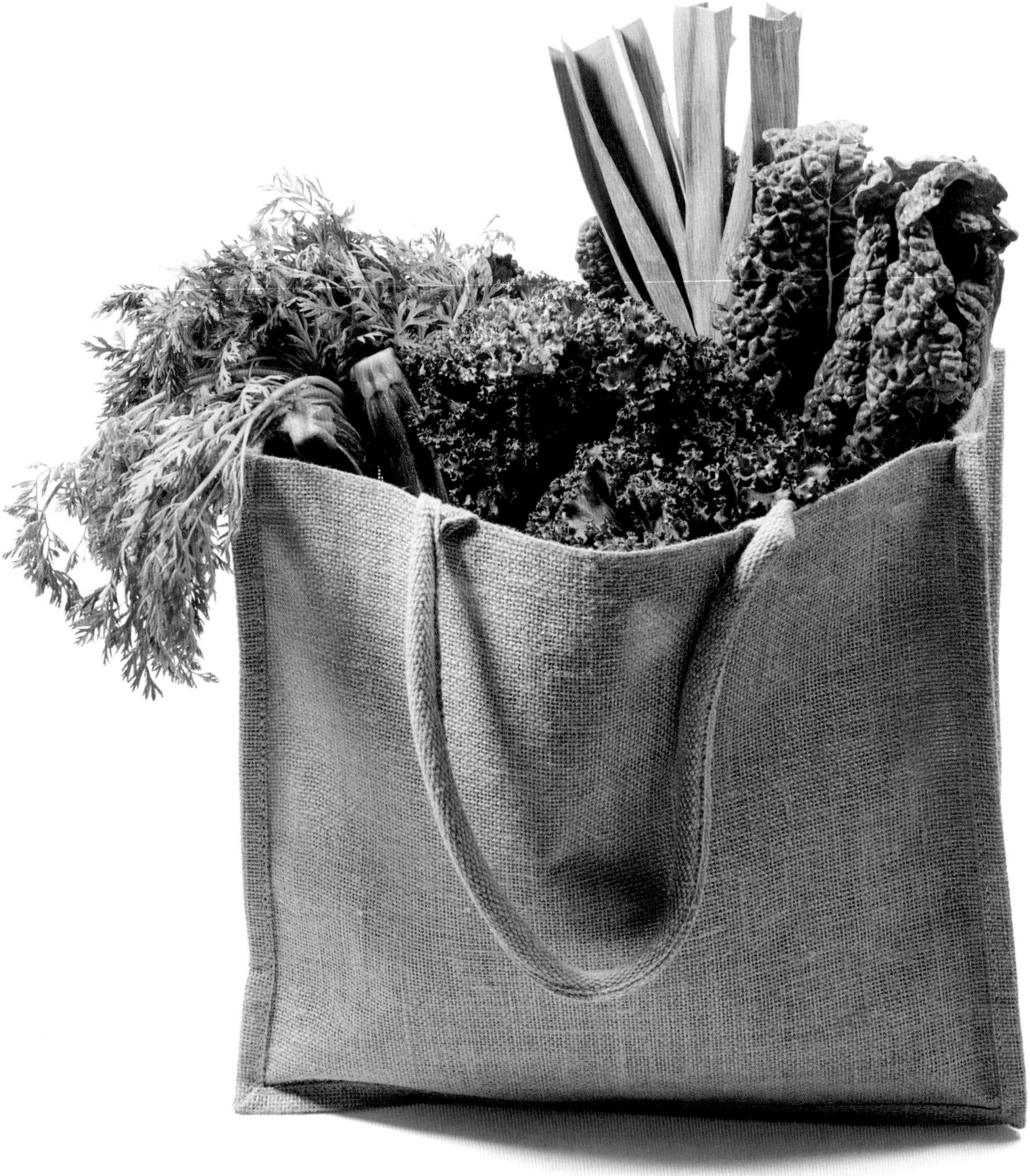

CHAPTER 1

The Benefits of Clean Eating

Step one in becoming a convert to clean eating is simply understanding how eating "dirty" processed food harms your body. You'll probably be pretty grossed out, and even a little outraged, which primes you perfectly for step two—learning how to choose whole and minimally processed foods that fight various diseases, optimize your metabolism, improve your appearance and energy, and even protect our oceans, air, and soil from dangerous pollution. This new understanding of how what you eat affects everything around you (and within you) will unleash you from the mental and physical grip of processed junk, and open you up to the possibility of a healthier, slimmer, more vibrant life.

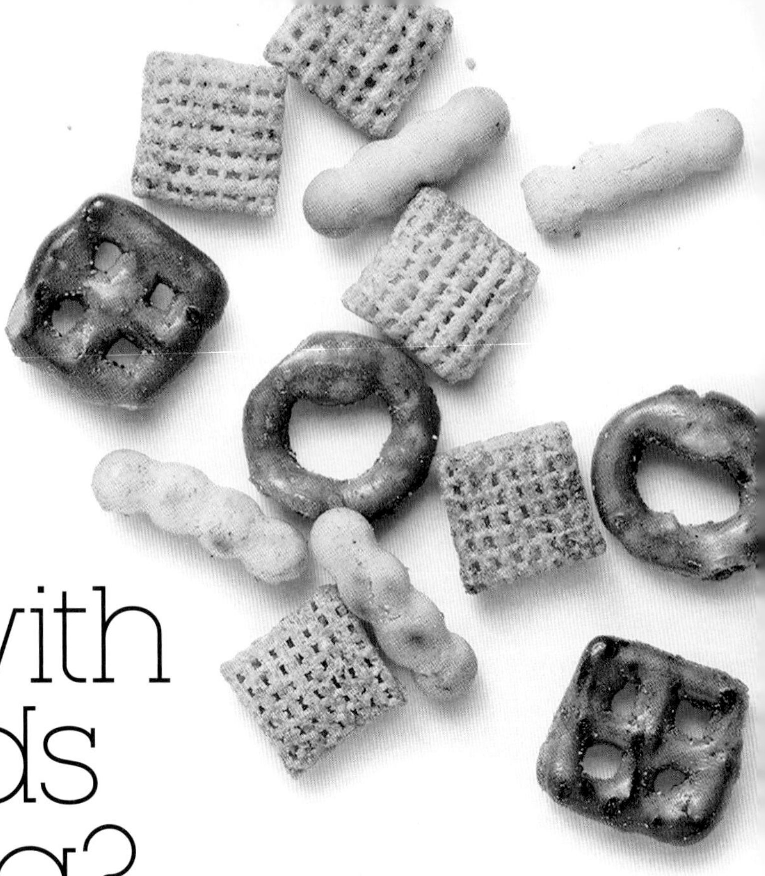

What's Wrong with the Foods I'm Eating?

In the last 100 years or so, Western society has gone from eating mostly whole foods to consuming mostly heavily processed and packaged foods—and the result has been more sugar, salt, refined carbohydrates, and trans fat (which didn't really exist in our food supply before the onset of processed foods) in our collective diets. All this junk, in turn, has made us fatter, sicker, more lethargic, and more dependent on prescription medications. It may seem innocent enough, but many of us don't even realize how our simple, everyday decisions—like reaching for that bag of potato chips instead of some fresh, crunchy carrots, or going for that box of sugary, white-flour crackers instead of a piece of warm, crusty whole-grain bread—are impacting our health in big, scary ways. Here's how highly processed foods are affecting your life—and your future.

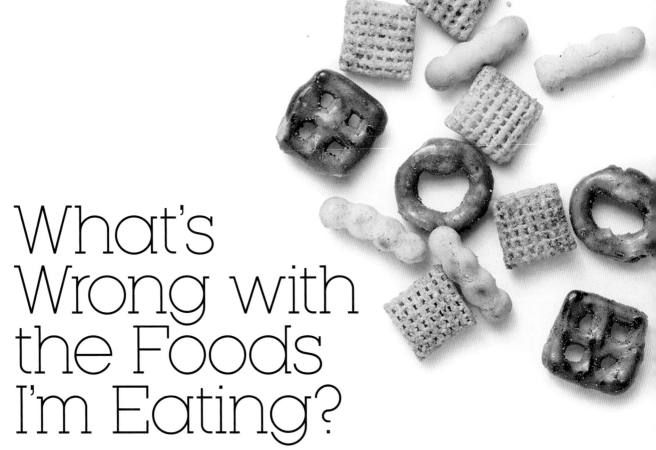

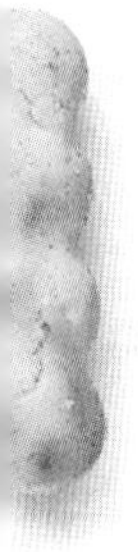

They're Dangerous to Your Health

Yep, you read that right: Lots of the packaged or processed foods that many of us eat every day are actually bad for our bodies and contain ingredients that can make us sick. Perhaps the most toxic ingredient is sugar, found in nearly every packaged food, even those you wouldn't think contain it, like pasta sauce, salad dressing, and canned soup. Then, there are additives that are actually toxic in large amounts—known and possible carcinogens used as preservatives, emulsifiers, and stabilizers. Let's not forget about artificial colors, sweeteners, and flavors, which have been linked to a bevy of health problems, including behavioral problems in children, obesity, even heart disease. Many "healthy" foods, like energy bars, sandwich meats, buttery spreads, and crackers, contain hidden trans fats, linked to heart disease, inflammation, and other major health problems—and even those that say they're trans fat–free can boast harmful amounts of it (learn how to spot sneaky trans fats on page 6). You want to talk about salt? Many processed foods will wallop you with upwards of half your recommended daily sodium intake in one serving. And you're getting all this sugar, chemicals, unhealthy fat, and salt without very many naturally occurring vitamins, minerals, fibers, and antioxidants, meaning you're just sucking up empty calories—and doing nothing for your health and well-being.

These are all reasons why consuming a typical Western diet, with large amounts of highly refined grains, high-sugar drinks and dairy products, and processed meats, has led to an increase in preventable illnesses like heart

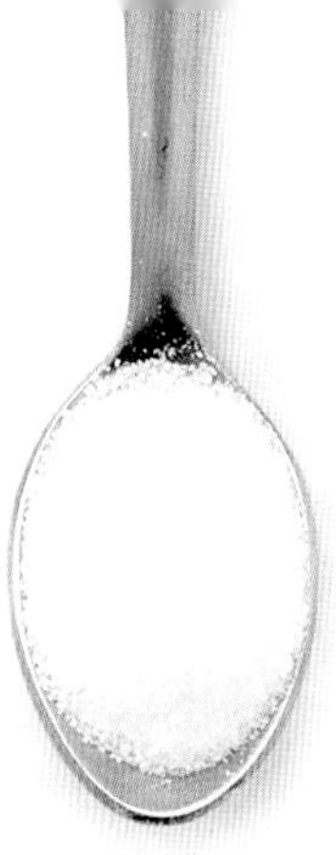

YOUR BODY ON SUGAR

One of the biggest toxins in the Standard American Diet (SAD) is sugar. Here's how getting too much (more than 24 grams for women and 36 grams for men) can mess with nearly every body part:

BRAIN: A sugar-loaded diet can rewire your brain's pathways, and up your risk of depression by 58%.

JOINTS: Sugar pumps inflammatory cytokines into your bloodstream, which can exacerbate arthritis.

HEART: Sugar inflames the linings of arteries, increasing your risk of stroke and heart attack.

SKIN: When you eat too much sugar, proteins incorporate it into skin structure, causing wrinkles.

GENITALS: Excess sugar impairs blood flow, upping women's risk of sexual arousal disorders.

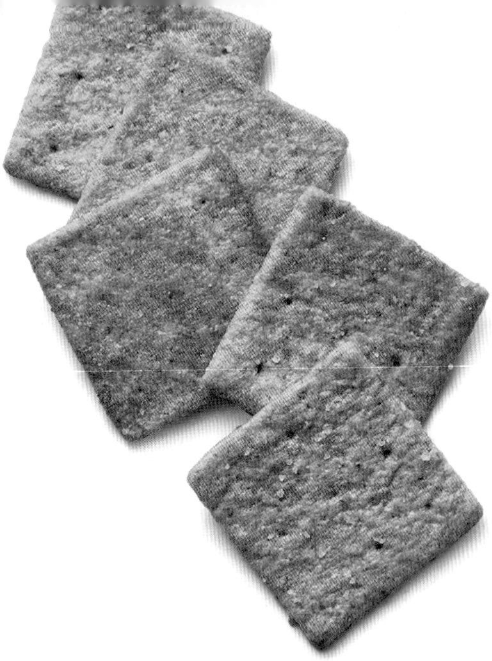

disease, diabetes, obesity, and some cancers. In particular, research has linked the Standard American Diet to high blood pressure, as well as heart disease, cancer, and diabetes. Yikes, right?! And while your genes and family history certainly play a role in your health, eliminating processed foods and committing to eating more whole foods are important steps to living a long, healthy life.

They Contribute to Weight Gain

Packaged and processed foods are actually extremely inefficient at powering you through the day. In fact, a diet full of these can make your weight skyrocket, and mood and energy levels plummet, because despite the calories, you're not actually being nourished. What you *are* getting when you down a soda, granola bar, or bagel is a shot of added sugar and refined carbohydrates—carbs usually made from wheat or corn that's been stripped of all nutrients (fiber, B vitamins, healthy oils) except for its highly digestible starch or sugar. These types of foods may not only contribute to heart disease, obesity, and diabetes, but their more immediate effects can be pretty dramatic, too—because they're quickly broken down, they spike blood sugar, which can result in ravenous cravings, fatigue, slower metabolism, bloating, and even mood swings. Whole grains like brown rice and whole fruits and veggies, on the other hand, leave all nutrients intact, and don't result in a blood sugar roller coaster.

What's really unfair, though, is that even savory stuff, like tomato sauce, salad dressing, crackers, and pizza, can contain added sugar, often in the form of high fructose corn syrup (HFCS), that will set you

SPOT SNEAKY TRANS FATS

The label on your box of multigrain crackers may claim to have 0 gram of trans fats, but don't be fooled. This lab-made fat that's been linked to diabetes and heart disease is still found in one in ten packaged foods, according to recent research, even if the label says it doesn't contain any. How can that be? Companies are allowed to say a food has 0 gram if it contains less than 0.5 gram per serving. Until 2018—when companies and restaurants will no longer be able to use trans fat in their foods—avoid products with "partially hydrogenated oils" in the ingredient list.

up to fail. While the fructose naturally found in fruit is easily recognized and broken down by the body, HFCS can only be metabolized by the liver, which breaks this sugar down directly into triglycerides and cholesterol that you end up storing in your liver and elsewhere in the body.

Of course, not all packaged and processed foods make you gain weight because they're loaded with calories and empty carbs—the artificial sweeteners in diet soda have been linked to weight gain, as well as the endocrine-disrupting phthalates and BPA in some food packaging, along with the residual hormones present in some animal products. Opting for whole foods and minimally processed packaged foods can help you avoid nearly all of this.

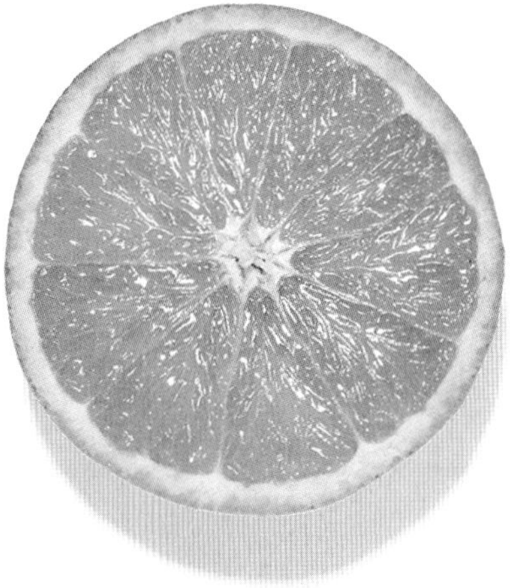

Whole Foods: The Benefits

Okay, enough of the doom and gloom!

It's easy—and delicious—to turn your health around and rectify the effects of the SAD. When you commit to eating mostly nutrient-dense, toxin-free whole foods, wonderful things start to happen. You will likely lose weight, your skin will be clearer and your hair fuller, you'll feel stronger and sleep better at night, you'll have more energy to exercise and do the things you love, and that's just the beginning. Eating more clean whole foods and less processed junk has been linked to improved digestion, lower blood pressure, healthier cholesterol levels, better mental health, and even mental clarity. Eating clean can help you prevent disease and even treat those illnesses that you may already be struggling with. After years of filling your body with toxins, trans fats, salt, sugar, and high fructose corn syrup, changing to a diet full of clean foods will likely result in increased energy and overall feelings of

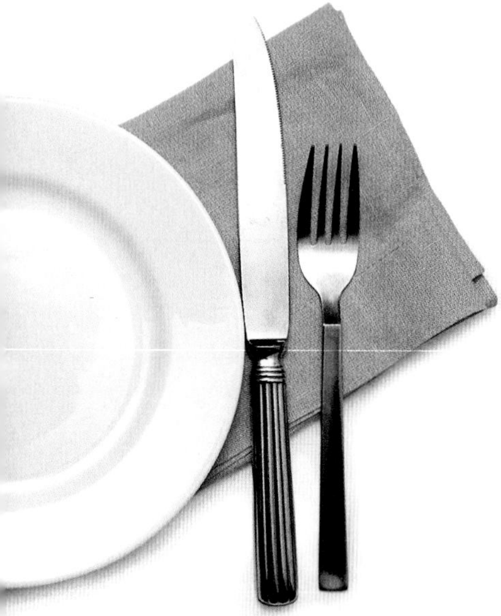

improved health. There are many ways clean eating can put you on the road to wellness—let's take a closer look.

They Help Keep You Slim

According to the Centers for Disease Control and Prevention, more than one-third of adults—or 78.6 million Americans—are obese. Obesity-related conditions include heart disease, stroke, type 2 diabetes, and most cancers. The good news? Many of these conditions are preventable, even reversible, by eating a diet of clean foods. Consuming a diet of mostly whole foods means you'll take in significantly fewer calories than you do on a diet of processed foods. Whole foods are also more "nutrient dense," which means they have more nutrients per calorie. For example, for the 30 calories in 1 cup of broccoli, you're getting a megadose of fiber, beta-carotene, vitamins C and B_6, potassium, antioxidants, and phytochemicals (healthy plant compounds). On the other hand, if you eat an "energy dense" food, one that is high in calories and low in nutrition, you'll get a lot less nutrition for a lot more calories: A bagel made from refined flour has more than 300 calories (not including toppings like cream cheese) and only trace amounts of vitamins and minerals. Not to mention, when you eat many processed and packaged foods, you'll also be ingesting things like preservatives, artificial sweeteners, chemicals from packaging, and pesticides that can mess with your hormones to stimulate appetite and slow metabolism.

Eating more nutrient-dense whole foods that are full of vitamins, minerals, phytochemicals, and antioxidants

WHAT IS MINDFUL EATING?

There's been a lot of buzz about mindful eating—that whole, "it's not all about what you eat, but how you eat it" mentality—that emphasizes slowing down and enjoying your meal. The perks: It may actually help you eat less and get you your optimal weight. But what exactly does it consist of? We could give you a dozen clever tips about dimming the lights and using a specific plate color, but essentially, it's all about slowing down to smell the pasta sauce. Simply focus on your food, not your phone; take mental note of how your meal tastes, feels, and smells; eat in a relaxed environment; and sit your butt down—no hovering over the kitchen sink!

will help crush cravings, rev up a slow metabolism, and trigger weight loss without feelings of hunger or deprivation. In fact, many people have a slower-than-optimal metabolism because they're low in essential nutrients such as magnesium, calcium, potassium, vitamin D, iron, and fiber—so when your body starts to regularly receive the right foods, your hunger signals and metabolism will respond accordingly. In addition to your body knowing it's receiving the nutrients it needs, the fiber, protein, and water found in clean foods help you feel full faster. These foods also take longer for your body to digest, so you'll be full for longer after eating a nutrient-dense meal or snack.

Perhaps one of the most positive benefits of clean eating is that you can eat more, and more frequently, without the negative results you'd get from eating processed foods. There's no dieting, starvation, or hunger strikes here: You can eat healthful foods whenever you want to and still lose weight.

They Reduce Inflammation

Sure, some inflammation is good—the acute kind is a form of self-protection, your body's immune response to a cut or pathogens entering the body. Chronic inflammation, however, the result of never-ending stress, being overweight, or a diet high in things like inflammatory sugar, trans fats, and various toxins, means that your body is constantly producing immune cells, which can damage the body. This inflammation has been associated with an increased risk of arthritis, diabetes, heart disease, high blood pressure, osteoporosis, and cancer. But while the wrong diet promotes excessive

WHAT'S MORE IMPORTANT: CLEAN EATING OR EXERCISE?

A proper diet and regular exercise are the two pillars of a healthy lifestyle. But that doesn't mean they're equally important when it comes to your weight, your disease risk, or how long you'll live. A recent editorial in the medical journal *BMJ* suggests that what you eat trumps how much you move. Why? Researchers point to the fact that during the past 30 years, physical activity rates haven't changed even as obesity and diabetes rates have skyrocketed. Sugar and refined carbohydrates, they say, are the biggest drivers of poor health and obesity. That said, regular exercise is *extremely* important if you want to live a long, healthy life. Many studies have shown physical activity safeguards your heart and brain from disease, including Alzheimer's; protects your joints; and even makes you more likely to stick to dietary changes.

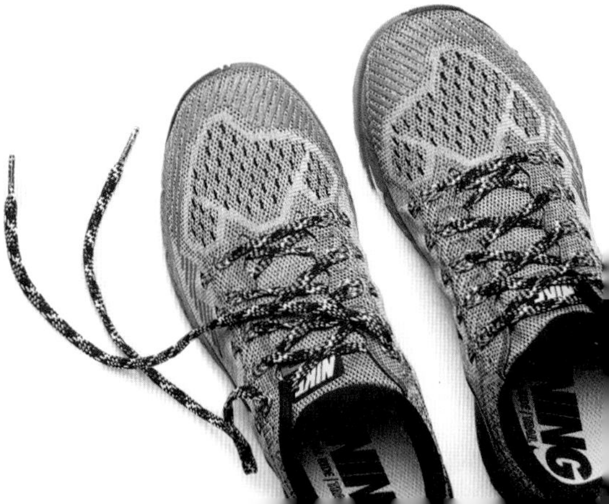

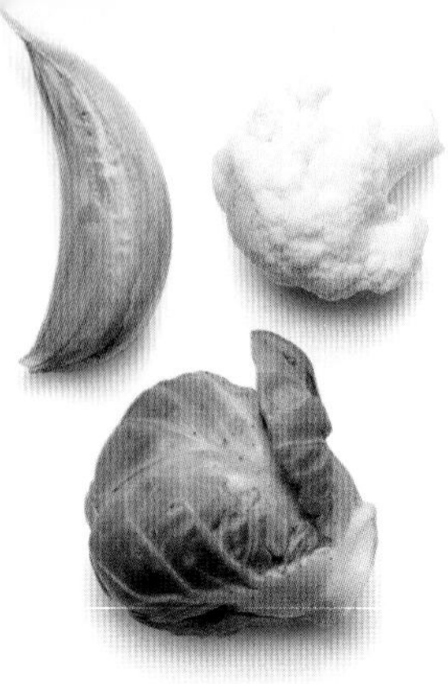

PHYTOCHEMICALS: WHERE TO FIND THEM

While fruits and vegetables offer many healthful benefits, the following foods are especially potent in a variety of health- and immune-boosting plant compounds called phytochemicals. What's interesting is that researchers think these compounds work best in synergy with each other—not isolated. All the more reason to eat a variety!

Apples
Blueberries
Broccoli
Brussels sprouts
Cabbage
Carrots
Cauliflower
Cherries
Cocoa powder
Garlic/leeks
Grapes
Kale
Parsley
Raspberries
Red onions
Tea
Tomatoes
Walnuts
Wine

inflammation, a diet rich in clean foods can help reduce it and its harmful effects on your body. The following foods in particular are anti-inflammatory powerhouses:

Spices and Herbs

Herbs and spices like basil, rosemary, thyme, oregano, turmeric, peppercorns, ginger, and cinnamon are loaded with all sorts of antioxidants that have even been found to reduce pro-inflammatory compounds that build up on meat during grilling. And ginger and turmeric, in particular, have been linked to joint pain relief. Add them to marinades, dressings, spice rubs, and teas for a dose of health and flavor.

Soy

Soy can reduce the inflammation marker C-reactive protein, which is linked to cardiovascular disease. Incorporate clean sources of soy into your diet, such as tempeh or edamame (recipes on pages 96–99).

Cold-Water Fish

Salmon, black cod, sardines, and anchovies are full of anti-inflammatory omega-3 fatty acids. Salmon is a particularly good choice—its rosy pink color comes from carotenoids, which also have anti-inflammatory properties.

Sweet Potatoes

Sweet potatoes are high in vitamins C and E and the carotenoids alpha- and beta-carotene, all of which reduce inflammation and promote healthy, vibrant skin.

Walnuts

Walnuts contain alpha-linolenic acid—an omega-3 fatty acid that reduces inflammation and is associated with a reduced risk of heart disease and diabetes.

Tea

Green, black, and white teas contain free radical–fighting catechins, which have recently been associated with reduced muscle inflammation and a speedier recovery after exercise. For unique ways to work hot and iced tea into your diet, go to page 232.

They Boost Your Immune System

Clean foods can give your immune system a powerful boost with an infusion of vitamins, minerals, and phytochemicals—naturally occurring chemical compounds in plant-based foods that are responsible for things like the vibrant color of blueberries and the pungent aroma of garlic. Together, these nutrients help halt cell damage and inflammation, and support your immune system by creating T cells, macrophages, and lymphocytes—the white blood cells that act as your body's first line of defense against disease.

They Help You Avoid Scary Allergic Reactions

A clean diet might just save your life—or at least save you a whole lot of discomfort if you suffer from a food allergy or sensitivity. Serious allergies to nuts, fish, soy, and dairy are on the rise as well as sensitivities to gluten, and these food triggers can end up in places you'd never expect them. Soy can be found in vegetable broth and chocolate bars; gluten can be found in salad dressing; and dairy can be found in seasoned chips, crackers, and popcorn. With

THE HIDDEN ALLERGEN IN YOUR GLUTEN-FREE FOODS

Ever hear of lupin? Probably not, but it should definitely be on your radar. Recently, the FDA released a warning about this legume, stating that it can cause allergic reactions ranging from a mild case of hives to full-blown anaphylaxis. The most susceptible populations: people with existing legume allergies, especially peanut allergies. The reason this news is troublesome is that lupin is popping up in an increasing number of foods, thanks to the onslaught of gluten-free products (apparently it makes a great substitute for gluten-containing flours)—yet people still have no idea what it is or that it may cause them harm. How to avoid it: Read your ingredient lists. Lupin is required by law to be listed as either "lupin" or "lupine."

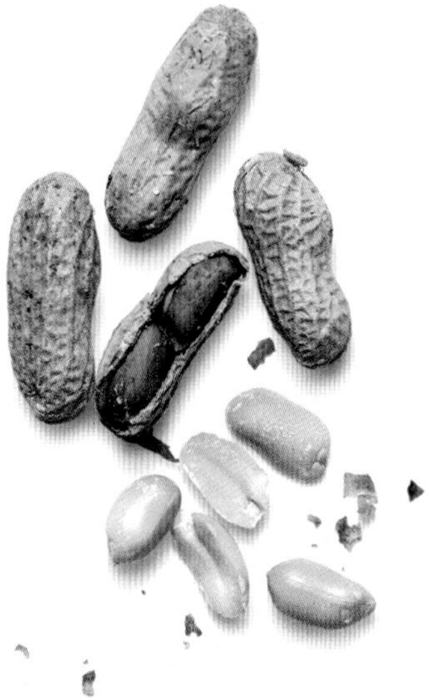

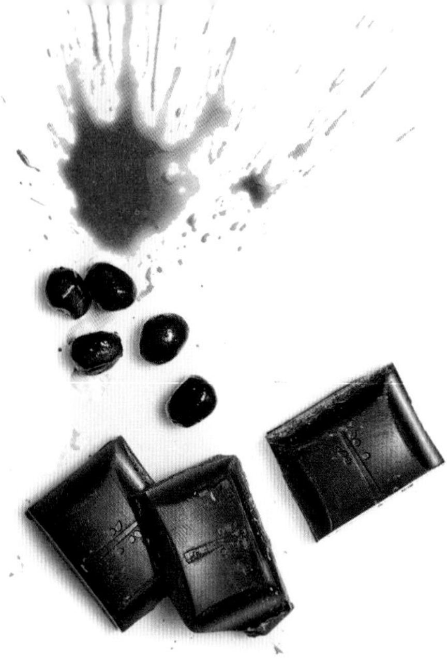

12 FOODS THAT BOOST YOUR MOOD

The joy you get from eating isn't simply a result of good flavor and mouthfeel—nutrients in certain foods can actually trigger the release of feel-good brain chemicals like dopamine. Luckily, plenty of clean foods fit the bill. Here are 12 blessed with compounds that lift your spirits:

- Clams
- **Walnuts**
- Flaxseed
- **Coffee**
- Radishes
- **Oysters**
- Pomegranates
- **Yogurt**
- Kefir
- **Shiitake mushrooms**
- Chocolate
- **Apricots**

whole foods, however, you know exactly what you're getting, so there's no need to pore over food labels. An orange is an orange, an apple is an apple, and your kale certainly doesn't contain peanuts. Of course, you still need to be label savvy with any packaged food, even if it's a relatively clean one, so read ingredient lists and be on the lookout for allergy warnings, which have to be listed if a product contains one of the eight major food allergens (milk, eggs, fish, shellfish, tree nuts, peanuts, wheat, and soybeans).

They Basically Replace Your Makeup

Ever hear that old myth about chocolate or pizza making you sprout pimples? Well, there might be something to the food-skin connection after all. While processed foods don't necessarily cause acne or other skin conditions, they can make an existing condition worse. Foods containing high amounts of sodium and trans fats can cause an increase in sebum production, which can clog pores and cause acne. Clean eating, on the other hand, minimizes exposure to these skin-sabotaging foods.

But the beautifying perks of good food go beyond clearing up a few zits. Worried about wrinkles? Let fruit be thy face cream—powerful phytochemicals in produce help combat skin-damaging free radicals that contribute to tired and dull-looking skin. Want full, lush hair? Beta-carotene, iron, zinc, vitamin C, and B vitamins—abundant in fruits, veggies, whole grains, and nuts—are good for your scalp and can strengthen hair. Iron actually strengthens hair follicles by infusing them with oxygen. And these same nutrients that liven up your locks can build strong, healthy nails that are pretty even without polish.

They Make You Happy

Nutrient-rich whole foods are basically edible Prozac. After a few weeks of eating clean, you may find yourself feeling happier and healthier, and having fewer dips in energy. Why? The vitamins, minerals, and phytochemicals in fruits, veggies, and other whole foods help cells do their job, so your body can operate more efficiently—in fact, a recent study found that people who eat seven or more servings of produce a day are happier and have better mental health. And eating complex carbohydrates and whole grains—as well as lean proteins and healthy fats—keeps your blood sugar leveled and keeps you satisfied for longer periods of time, so you can avoid getting "hangry" and resist the temptation for a midafternoon cookie or coffee pick-me-up.

CLEAN EATING IS GOOD FOR THE PLANET

The perks of clean eating don't stop at you—these healthy habits are also good for the planet. Clean, organic foods are grown without pesticides and chemicals that can end up in our waterways and drinking supply; fruits and vegetables require little to no packaging, resulting in less waste; and locally produced food doesn't have to travel hundreds of miles to reach your plate, resulting in less pollution. Local foods can often be purchased and eaten shortly after they are harvested, resulting in fresher, more flavorful, more nutritious food for you. Local produce is also inherently seasonal, so you'll be enjoying fruits and vegetables at their peak.

In buying local produce, meats, dairy, and eggs, you're also putting money directly into your community: You're supporting local farmers and encouraging the production of more quality local food.

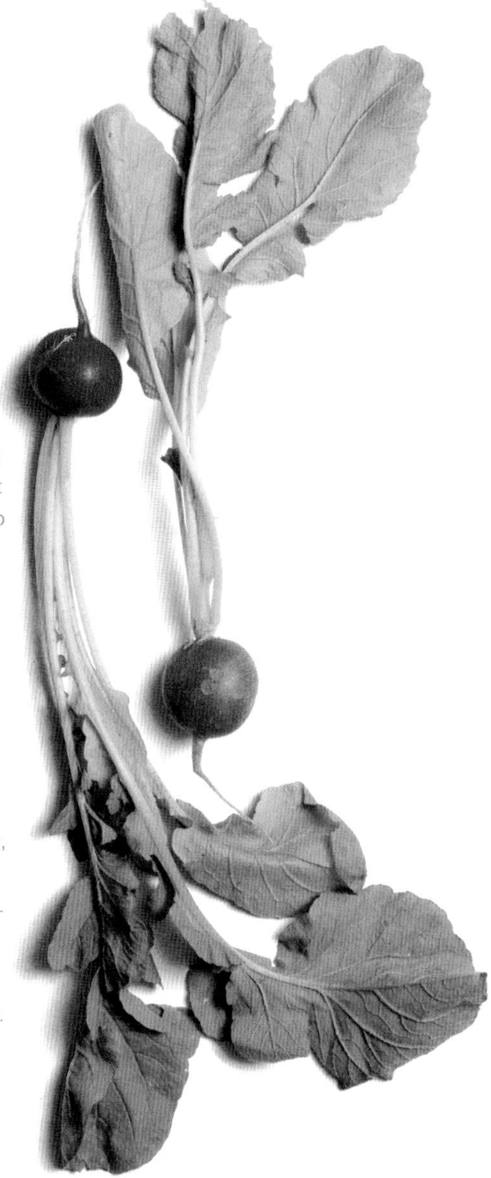

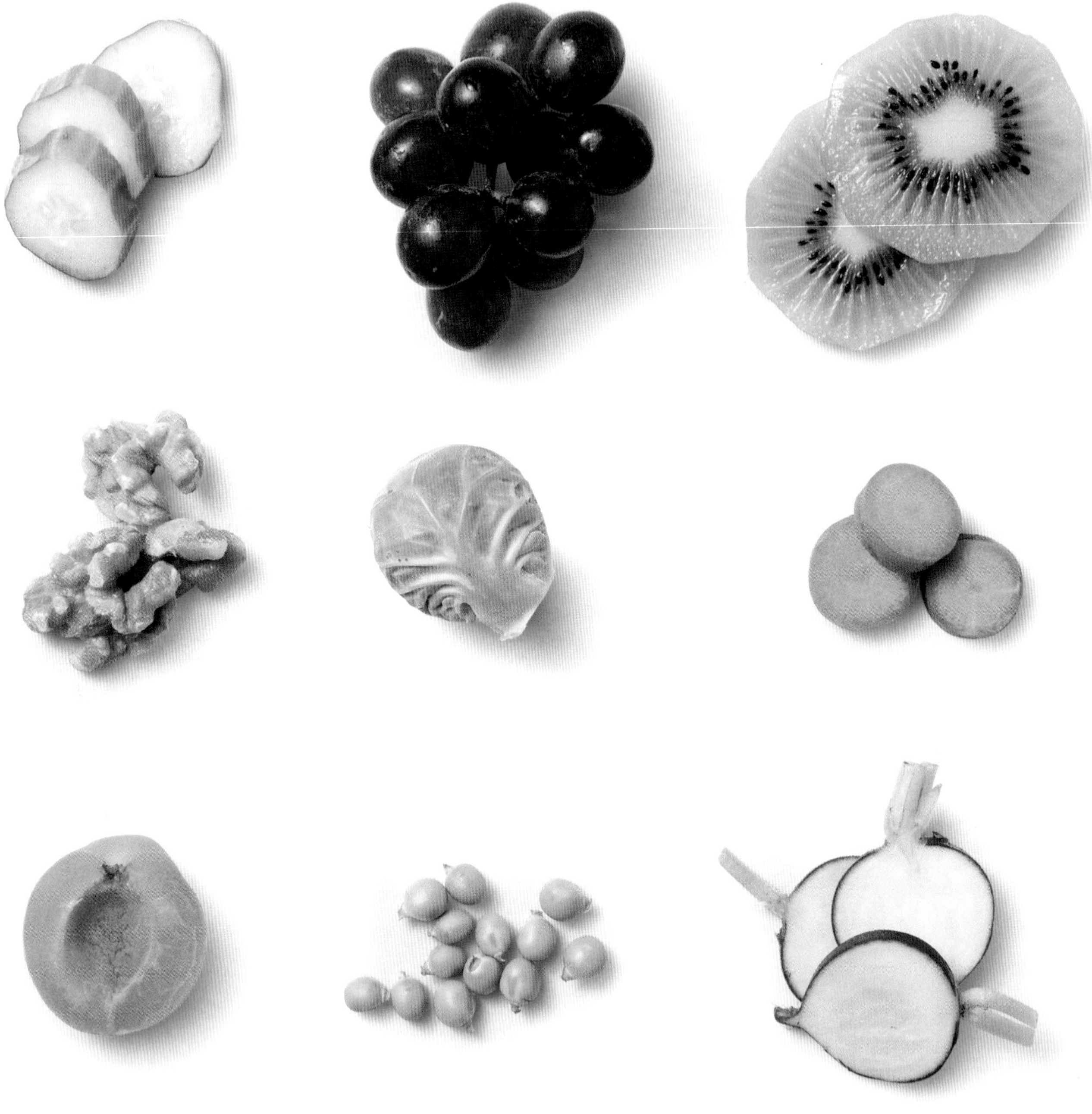

CHAPTER 2

The Basics of Clean Eating

Starting a new journey is exciting, but also a bit scary. You've made a conscious choice to stop filling your body with chemicals, preservatives, sugar, fat, and salt and to start treating yourself to the healthiest foods on the planet. But maybe making it all happen freaks you out, especially since so many companies are trying to fool you with their savvy "health food" marketing. You can relax though. Here, you become a clean food detective: After this chapter, you'll know how to differentiate the meaningless claims and labels from the truly important ones, steer clear of dangerous food additives, and find the best deals on fresh local fare. You'll also learn how to focus your attention away from what you're "missing out on" and onto a delicious world of whole foods that you can eat without counting calories. Now, let's get to know the basics of eating clean.

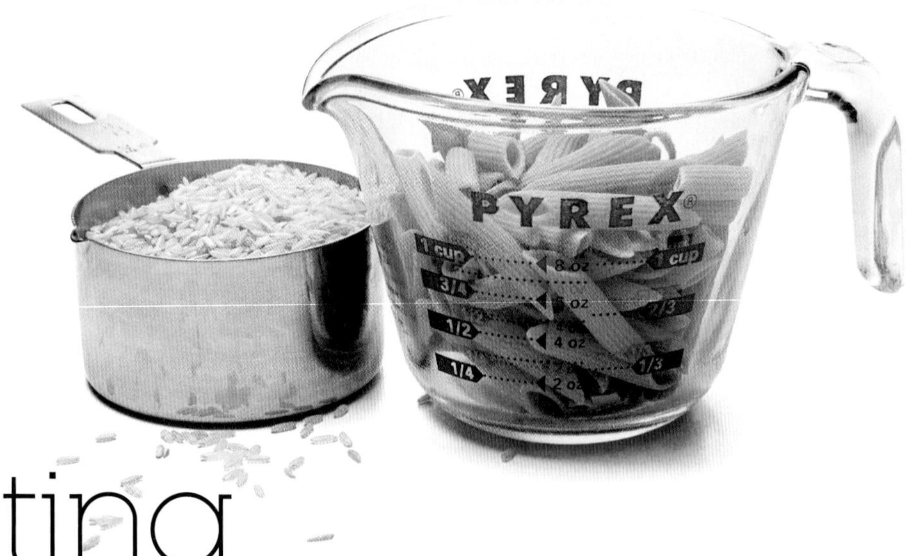

Stop Counting Calories

Remember: Clean eating isn't a diet. The parameters we lay out here are flexible guidelines meant to help you find the foods you'll personally thrive on—every *body* is different, after all. But one thing we're pretty adamant about is that you should stop counting calories. The reason: It's unnecessary and even counterproductive. As you start to cut out the junk and embrace truly nourishing foods, you'll get better in tune with your body and understand how much you need of certain foods to feel satisfied, energized, and healthy—in other words, you'll naturally self-regulate. Counting calories, on the other hand, has you focusing on a number, and often results in you feeling guilty when you don't clock in where you should at the end of the day.

If you lack confidence in your ability to self-regulate, understand that it develops over time. In the beginning, there are certainly strategies that can really help you tune into your food and your body so you don't overdo it. One is to eat mindfully—chew slowly, focus on how your food smells and tastes, and eat until you're nearly full. Another is to rethink what you consider a serving size. It has become a huge challenge to eat reasonable portions because we live in an age of

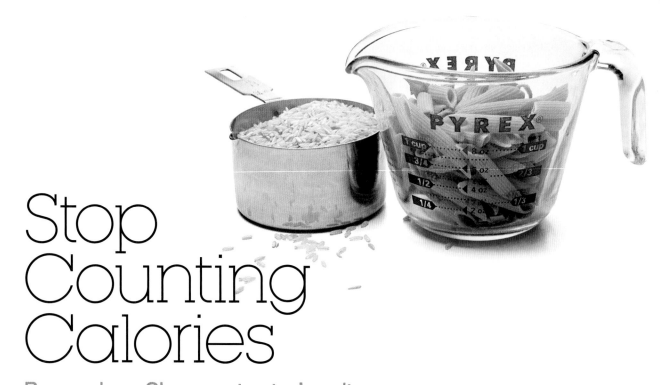

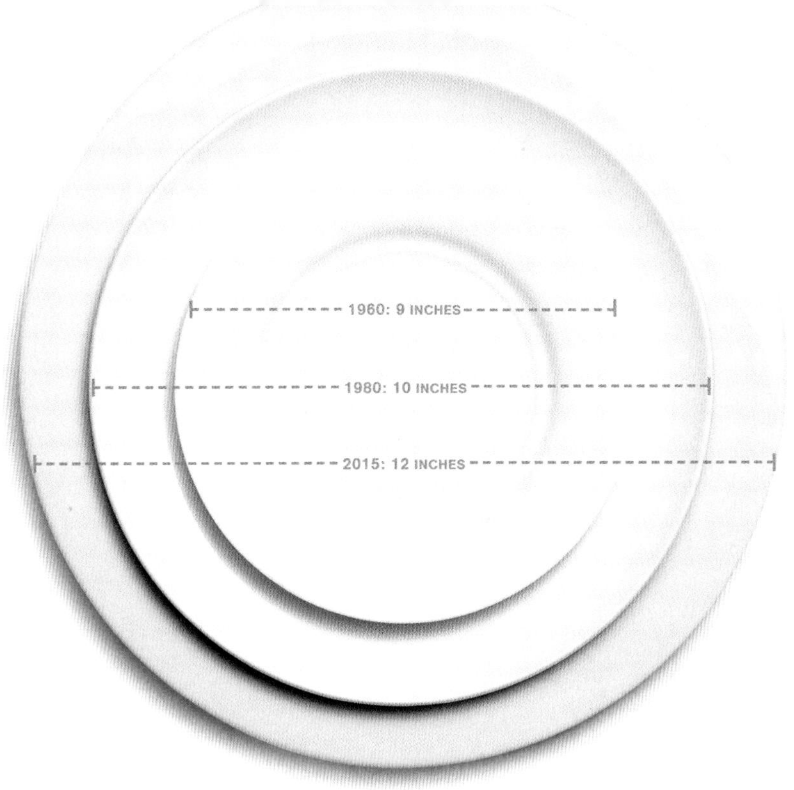

EVOLUTION OF THE DINNER PLATE

Fun fact: In the 1960s, the diameter of the average American dinner plate was 9 inches. In the 1980s, 10 inches. And today, 12 whopping inches. So, is it a coincidence that the average American today is 24 pounds heavier than in 1960, or that obesity rates have more than doubled in the past 35 years? Well, we're not saying plate size is everything, but it's certainly something to think about.

"bigger is better," but one of the simplest things you can do is to use smaller dinner plates. Instead of just mind*less*ly mowing down whatever's on your giant 12-inch-diameter dinner plate, a smaller plate (with its more reasonable amount of food) makes you more mind*ful*, forcing you to pause and ask yourself if you really want seconds.

Focus on Whole Foods

Take a close look at what's in your kitchen. It's time to say good-bye to highly processed convenience foods and fill your pantry and fridge with fresh, nutritious whole foods. As you begin your clean-eating journey, you'll want to stock up on a variety of fruits and vegetables, whole grains, nuts and seeds, lean proteins, and healthy fats. These will be the pillars of your new diet and lifestyle.

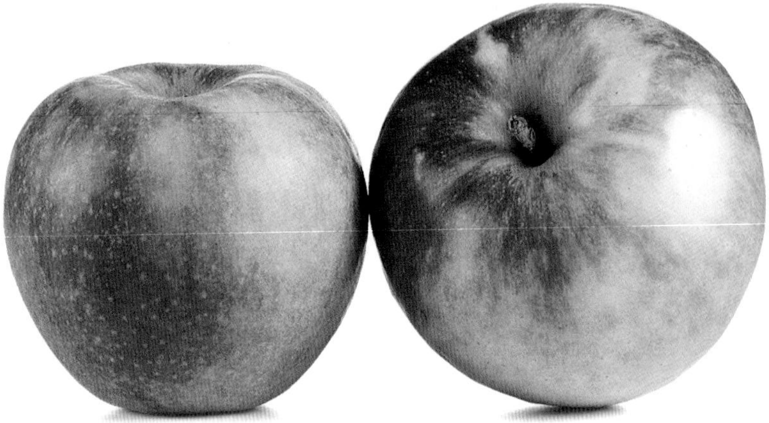

Eat Organic (as Much as Possible)

Want to hear something gross? There are more than 600 chemicals currently registered for agricultural use in the United States, and billions of pounds of these chemicals are used on produce each year—working out to about 16 pounds per person per year. The real kicker: Most of these chemicals weren't subject to extensive testing before being deemed safe. A pretty compelling case for eating organic, isn't it?

While you don't have to eat strictly organic, buying organic (or from small local farmers and producers who you know don't use chemicals) whenever possible is a good idea: Per the USDA, organic produce must be grown on land that has been free of all banned fertilizers and pesticides for the past 3 years; has never been fertilized with sewage sludge (treated human waste) or chemical pesticides and fertilizers; has never been treated with irradiation to kill bacteria; and has not been grown from genetically modified seeds. When it comes to processed organic foods, the USDA prohibits them from containing artificial preservatives, colors, or flavors and requires that the product be made up of 95% organic content. If the label says "contains organic ingredients," it must be 70% organic. Conventional fruits and vegetables, and packaged foods, on the other hand, have often been grown from low-nutrient soils, and come into contact with pesticides, fungicides, herbicides, and sewage sludge.

Now that you know why you should eat organic, you may still be balking over the cost. It's true, organic is more expensive, but there are ways to get your hands on the good stuff without all the stress on your wallet. Here are some money-saving strategies:

- **Shop at your regular grocery store:** You don't have to start shopping at a high-end market or natural food store to get organic foods. Chain stores like Target, Wal-Mart, Costco, Safeway, and Kroger all carry their own reasonably priced lines of organic foods.
- **Buy in bulk:** Organic oats, brown rice, dried beans, nuts, and seeds are usually cheaper in bulk because you're avoiding all that packaging. To figure out just how much you'll save—and if it's worth it—compare the unit price of bulk and individually packaged items.
- **Enjoy in-season produce:** Locally grown, in-season fruits and vegetables are cheaper since there are essentially no transportation costs. Bonus: Eating seasonally forces you to switch things up in the kitchen and ensures that you're getting a variety of health-boosting nutrients.
- **Consider a CSA:** A CSA (Community Supported Agriculture) involves buying shares of a local farm and, in return, getting a weekly box of fresh produce. These collectives are great for your wallet and community.
- **Eat less meat:** While lean animal proteins are certainly a healthy component of clean eating, they're one of the most expensive organic foods you can buy. Consider eating a few meatless meals a week to save on costs. Instead, experiment with delicious organic plant-based recipes featuring vegetarian proteins like tempeh, lentils, and chickpeas.

Organic Produce

It's long been debated whether or not organic produce packs a bigger nutritional punch than conventional. For a while, scientists said they were equals, but that all changed upon the publication of a recent study in the *British Journal of Nutrition*. After reviewing 343 studies, researchers concluded that, on average, organically grown crops contained higher levels of antioxidants, likely because they've been grown in more nutrient-rich soil that hasn't been depleted

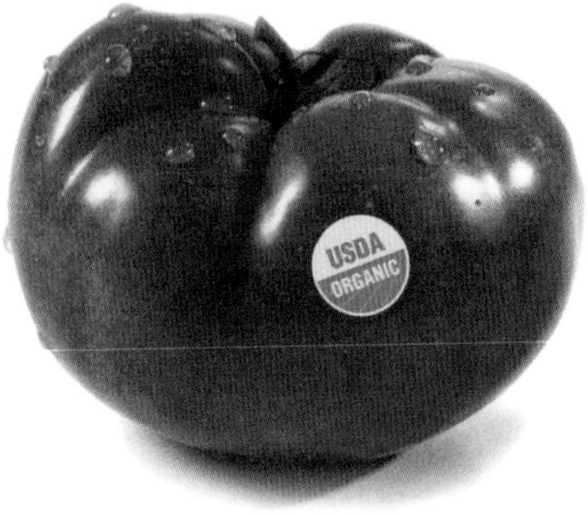

GET STICKER SMART

An organic, conventional, and genetically modified zucchini can all look pretty darn identical. So how are you supposed to tell the difference? It's simple: Look at the sticker. They may be annoying to remove, but printed on each you'll see the PLU (price lookup) code—a number that reveals how it was grown. Conventional produce grown with pesticides always start with 3 or 4, while organic produce starts with 9, and genetically modified produce will start with an 8.

of its benefits with years of chemical pesticide and fertilizer use. (Bonus: Because they're grown in such well-nourished soil, organic fruits and veggies tend to taste fresher and more flavorful, too!)

While buying all organic produce may not be realistic for you, it's important to at least buy organic when it really counts. This means buying organic versions of fruits and veggies that tend to have the highest pesticide residue (even after they're washed) when grown conventionally. Not sure what these are? The Environmental Working Group prepares "Clean Fifteen" and "Dirty Dozen Plus" lists, which reveal the cleanest and dirtiest of the conventional crowd. Of course, eating conventionally grown produce is better than not eating fruits or vegetables at all.

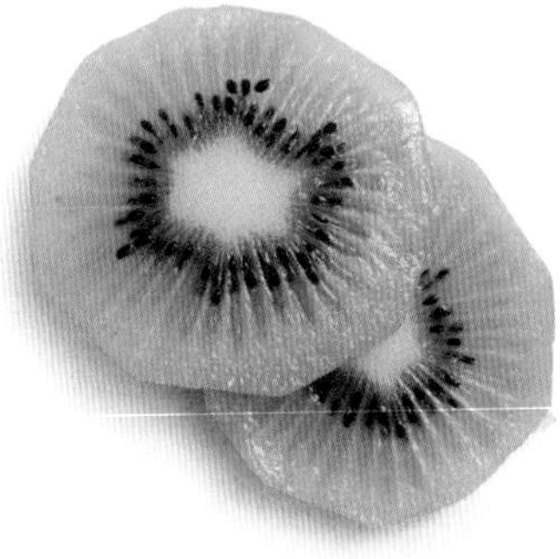

CLEAN FIFTEEN
(okay to buy conventional)

- Avocados
- **Sweet corn**
- Pineapples
- **Cabbage**
- Sweet peas (frozen)
- **Onions**
- Asparagus
- **Mangoes**
- Papayas
- **Kiwi**
- Eggplant
- **Grapefruit**
- Cantaloupe (domestic)
- **Cauliflower**
- Sweet potatoes

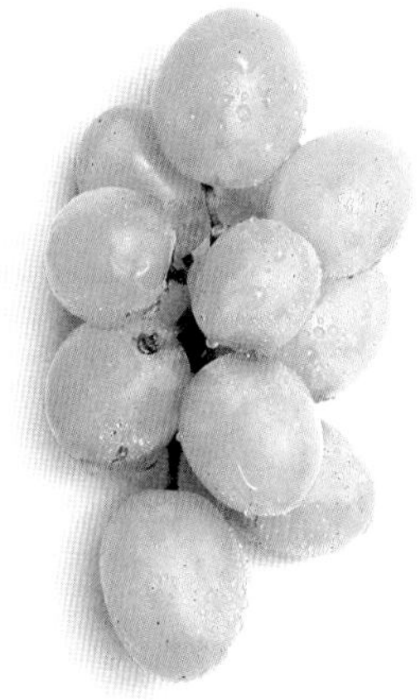

THE DIRTY DOZEN PLUS
(always buy organic)

- Apples
- Peaches
- Nectarines
- Strawberries
- Grapes
- Celery
- Spinach
- Sweet bell peppers
- Cucumbers
- Cherry tomatoes
- Snap peas (imported)
- Potatoes
- Hot peppers
- Kale/collard greens

Organic Animal Products

A good chunk of the pesticides that the average American consumes comes from conventionally produced meat and dairy products. You might wonder *how*, since farmers aren't exactly spraying their cows and chickens with Roundup, but it's because these animals are being fed grains made from crops that have been heavily treated with chemical pesticides. This is then passed on to you when you fire up the grill and cook your favorite cut of steak.

Beyond pesticides, an additional concern of eating nonorganic animal products is the growth hormones being pumped into farm animals. Farmers give sex hormones and growth hormones to cattle to increase meat and milk production. Some of these hormones are then passed to you, as it's not possible for them to be broken down in cows' digestive systems. The growth hormones rBHG and rBST are particularly concerning, as they've been linked to cancers in women.

Perhaps even scarier than pesticides and hormones is the widespread use of nontherapeutic antibiotics to make animals gain weight faster. This has actually reduced the effectiveness of some antibiotics that are essential for treating infections in both livestock and humans.

Do you need more of a reason to pick organic animal products? We hope not! Rest assured that they'll be free of all the junk mentioned above.

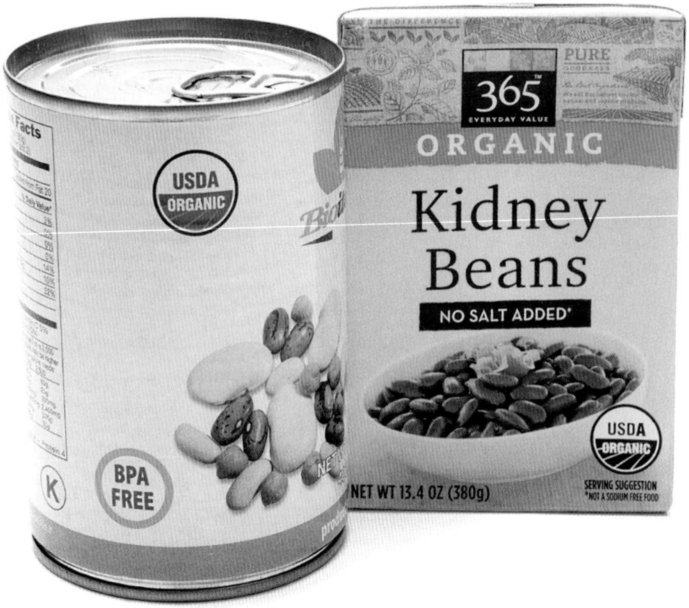

Choose Clean Packaged Foods

In a busy day full of work and errands, a trip to the supermarket should be one of the simpler tasks we perform. But with stores stocking more choices than ever—and with food labels making claims for everything from "more protein" to "added antioxidants"—shopping can be overwhelming. While your commitment to clean eating will ultimately make shopping easier, navigating the supermarket can feel like a challenge at first. So in the meantime, try to remember that the concept behind clean eating is very simple: Focus on whole, unprocessed foods that contain no chemicals or other ingredients.

Also understand that, yes, sometimes it's perfectly healthy to buy food in a package. While ideally you'll strive to fill your diet with fresh fruits and vegetables and lean proteins, there are times when you may want to buy food that comes frozen or in a can or box. For example, while broccoli fresh from the farmers' market may be the healthiest pick, you'll want to have some frozen, prechopped broccoli on hand for a meal in a pinch. Tetra Paks of cooked beans, a box of whole-grain pasta, and yogurt can also be smart, minimally processed packaged choices. Of course, sometimes it's hard to determine which packaged picks are best. That's why knowing what to look for on the label can make a big difference in ensuring that these foods are as healthful as they possibly can be. Keep reading—we'll arm you with the info to pick only the good stuff.

Scrutinize Food Claims

Eating whole foods is generally the best way to ensure you get all of your essential vitamins and nutrients, but today many packaged foods are claiming big additional health benefits. Protein is being added to everything from waffles and cereal to juice. Food packages are tempting us with claims of antioxidants and omega-3s. Probiotics are now in chocolate. What does this all really mean?

As for protein, many foods add soy protein isolate, which is often made from genetically modified soybeans that have undergone some pretty extreme processing with the chemical hexane before they resemble anything close to the protein powder that's added to packaged foods. A better choice would be foods fortified with whey or pea protein concentrate, both of which tend to be less processed.

What about antioxidants? Well, at this point, there's not enough research to say whether antioxidants, such as resveratrol, eaten out of the context of the foods they are found in naturally in foods are beneficial. Probiotics—good bacteria that occur naturally in some dairy and fermented

SHOP CLEANER AT THE SUPERMARKET

Stick to your shopping list so you won't be tempted by processed foods. Some grocery stores, like Wegman's, even have smartphone apps that automatically organize your list by aisle, so you save time and avoid impulse buys.

Have a light meal or snack before you go shopping. It's easier to slip and make a bad choice if you're hungry. Some research even suggests that chewing mint gum as you shop offers the same benefit.

Stick to the outside perimeter of the store, where whole foods are generally kept, as much as possible. The center aisles tend to contain the processed foods.

Resist chocolate and candy while you're at the checkout. You made it that far! You are strong enough to resist.

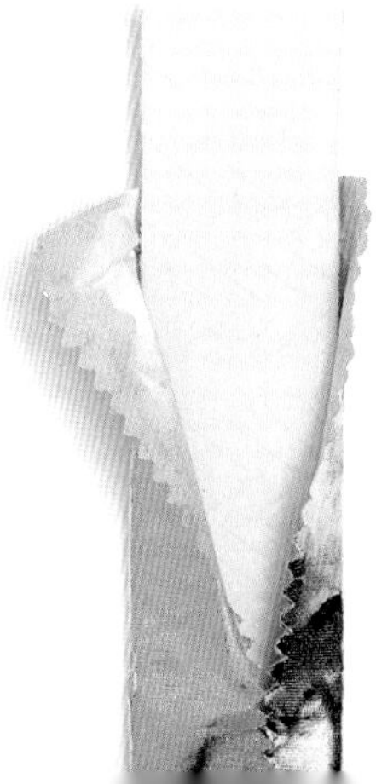

vegetables, and that can be added to other packaged foods—may be helpful, but different strains benefit different health concerns. If a particular strain found in a food isn't right for you, you won't be receiving any additional perks. Omega-3s, now being pumped into everything from granola bars to ice cream, won't do you much good unless they're in the form of DHA and EPA—the kind found in fish.

Basically, you don't want to seek out packaged foods for these nutrients. Stick to whole, unprocessed foods that will naturally bring everything from antioxidants to omega-3s into your diet without any extra junk.

Deciphering "Healthy" Food Terms

All those labels and health claims can be confusing. Here, we break down some of the most common, what they actually mean, and whether or not you should bother.

ORGANIC: For produce, this term means plants weren't grown from genetically modified seeds; were not grown with pesticides, herbicides, or sewage sludge; or were not irradiated. For meats and poultry, this means that animals were fed organic feed with no animal byproducts, were not given antibiotics or hormones, and had some (but not necessarily much) access to the outdoors. For a packaged food to be labeled "organic," it must be made up of at least 95% organic ingredients, while a label stating "made with organic ingredients" must contain 70% organic ingredients. It's good to look for this label when budget permits, but you can also buy from small local producers and farmers who you know follow good practices but may not have the revenue for organic certification.

CAGE-FREE: For eggs, the term "cage-free" means the hens are not confined to cages—but they do not necessarily have access to an outdoor space. While this isn't ideal, it does give them a chance to spread their wings and lay eggs in nest boxes, which is closer to their natural behavior. Unless they're organic, cage-free hens can still be fed grains made from genetically modified crops that have been heavily treated with chemical pesticides, which can then be passed on to you. Because there's no mandatory third-party auditing for the term "cage-free," look for the term along with a third-party certification seal such as "Certified Humane" or "Animal Welfare Approved."

FREE-RANGE: Found on poultry and egg packaging, this term means that hens have access to the outdoors—though the amount, duration, or quality of that outdoor time is not specified. Unless certified organic, free-range animals may still be given antibiotics and pesticide-riddled feed. These are a slightly better option than cage-free, but again, there's no mandatory third-party auditing for the term "free-range," so look for the term along with a third-party certification seal such as "Certified Humane" or "American Humane Certified."

PASTURE-RAISED: This term can apply to all kinds of meat as well as eggs. Pastured animals are often reared on grassland, where they're able to eat a diverse diet of grass, bugs, and other natural vegetation that lends their meat (or dairy) a richer flavor and higher levels of nutrients, including omega-3s. This label can mean great things for your meat and eggs, but, unfortunately, there's no mandatory third-party auditing for the term "pasture-raised," so it's best to buy pastured meats and eggs from a local producer who can offer details on their practices. Or buy from a brand that's been voluntarily pasture-raised and certified by a reputable third party—"Certified Humane" or "American Humane Certified" will appear on the packaging if that's the case.

GRASS-FED: The USDA has defined grass-fed beef, bison, lamb, goats, and dairy as coming from animals that ate 100% grass (which means no corn or soy) and enjoyed continuous access to pasture. But there are some loopholes, so look for products from farmers certified by the American Grassfed Association, which has even stricter standards on "grass-fed" than the USDA.

NATURAL: Natural refers to a product that is made without artificial flavors, colors, or other synthetic substances. However, "natural" foods can still contain other potentially damaging ingredients such as high fructose corn syrup and "natural flavors," which, in reality, are flavors produced in a laboratory. Even worse, a recent study by Consumer Reports found that many "natural" products contained genetically modified ingredients. Don't buy a packaged food based on a "natural" claim. Inspect the ingredients and make sure you recognize what you see.

NO HORMONES: A "no hormones" label on meat and dairy products means that hormones were not used during production. It should be noted that the USDA already prohibits the use of hormones on pork and poultry, so no need to seek out the label for those products.

NO ANTIBIOTICS: This claim means that no antibiotics were used in the production of the product. It may be found on labels for meat or dairy products. This is a good thing, as antibiotic use in animals has been linked to drug resistance; but if you're going to shell out more money for

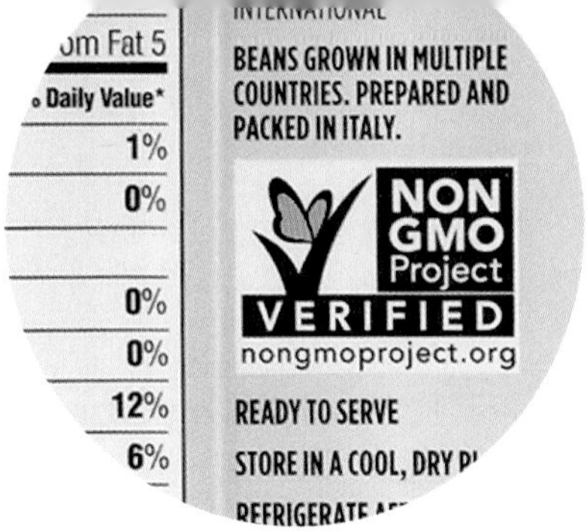

THE LABEL THAT'S ALWAYS WORTH THE EXTRA CASH

Many experts believe all food, whether organic or not, should have a non-GMO label—or more specifically an NGP (Non-GMO Project) seal, the strictest non-GMO seal in the world, which features a little orange butterfly sitting on piece of grass that looks like a checkmark. Any product with this little sticker not only has zero genetically modified (GM) ingredients, it also doesn't contain any ingredients derived from animals raised on GM feed. And since some food manufacturing processes can destroy detectable GMO DNA, the NGP uses accredited labs to analyze all ingredients individually in a product before being added to food—talk about strict! Compare this to the National Organic Standard (NOS), which doesn't require regular testing of organic products for the presence of GM species; or "non-GMO" or "GMO-free" labels, which aren't third-party verified.

meat, you might as well go organic.

CERTIFIED HUMANE: "Humane conditions" refers to the environment in which the animals were raised. This means that the animals had access to enough space to allow freedom to move, and were not treated with artificial growth hormones or antibiotics to increase weight. This is a good label—not only for your conscience, but for your health, too. "Certified Humane" has three levels of certification: regular (cage-free), free-range, and pasture-raised.

HEART-HEALTHY: The American Heart Association's Heart-Check program's standard certification requires that a product have less than 6.5 grams total fat, 1 gram or less saturated fat (or less than 15% of total calories), less than 0.5 gram trans fats, and 20 milligrams or less cholesterol per serving; and less than a certain amount of sodium, depending on the food category. It must also contain 10% or more of the daily value of one of six beneficial nutrients (vitamin A, vitamin C, iron, calcium, protein, or dietary fiber). Because of its emphasis on reducing fat intake, when mounting research is devilifying most quality fats, this label should be taken with a grain of salt. Look at the ingredient list and nutrition panel instead.

HIGH-FIBER: If a food label states "high-fiber," the product must have at least 5 grams of fiber per serving, according to the Whole Grains Council. Most whole grains typically contain just 0.5 to 3 grams of fiber per serving, so you'll most likely see the "high-fiber" label on processed foods to which manufacturers have added extra fiber in the form of resistant starch, inulin, or cellulose. If you're eating a diet rich in whole foods with plenty of veggies and grains, you don't need to bother with this label.

RAW: You'll often see this label on juices, fermented drinks and vegetables, and dairy. Essentially, it means the product was not cooked or heated to a temperature that destroys beneficial nutrients and enzymes. For things like kombucha, kimchi, and sauerkraut, this is important, as it means the product has retained its probiotic benefits. For juices, the benefits are more up for debate, as pasteurized juice still retains many vitamins and minerals. And for milk, the benefits may not outweigh the risk of foodborne illness.

NON-GMO, GMO-FREE: These terms, meant to imply that there are no genetically modified organisms in a food product, are not regulated. The only labels to feel good about when trying to avoid GMOs are Certified Organic and Non-GMO Project Verified.

Check the Ingredients

When scanning a label, you need to ask yourself if most items in the ingredient list are whole foods. A good rule of thumb: The fewer ingredients, the better. Take, for example, organic quinoa pasta. The ingredient list simply reads *whole grain kamut wheat, whole grain quinoa*—two whole, clean foods. While this pasta is minimally processed (the kamut and quinoa were ground into a flour beforehand), it still contains all parts of the grain and counts as a clean food.

Some foods, however, have excessively long ingredient lists. Let's take a look at a cereal bar. It doesn't sound like a bad choice—especially since the package boasts that it "contains whole grains" and is "low fat." A closer look, however, reveals something different:

WHOLE GRAIN OATS, ENRICHED FLOUR (WHEAT FLOUR, NIACIN, REDUCED IRON, VITAMIN B_1 [THIAMIN MONONITRATE], VITAMIN B_2 [RIBOFLAVIN], FOLIC ACID), WHOLE WHEAT FLOUR, SOYBEAN AND/OR CANOLA OIL, SOLUBLE CORN FIBER, SUGAR, DEXTROSE, FRUCTOSE, CALCIUM CARBONATE, WHEY, WHEAT BRAN, SALT, CELLULOSE, POTASSIUM BICARBONATE, NATURAL AND ARTIFICIAL FLAVOR, CINNAMON, MONO- AND DIGLYCERIDES, SOY LECITHIN, WHEAT GLUTEN, NIACINAMIDE, VITAMIN A PALMITATE, CARRAGEENAN, ZINC OXIDE, REDUCED IRON, GUAR GUM, VITAMIN B_6 (PYRIDOXINE HYDROCHLORIDE), VITAMIN B_1 (THIAMIN HYDROCHLORIDE), VITAMIN B_2 (RIBOFLAVIN), FILLING: INVERT SUGAR, CORN SYRUP, APPLE PUREE CONCENTRATE, GLYCERIN, SUGAR, MODIFIED CORN STARCH, SODIUM ALGINATE, MALIC ACID, METHYLCELLULOSE, DICALCIUM PHOSPHATE, CINNAMON, CITRIC ACID, CARAMEL COLOR.

Now that's definitely not a clean food. It's packed with foods that aren't whole, as well as preservatives, several types of sugars, artificial flavors, and a potentially carcinogenic artificial color—sounds like a bad

THE DIFFERENT NAMES FOR SUGAR

Agave syrup
Barley malt
Beet sugar
Brown rice syrup
Brown sugar
Buttered syrup
Cane sugar
Caramel
Carob syrup
Coconut sugar
Corn syrup
Date sugar
Dextran
Dextrose
Evaporated cane juice
Fructose
Fruit juice
Fruit juice concentrate
Glucose
Glucose solids
Golden syrup
Grape sugar
High fructose corn syrup
Honey
Invert sugar
Lactose
Malt syrup
Maltodextrin
Maltose
Mannitol
Maple syrup
Molasses
Raisin juice concentrate
Raw sugar
Refiner's syrup
Rice/rice bran sugar
Sorbitol
Sorghum syrup
Sucrose
Sugar
Turbinado sugar

science experiment, doesn't it?

You should also understand that ingredients are listed from the highest to lowest amounts. Meaning: If some form of sugar is the first ingredient, that's probably a pretty high sugar food. But, just because an ingredient is listed last doesn't mean you're consuming a small amount of it either—it's all about how it stacks up to the other ingredients. All the more reason to always look at your ingredient list in conjunction with the nutrition facts panel.

Beware of Hidden Sugars

Sugar is everywhere. Even if you don't eat dessert, it's possible that you're shoveling down the sweet stuff without realizing it—even foods marketed as healthy, like oatmeal and spaghetti sauce, can pack a hefty dose. Fortunately, a commitment to eating clean whole foods can drastically cut your sugar intake. But, for those occasions that call for packaged foods—and yes, they do exist—it's important to be vigilant about reading food labels. Food manufacturers are catching on to the fact that sugar is a concern, so naturally, they're starting to list it under one of its many aliases to confuse you. Familiarize yourself with all the different names for sugar.

Steer Clear of Funky Additives

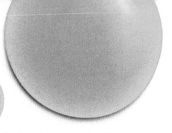

Get this—many of the additives in packaged snacks and meals haven't actually been tested by the US Food and Drug Administration (FDA) because they fall on the "generally recognized as safe" list. Per the FDA's GRAS Notification Program, substances that are "generally recognized, among experts qualified by scientific training and experience, to be safe under the conditions of their intended use," are excluded, and do not require FDA testing and approval. This system makes sense for benign additives like basil and black pepper, but there are enormous loopholes that basically allow manufacturers to deem potentially risky additives safe without any oversight.

This is just plain dangerous—some of the most common additives in processed foods have been linked to health issues such as cancer, hyperactivity in children, heart disease, dizziness, headaches, anxiety, obesity, and depression, just to name a few. These additives can be hard to avoid, but clean eating promotes a diet of whole foods that are naturally additive-free. Of course, you're going to pick up a packaged food now and then, so for those instances, here are some common additives with potentially sketchy side effects that you may want to avoid:

ASPARTAME: An artificial sweetener found in "diet" or "sugar-free" products such as diet soda, sugar-free gum, sugar-free desserts, chewable vitamins, cough syrup, toothpaste, and even cereal. This, along with other artificial sweeteners, has been associated with health problems such as obesity, headaches, and some types of cancer. Mounting research also suggests artificial sweeteners can lead to an unhealthy ratio of the good to bad bacteria in our guts that play a role in everything from metabolism to mood.

HIGH FRUCTOSE CORN SYRUP: A sweetener found in processed foods such as breads, candy, yogurts, salad dressings, canned vegetables, and cereals. This processed version of fructose is toxic to the liver, and too much promotes insulin resistance, a risk factor for diabetes and heart disease.

MONOSODIUM GLUTAMATE (MSG): A flavor enhancer found in some Chinese food, potato chips and snacks, cookies, seasonings, canned soup, frozen meals, and lunchmeats. This additive is a common migraine trigger and goes hand in hand with high amounts of sodium—it's 21% sodium itself.

TRANS FAT: Lab-produced fats found in processed foods such as margarine, chips, crackers, baked items, and fast foods. These are used to extend shelf life and improve texture of foods, and have been strongly linked to heart disease and diabetes. Luckily, the FDA recently ruled that added trans fat will phased out of most packaged and restaurant foods by 2018.

FOOD DYES, BLUE #1 & #2, RED #3 & #40, YELLOW #5 (TARTRAZINE) & #6: Artificial colors found in fruit cocktail, maraschino cherries, ice cream, candy, baked goods, American cheese, macaroni and cheese, and more. Several of these petroleum-based dyes have been linked to hyperactivity in children and cancer in lab animals.

CARAMEL COLOR: A widely used food coloring found in sodas, beer, brown bread, chocolate, cookies, donuts, ice cream, and pickles. Some caramel color is processed with ammonia, which results in the production of the potentially carcinogenic compound 4-methylimidazole.

SULFITES: Preservatives and flavor enhancers found naturally in wine and beer and added to soft drinks, juice, dried fruit, condiments, and potato products. The FDA estimates that about 10% of the population is sensitive to these sulfur-based compounds with symptoms ranging from mild hay fever to life-threatening anaphylaxis.

SODIUM NITRITE: A synthetic preservative found in processed meats such as hot dogs, lunchmeats, bacon, and smoked fish. Some animal research suggests that these morph into carcinogenic compounds in the body, but that's still up for debate. Natural sodium nitrates in the form of celery powder found in many "uncured" meat products may be safer.

BHA AND BHT: Preservatives found in potato chips, gum, cereal, frozen sausages, enriched rice, lard, shortening, candy, and Jell-O. These are manufactured from petroleum, and the National Institutes of Health reports that, based on animal studies, BHA is likely a human carcinogen; BHT has been linked to cancer to a lesser degree.

POTASSIUM BROMATE: A flour-bulking agent found in breads and rolls, bagel chips, wraps, and bread crumbs. This is used to strengthen dough and shorten baking time but may cause kidney or nervous system disorders and gastrointestinal discomfort.

HOW TO SELECT A CLEAN PACKAGED FOOD

Yes, prepping and cooking foods from scratch is always the cleanest bet, but there are times when you'll need to rely on a package. Even if you don't have time to scrutinize every detail on the label, you can still end up with safe and healthy options if you follow these basic guidelines:

- The product shouldn't contain genetically modified ingredients (GMOs). Seek out foods with the Non-GMO Project (NGP) seal. This seal is found on foods that have been vetted through the Non-GMO Project, the only third party that verifies products for GMO avoidance.
- Stick to product with less than 15 grams of sugar per serving, with most of that sweetness coming from real foods like fruit, not added sugars.
- A snack should have less than 200 milligrams of sodium per serving, and a meal less than 400 milligrams, so you remain on track to stay within the recommended daily sodium limit of 2,300 milligrams (or 1,500 milligrams if you're over 51).
- Try to only buy food that comes in BPA- and BPS-free cans—these two endocrine-disrupting chemicals can leach into food and may contribute to obesity, cancer, and reproductive problems.

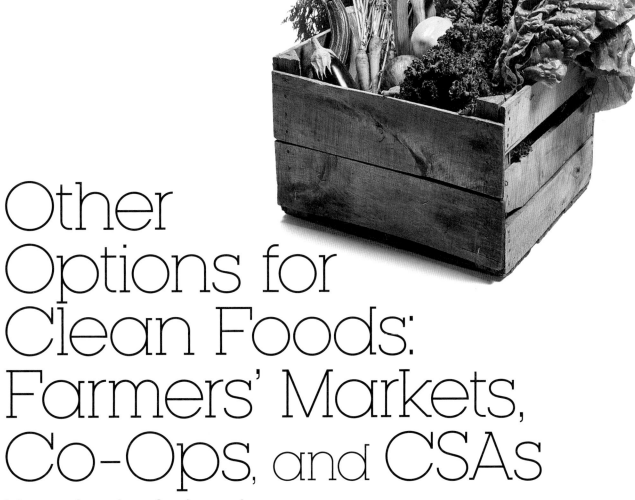

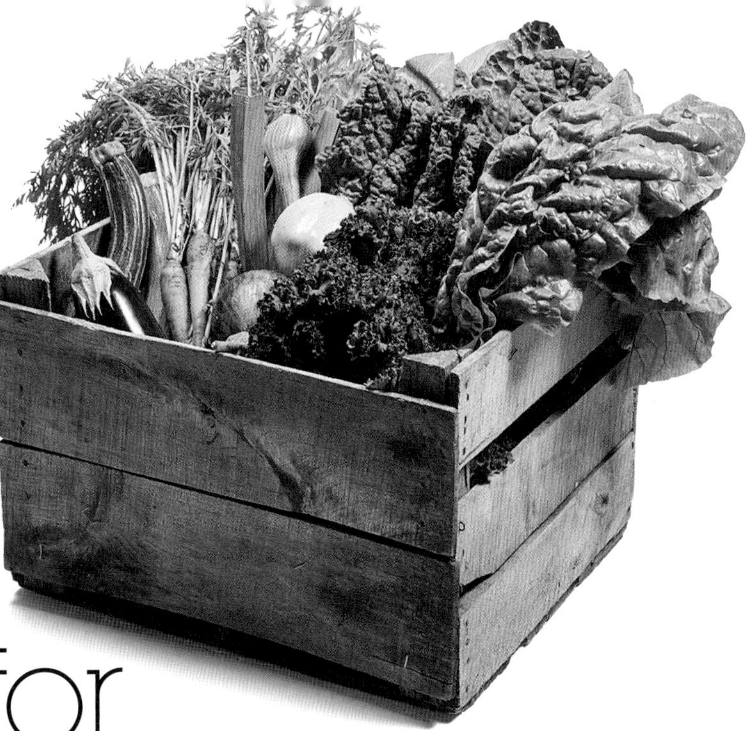

Other Options for Clean Foods: Farmers' Markets, Co-Ops, and CSAs

It's not hard to find produce, whole grains, meats, and poultry: Modern-day supermarkets have all the basics, even if they had to be imported from Ecuador. But if you're looking for high-quality, in-season products (and we know you are), break with convention and take advantage of some of your local clean food suppliers. They'll meet your high standards and support your local economy simultaneously. Here are some options.

Join a Nearby Co-Op

Concerned about the cost of going organic? See if there's a food co-op located in your community. This is essentially a member-owned grocery store that focuses on whole foods, including organic produce, dairy products, and meats. Typically, a small membership fee is paid in exchange for shares in the co-op (some co-ops keep costs low by requiring members to work short shifts as well). Members are then offered a significant discount on food—in many cases, just slightly above cost.

Invest in a CSA

CSA stands for "Community Supported Agriculture." When you buy shares of a CSA, you are investing in a community farm and receiving produce in exchange—usually a weekly box of produce (some farms may offer eggs, dairy, and meats as well). Some CSAs ask members to pick up their food from a central drop-off, while others deliver directly to your home. In addition to the great food, you're boosting your local economy and shrinking your carbon footprint (win-win-win!).

Find a Farmers' Market

Farmers' markets go way beyond produce—most offer fresh eggs, dairy products, meats, and a variety of artisanal jams, breads, and baked goods. They also happen to be the perfect place to socialize with fellow foodies, or pick your farmer's brain about what apples will work best in your pie, or how the heck to cook kohlrabi. As more markets pop up around the country, chances are you've got a few options near you. Locate them at localharvest.org.

Grow Your Own

Maybe you're the DIY type. Or maybe you just hate spending money. Either way, growing your own organic veggies could be the solution. Bonus: It's totally therapeutic—research finds gardening to be a simultaneous workout and stress reliever. Some of the hardest veggies to screw up, even if you're a notorious plant murderer, are salad greens, tomatoes, cucumbers, carrots, radishes, green beans, zucchini, and summer squash. Even easier, and totally doable in winter, are microgreens—you can grow them right on your windowsill. Here's how:

1. Buy organic sprouting seeds from online retailers like Sprout People (sproutpeople.org).

2. Re-use plastic berry containers to plant them—cut off the lid and poke holes in the bottom for drainage. Place the top lid under the container for use as a drainage tray.
3. Fill containers three-fourths full with organic potting soil, scatter the seeds on top, and cover with a thin layer of soil. Place on a sunny windowsill and water daily.
4. When the plants are 1 to 2 inches tall (7 to 10 days), your microgreens are ready. Cut them slightly above the soil line. (Don't worry, they'll keep growing!)
5. Add to salads and sandwiches, blend into pesto and smoothies, or use them as a garnish for soups and pasta.

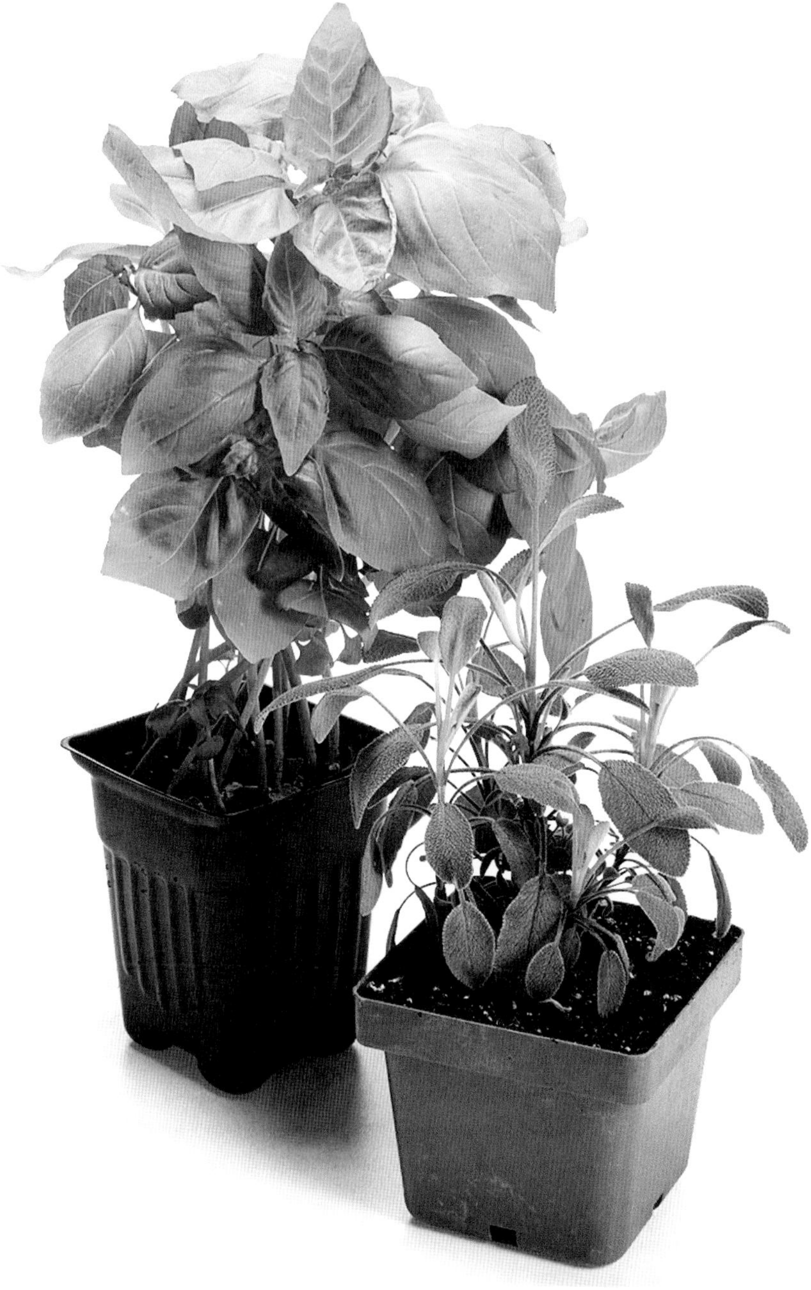

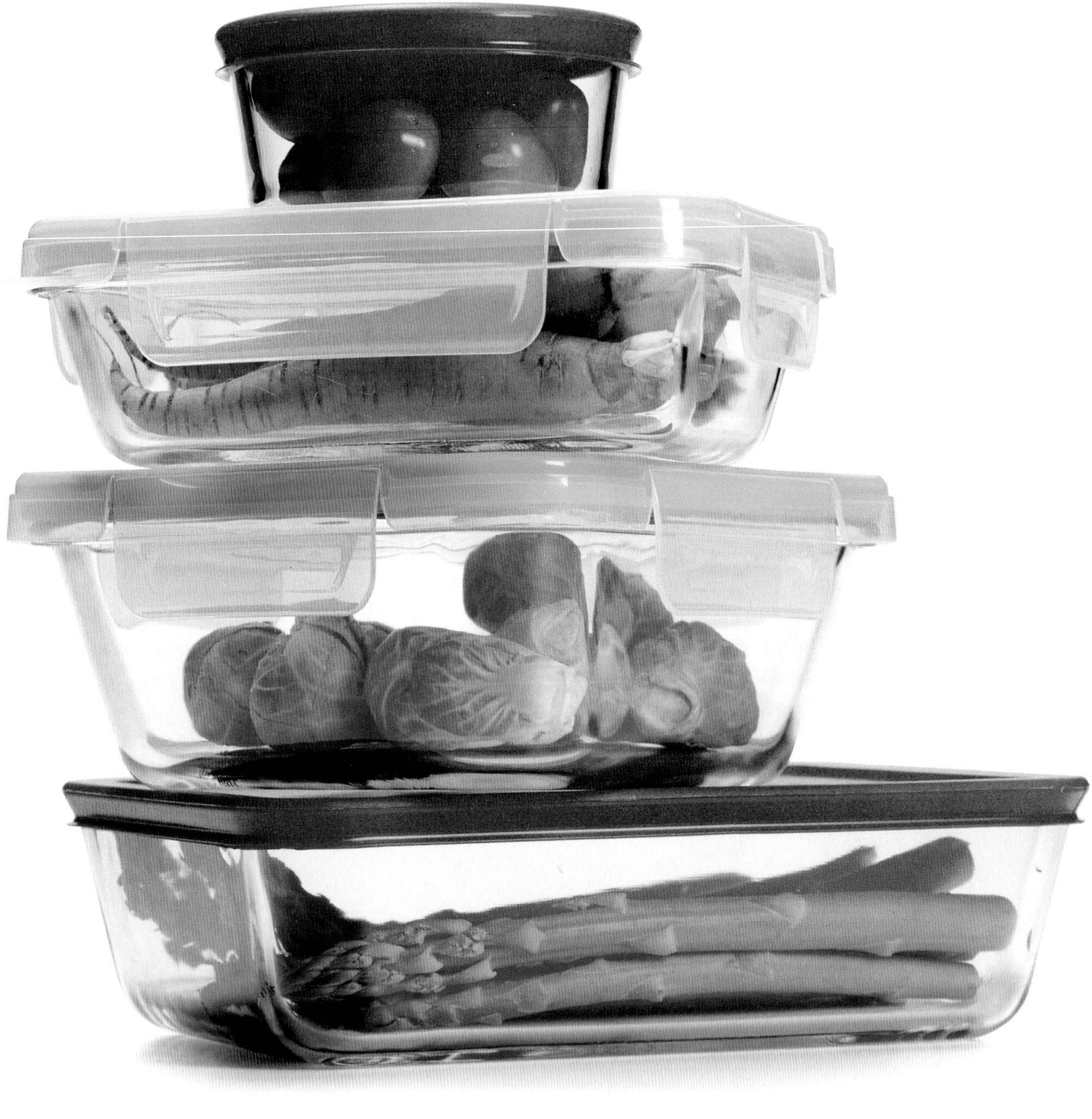

CHAPTER 3

A Clean Lifestyle

Now that you know how to locate clean, healthy foods, the next step is actually incorporating them into your life—otherwise known as the part that counts. It's easy to feel overwhelmed by your meal choices and the bounty of whole foods in your refrigerator and pantry, but armed with the right strategies—killer snack ideas, tips for eating well on the go, ideas for giving leftovers new life, learning how to cook once and eat all week, and more—you'll set yourself up for nothing but success.

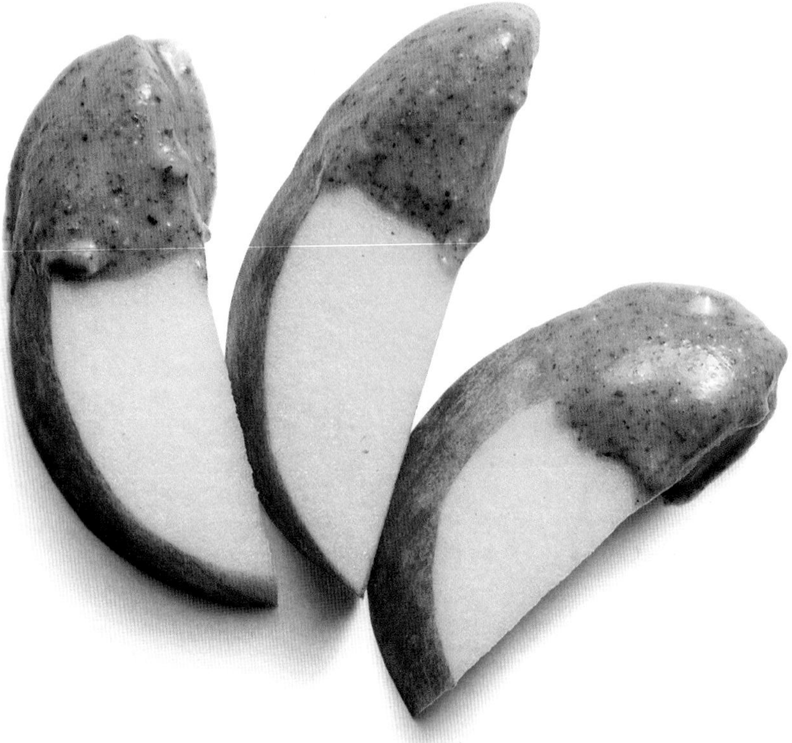

Snack Smarter

You know you should eat mindfully, sans any distractions, whenever possible—but sometimes you have no choice but to inhale a snack between work and yoga. That's okay, but it's not permission to compromise on quality (back away from the vending machine!). Nourishing grab 'n' go snacks can easily be made from unprocessed whole foods—all it takes is a little prep work and creativity, and lots of portable food containers. The reward is pretty great, too. Once you start experiencing the increased energy and satisfaction that comes from replacing nutrient-devoid granola bars with nourishing veggies and hummus, trail mix, and roasted chickpeas, you'll never look back. Here are some snacks to keep you eating clean despite a busy schedule:

- Sliced carrots and celery with nut butter or hummus
- Apples, pears, and bananas with nut butter
- Leftover turkey or chicken wrapped in a lettuce, kale, or Swiss chard leaf and secured with a toothpick
- Hard-boiled eggs—make a bunch on the weekend to eat throughout the week.
- Single portions of healthy trail mix—nuts and dried fruit are all you need.
- Homemade roasted chickpeas made with a dash of salt and rosemary
- Whole-grain toast, slathered with nut butter and topped with a sliced banana
- Cottage cheese topped with fresh pineapple, grapes, strawberries, or blueberries
- Whole wheat toast slathered with mashed avocado and finished with red-pepper flakes
- Homemade Chili-Lime Kale Chips (page 188)
- A few Medjool dates sliced lengthwise and filled with peanut butter, or filled with goat cheese and wrapped in uncured prosciutto
- Popcorn drizzled with olive oil and seasoned with herbs and black pepper
- DIY instant oatmeal—organic quick oats, cinnamon, raisins, and a sprinkle of brown sugar
- Grass-fed beef jerky and a piece of fruit

Anatomy of a Clean Lunch

Lunch is arguably the most difficult meal to eat clean. You're usually away from home and your well-stocked pantry, and often confronted with less-than-awesome cafeteria or fast-food options—not to mention your coworker's famous chocolate chip cookies that she feels the need to make on a biweekly basis. That's why packing your own lunch is key in maintaining a clean diet. But it's not as simple as throwing whatever you have in a paper bag. Here, we'll explain just what a clean, healthy, filling lunch looks like along with some quick and easy ideas:

- For maximum nutrition and to stay fuller for longer, pack lunches that contain a lean protein (chicken, tempeh, tuna salad), some high-quality fat (nuts, seeds, avocado), and complex carbs (fruits, veggies, quinoa, brown rice).
- Don't kid yourself—you can't get through the day without snacks. Toss a few high-nutrient picks in your lunch box, like the ones on

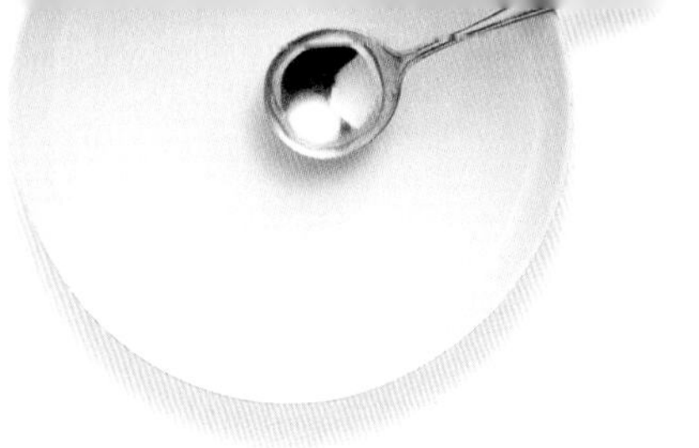

SOUP'S ON!

Did you buy more kale and carrots than you could eat in a week? To avoid waste and make the most of the produce you have on hand—even if it's starting to wilt—try making a big soup with your leftover vegetables at the end of each week. You can use nearly any combo of veggies and legumes with a low-salt, organic stock to create a delicious, healthy soup and give your sad-looking produce new life.

page 37, so you don't end up at the vending machine.

- Hydrate! Pack a big water bottle and set it right on your desk at work. Refill it a few times each day, so you're not tempted to drink a soda or juice. Can't take it flat? Stock up on some naturally flavored seltzer.
- Build a cleaner sandwich by making it on whole-grain bread and loading it with fresh veggies, a clean version of your favorite protein, and a low-sugar condiment.
- Build a "kitchen sink" salad—load up a large portable container with your favorite organic greens along with whatever veggies, protein, nuts, and dried fruit you have on hand. Top it all off with a simple homemade vinaigrette of oil, vinegar, and herbs.
- Get unconventional with your lunch. Want a lower-carb sandwich? Wrap up your protein in a kale or Swiss chard leaf. Want to skip the sandwich altogether? Top a roasted sweet potato with leftover veggies and a drizzle of olive oil for a clean take on a loaded baked potato.

Embrace Big-Batch Cooking

The key to cutting down time spent in the kitchen? Doubling recipes! It requires little extra effort up front, but will save you loads of time later in the week. Simply whip up a big meal on Sunday, then save leftover portions for lunches and dinners over the next few days. Alternatively, you can freeze them for later to create your own healthy version of a TV dinner. In addition to making one big meal, weekends are the perfect time to cook up a few staples that will work double or triple time for you during the week—a big batch of beans can be used in salads, soups, and chili; a roasted chicken can be dinner one night, incorporated into a salad or sandwich the next, and then turned into a stock; a medley of roasted or steamed vegetables can be tossed into stir-fries and frittatas. As you become accustomed to cooking with clean foods, you'll start to see how some have great multitasking potential.

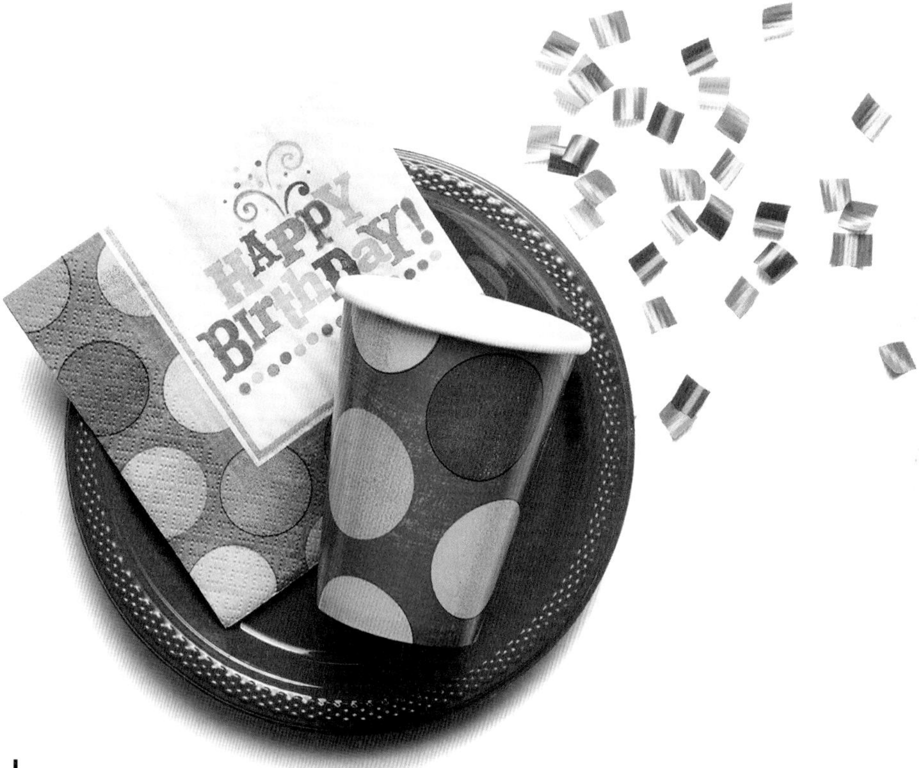

Learn Tricks to Eat Clean Anywhere

You've stocked your pantry and fridge with only clean, healthy options. You've been eating fruits, vegetables, lean proteins, and healthy grains and are feeling great. So what happens when you're invited to a dinner party, baby shower, or even just a nice dinner? Luckily, eating clean is not a "diet" in the standard sense. Instead, it's a way of life—and one that you can easily adapt to most every situation you find yourself in.

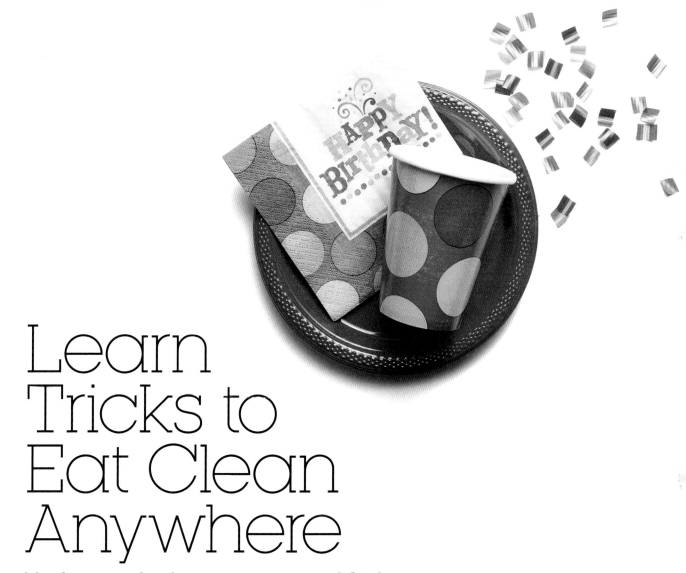

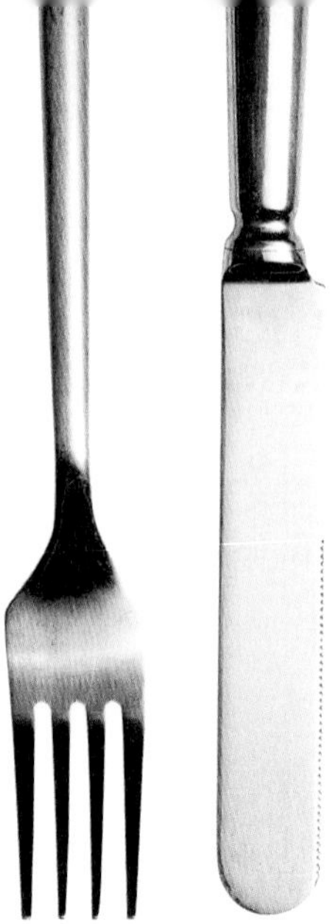

EATING OUT? SIT HERE

When you're eating out, sit at a high table close to a window—both factors can help you eat less and eat healthier, according to research done by Brian Wansink, PhD, director of Cornell's Food & Brand Lab. In Wansink's experiments, people sitting by windows or at high tables ordered healthier food and tended to skip dessert and alcohol compared to people sitting in dimly lit booths. Why? Being more visible and sitting in a more upright, alert position may make you more tuned into your hunger and food choices, making you less likely to indulge in something you know you should probably skip.

Eating Clean at a Restaurant

Obviously, restaurants are designed to get you excited about ordering food, and lots of it. But knowing what to look for on the menu can help you stay on track. Opt for dishes that feature a protein and vegetables, but not heavy processed starches like pasta. Seek out items described as baked, broiled, poached, or steamed, and avoid foods described as crispy, battered, breaded, fried, Alfredo, au gratin, Parmigiana, carbonara, or smothered. If there's sauce or salad dressing, ask what's in it and if you can have it on the side.

Another strategy: Ask for clean substitutions. You may be able to get fruit salad or mixed greens with an omelet instead of the go-to greasy home fries, or a green salad with a sandwich instead of French fries. As you grow accustomed to your clean-eating lifestyle, it will become easier to identify good choices at restaurants. And if you choose to "cheat" with something that doesn't classify as clean, don't sweat it, but do take note of how you feel after the meal. As your body becomes more accustomed to whole, unrefined foods, you'll likely find that heavy, processed foods make you feel sluggish, bloated, or even sick. Don't be surprised if you stop craving them altogether!

Eating Clean at a Party

Now this might seem impossible—*are those maple bacon mini cupcakes over there?!* But you've got this. Just remember, you are in control of what you put in your mouth. If there are clean choices available, like crudités or maybe light appetizers such as fruit slices and Cheddar, opt for those (and you can always bring your own dish, or stash some nuts in your purse). Pass on chips and creamy dips, heavy dishes like lasagna and casseroles, and sugary desserts. If you're going to drink alcohol, choose a glass or two of wine over hard liquor, and be sure to drink plenty of water as well—a seltzer with lime can feel more festive while still keeping calories close to zero. And keep in mind that enjoying a party is about the people, not the food. Have fun socializing with the other guests, talk about the dish you brought or your foray into healthy cooking, and pass on eating a full meal until later if there aren't any clean options available. But if you do indulge, just be sure to savor it—treats are certainly okay *in moderation*.

CLEAN FOOD STORAGE 101

Don't go through the trouble of making awesome clean meals only to toss them in a chemical-leaching container. A recent study found that there really are no "safe" plastics. Nearly all plastic containers tested exhibited some kind of estrogenic activity (yes, even BPA-free plastics), and things like heating these containers and loading them with acidic foods like tomato sauce caused them to leach even more chemicals into food. Your safest bet? Forgo storing your food in plastic altogether. Instead, use containers with a glass, stainless steel, or ceramic base and a plastic lid that doesn't come in contact with food (canning jars or recycled glass peanut butter jars will work!); buy foods like produce and nuts in bulk that you can store in your own plastic-free containers; and use reusable produce bags, like the ones from ecobags.com—typical flimsy produce bags can leach chemicals into your berries and broccoli.

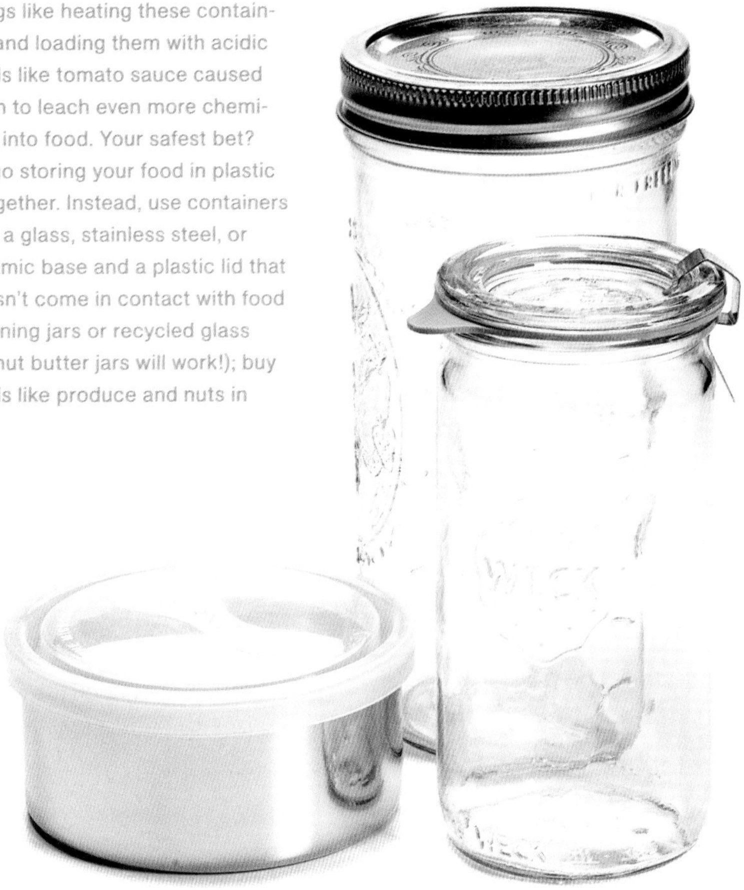

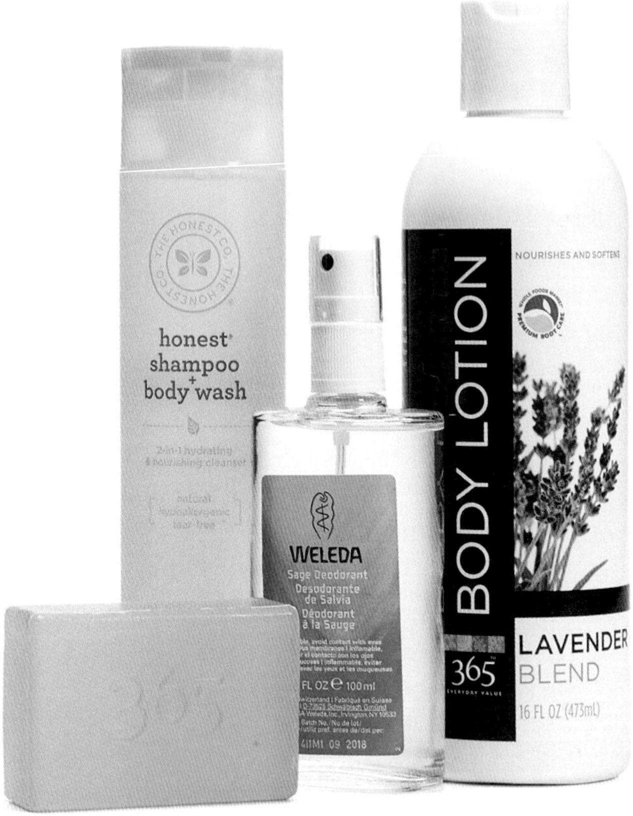

Clean Beauty Products

We hardly give our makeup routine a second thought, but after food, that might just be our biggest opportunity to avoid direct contact with some pretty funky ingredients. A disheartening amount of beauty products actually contain potential carcinogens, skin irritants, and byproducts of petroleum. Scary stuff! Read your labels and avoid products that contain these additives.

- **PHTHALATES:** Once these endocrine disruptors enter your system, they mimic hormones like estrogen and have been linked to early menopause. You'll find them in perfumes, lipstick, lotions, makeup, nail polish—anything with "fragrance" or "parfum" in the ingredient label (you'll never see "phthalates" there). Choose organic or phthalate-free products instead.
- **PARABENS:** These preservatives prevent bacteria, yeast, and mold from growing in your makeup, but they also mimic estrogen and could increase your risk of breast cancer. You'll find them in anything that ends in "–paraben" on the ingredient label—especially in deodorant, moisturizer, and makeup. Choose organic or paraben-free products instead.
- **FORMALDEHYDE-RELEASING PRESERVATIVES:** Certain preservatives in hair and skin products meant to keep bacteria at bay release the probable human carcinogen formaldehyde. You'll find them in shampoos, conditioners, moisturizers, cleansers, hand cream, hair gel, and shaving cream. Choose products labeled organic or preservative-free instead.
- **DBP (DIBUTYL PHTHALATE):** This chemical can be absorbed through skin or via inhalation and has been linked to birth defects in animals. You'll find it primarily in nail polish to make it flexible and stand up to chipping. Choose "3-free" or water-based products, which are free of a trifecta of dangerous nail polish ingredients, instead.
- **SULFATES:** These harsh detergents can strip the hair and skin of natural oils. You'll find them in shampoos, facial cleansers, body washes, or any other product that's meant to get sudsy. Choose sulfate-free products instead.
- **TOULENE:** Exposure to this neurotoxicant during pregnancy may cause developmental issues. You'll find it in nail polishes, synthetic fragrances, and hair dye. Choose "3-free" or water-based products instead.
- **PETROLEUM-BASED CHEMICALS:** Some petroleum derivatives may slow cell turnover—a process that's necessary for new, younger-looking skin. You'll find them in deodorant, aftershave, lotion, hair gel, and shampoo. Choose organic or petroleum-free products instead.
- **BUTYLATED HYDROXYANISOLE (BHA):** BHA is a preservative that's listed as a possible carcinogen. You'll find it concealer, mascara, blush, eyeliner, lip-gloss, and even diaper cream. Choose organic or preservative-free products instead.

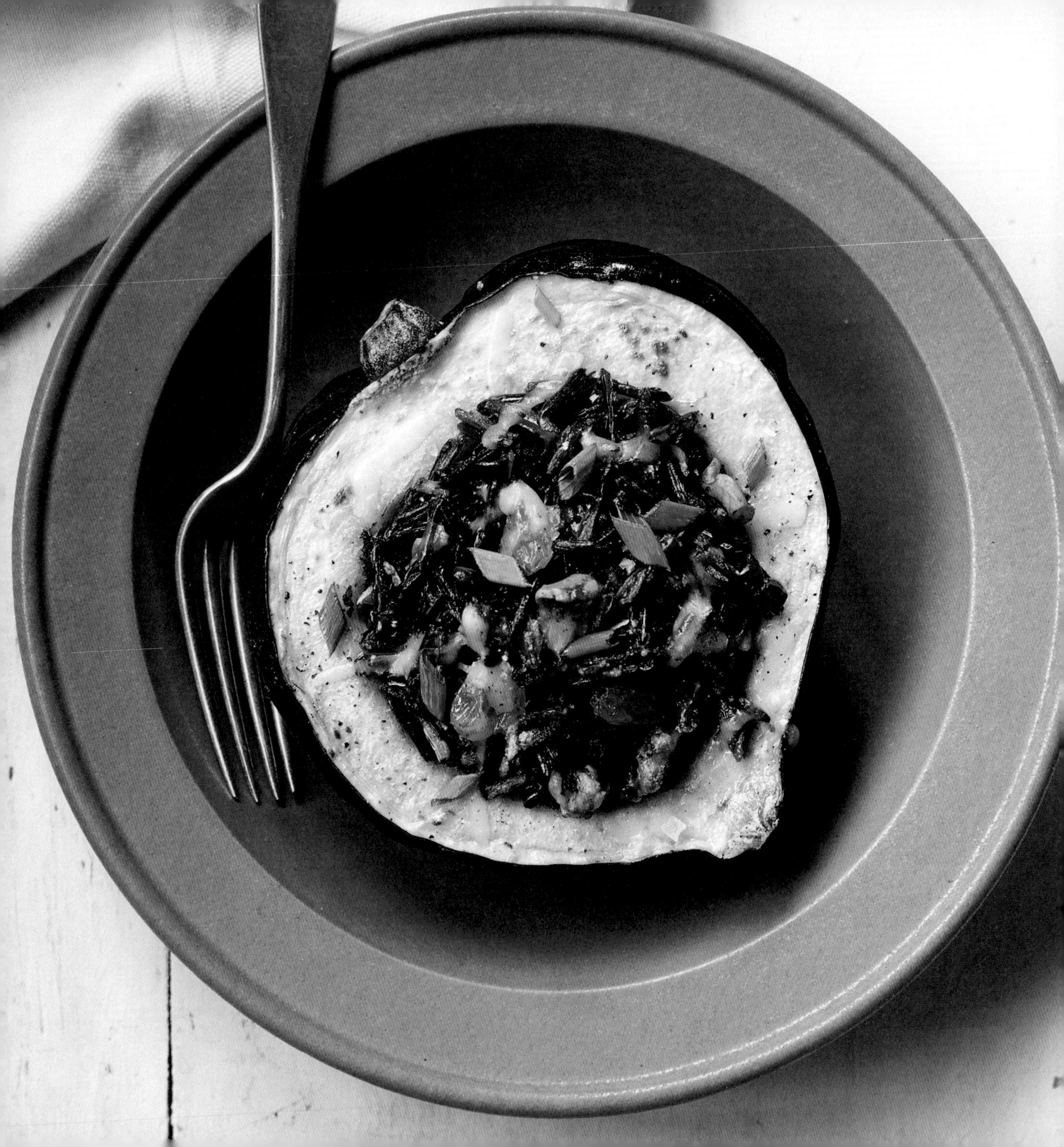

PART 2

The Ultimate Clean Foods (Plus Recipes!)

Sure, you've got the clean-eating basics down, but maybe you still have questions about putting your newfound knowledge into practice. Can I still have dessert? What kind of milk is best for me? Is pasta okay? What do I drink if I don't want water? This next part will explore some of these more complicated questions, help you navigate the grocery store, and ensure you have the best possible chance of eating clean and staying lean for good.

Packaged Fruit

Let's start with our juicy stand-in for all fruit—packaged peaches. As it turns out, frozen fruits without added sugar can actually have *more* nutritional value than their fresh counterparts. See, convenience doesn't always mean compromising.

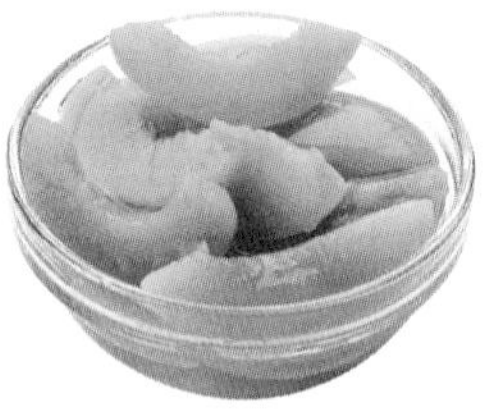

✷

NOT CLEAN

CANNED PEACHES IN SYRUP

Peaches in syrup are basically low-nutrient sugar bombs. Thanks to the addition of corn syrup, they have more sugar than either frozen or canned-in-juice varieties. Another bummer: The high heat used in the canning process degrades those powerful antioxidants.

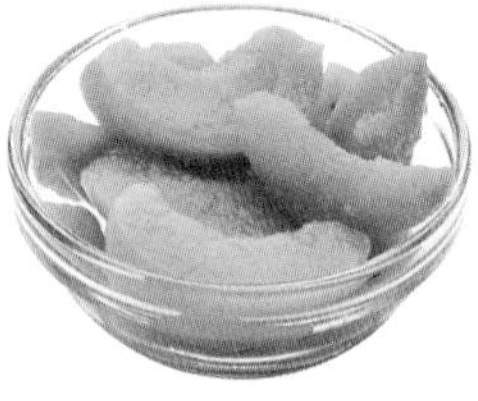

✷✷

CLEAN

CANNED OR JARRED PEACHES IN 100% JUICE

Peaches in 100% juice may contain some of the nutritional benefits of fresh and frozen such as antioxidants beta-carotene, vitamin C, and vitamin E, as well as B vitamins like folate. The big difference, though, is that they lack flavor.

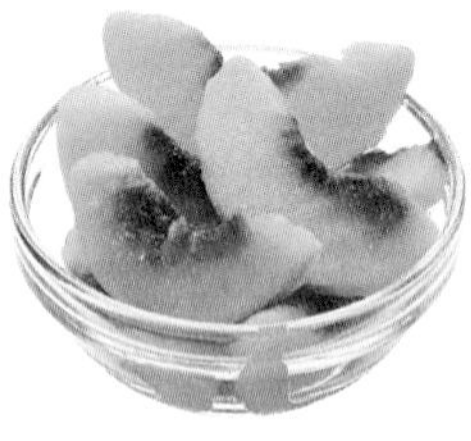

✷✷✷

CLEANEST

ORGANIC FROZEN SLICED PEACHES

Frozen fruits are frozen just after they're harvested—at their nutritional peak—so their vitamins, minerals, and antioxidants are locked in and won't be depleted as they sit in the freezer. Bonus: They're insanely versatile. Blend them with yogurt for a protein-packed smoothie; bake them with oats, cinnamon, and a drizzle of olive oil for dessert; or simply use a few to top off your morning oatmeal.

SPICED PEACH BUTTER

2 pounds frozen sliced peaches
½ cup honey
1½ teaspoons cinnamon
¼ teaspoon nutmeg
¼ teaspoon ground ginger

1. PLACE the peaches and ¼ cup plus 2 tablespoons water in a medium saucepan and cook over medium heat, stirring occasionally. Once it begins to boil, reduce the heat to low. Simmer until the peaches are soft, about 20 minutes. Add the honey and spices.

2. BLEND the peach mixture in a food processor or blender until smooth.

3. RETURN the peach mixture to the saucepan and cook over very low heat, stirring frequently, until thick enough that it doesn't run off a spoon when turned upside down, up to 2 hours. Place in a small jar and store in the refrigerator.

MAKES ABOUT ¾ CUP ||| Prep time: 35 minutes |||
Total time: 2 hours 35 minutes

Keep it Fresh!

Want to eat fresh peaches year-round without leaving a big carbon footprint? Freeze 'em yourself when they're in season! Simply halve, pit, and slice them into wedges. Place them on a parchment-lined baking sheet, freeze until firm, then transfer to a freezer bag and label. Voilà! Your summer's bounty preserved at its peak.

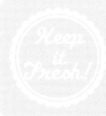

MINTY PEACH & HEMP HEART SMOOTHIE

2 cups frozen sliced peaches

1½ cups unsweetened plain almond milk

⅓ cup hemp hearts

¼ cup chopped Medjool dates

1 tablespoon vanilla extract

2 tablespoons finely chopped fresh mint leaves, plus sprigs for garnish

COMBINE the peaches, almond milk, hemp hearts, dates, vanilla, and chopped mint in a blender and process until smooth and frothy. Garnish with mint sprigs.

MAKES 2 SERVINGS ||| Prep time: 5 minutes ||| **Total time: 6 minutes**

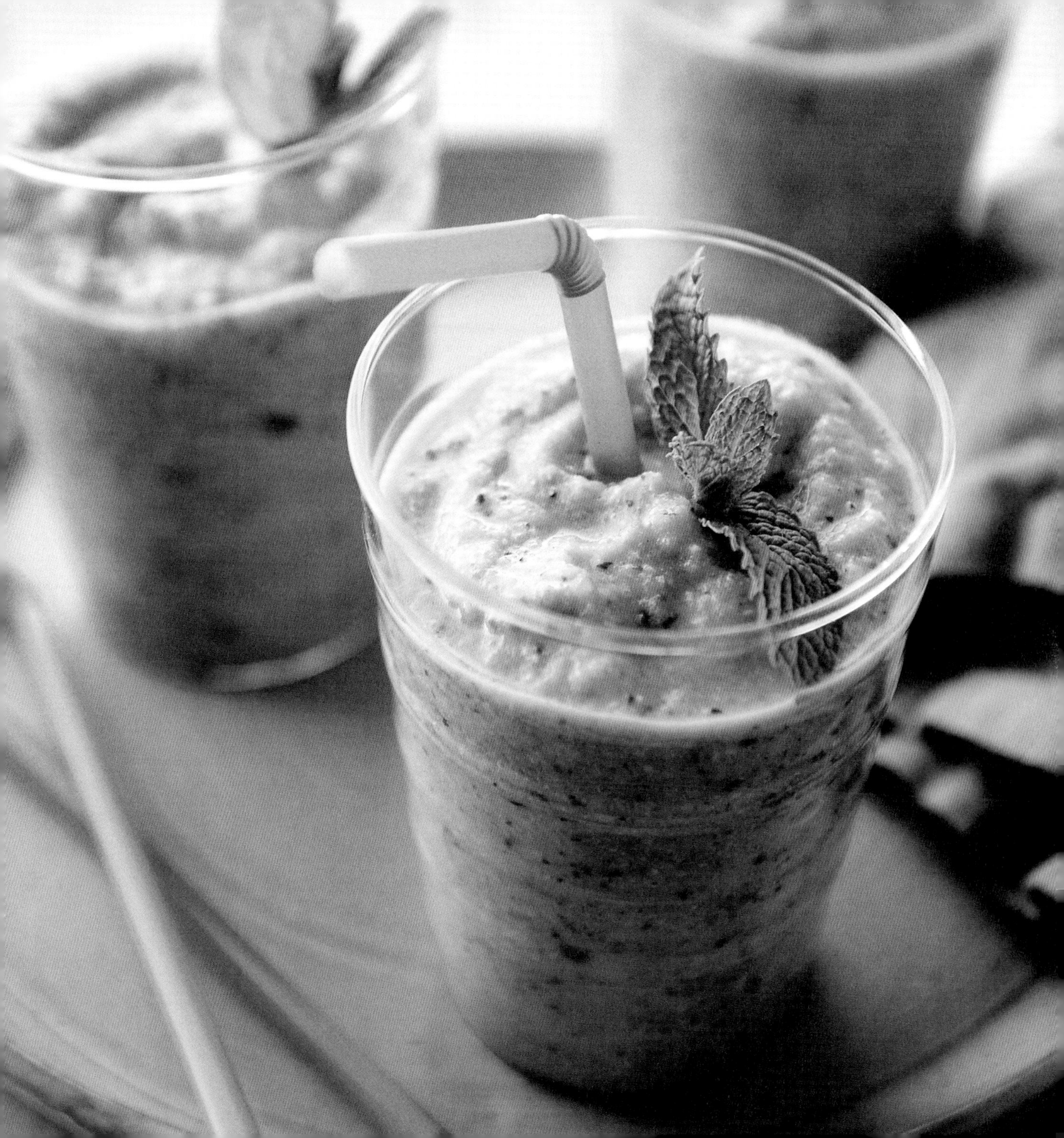

GRILLED THYME CHICKEN WITH QUINOA-PEACH SALAD

MARINADE AND CHICKEN

- **1 teaspoon chopped fresh thyme**
- **1 teaspoon minced garlic**
- **2 teaspoons extra virgin olive oil**
- **1 tablespoon fresh lemon juice**
- **⅓ cup low-sodium chicken broth or dry white wine**
- **½ pound boneless, skinless chicken breast**

SALAD

- **1 tablespoon chopped fresh thyme**
- **1 teaspoon minced garlic**
- **½ teaspoon grated lemon zest**
- **1 tablespoon fresh lemon juice**
- **2 teaspoons extra virgin olive oil**
- **½ teaspoon Dijon mustard**
- **1 cup frozen sliced peaches, thawed and cut into ½-inch pieces**
- **1 cup cooked quinoa**
- **¼ cup finely chopped unsalted dry-roasted almonds**

1. MARINATE the chicken: Combine the thyme, garlic, olive oil, lemon juice, and broth in a large zip-top plastic bag (or a shallow nonporous dish). Add the chicken and seal the bag (or cover the dish) and turn to coat. Marinate in the refrigerator for 2 hours.

2. PREPARE a grill for covered grilling at medium heat (or heat a stove-top grill pan over medium-high heat). Lightly oil the grill surface when ready to cook. Carefully place the chicken on the grill surface and grill until the center is no longer pink and the internal temperature reaches 165°F, about 8 minutes per side. Let stand for a few minutes before cutting into small chunks.

3. PREPARE the dressing: Whisk together the thyme, garlic, lemon zest, lemon juice, olive oil, and mustard in a small bowl. Add salt and pepper to taste.

4. TOSS together the chicken chunks, peaches, quinoa, almonds, and dressing in the bowl. Cover and chill in the refrigerator for 1 to 2 hours before serving.

MAKES 2 SERVINGS ||| Prep time: 30 minutes ||| **Total time: 35 minutes + 3 to 4 hours marinating and chilling time**

Packaged Vegetables

Popeye didn't eat it for nothing. Spinach is our stand-in for veggies because it is one of the most nutrient-dense greens you can find—in addition to a healthy dose of vitamin C, it's packed with vitamin K, which will helps keep your bones healthy; lutein, which helps prevent cataracts and macular degeneration; and twice the iron of most other greens—but if you're not buying fresh, you may not reap the benefits.

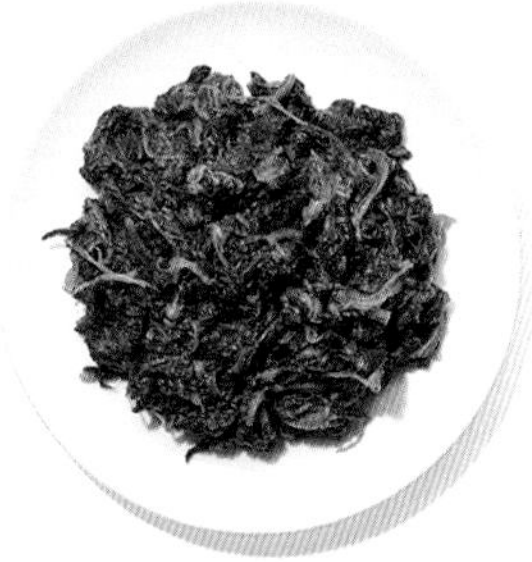

*

NOT CLEAN

CANNED SPINACH

Sure, a can of spinach is far from junk food and may still provide some health benefits, but you're going to lose out on taste and texture, and add a bunch of unwanted sodium to your diet.

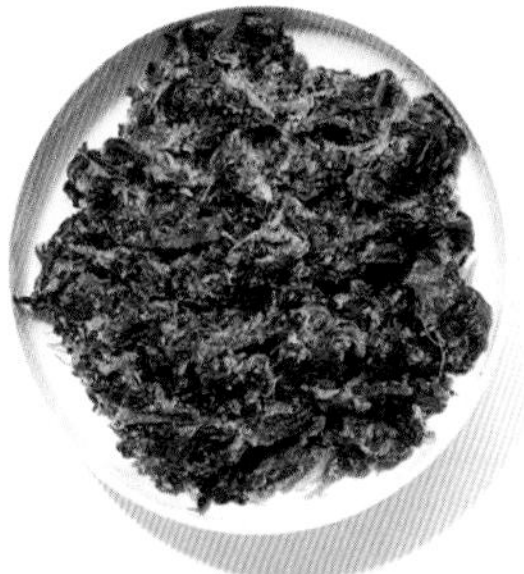

**

CLEAN

FROZEN SPINACH

While some frozen fruits and veggies can actually have a higher nutritional value than their fresh counterparts, a study by the Frozen Food Foundation found that frozen spinach had less vitamin C than a fresh bunch.

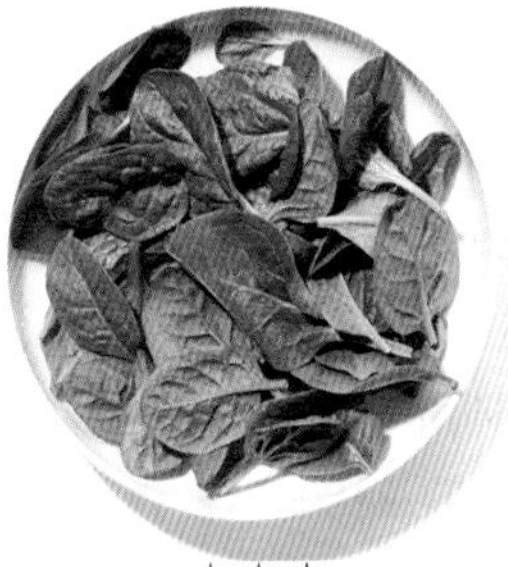

***

CLEANEST

ORGANIC BAGGED SPINACH

A bag of washed and ready-to-eat fresh spinach retains the most nutrients and is far more versatile than other forms—use it to quickly prepare salads and soups, sauté and use as a base for your protein, or whip it into a smoothie.

SPINACH, APPLE & CHIA SMOOTHIE

- ½ avocado, pitted and peeled
- ½ medium banana, frozen
- 2 Granny Smith apples, chopped
- 2 large handfuls spinach
- 2 tablespoons chia seeds
- 1 teaspoon vanilla extract
- 1 cup ice cubes
- 1½ cups unsweetened plain almond milk or milk of your choice
- 1 teaspoon honey (optional)

PLACE all the ingredients in a blender and process on high speed until smooth, about 2 minutes. Pour into 2 glasses and serve immediately.

MAKES 2 SERVINGS ||| Prep time: 5 minutes ||| **Total time: 5 minutes**

INDIAN-SPICED LENTILS WITH SPINACH & RED ONIONS

- 1 tablespoon grapeseed oil
- ½ cup finely chopped red onion
- 2 tablespoons golden raisins
- 1 teaspoon minced garlic
- ¾ teaspoon minced fresh ginger
- ½ teaspoon minced fresh serrano chile
- 1½ cups low-sodium vegetable broth
- ½ cup lentils, rinsed
- ½ teaspoon ground cumin
- ¼ teaspoon garam masala
- ¼ teaspoon turmeric
- 1 bag (5 ounces) spinach, chopped
- Fine sea salt and black pepper
- 1½ cups cooked brown rice or quinoa
- ¼ cup finely chopped cilantro (optional)

1. HEAT the oil in a medium skillet over medium heat. Add the onion and raisins and cook until the onion is lightly browned, about 10 minutes.

2. STIR in the garlic, ginger, and serrano. Cook for 1 minute, then stir in the broth, lentils, cumin, garam masala, and turmeric. As soon as the lentil mixture starts to boil, reduce the heat to low and simmer for 25 minutes.

3. ADD the spinach and a dash of salt and pepper. Cover and cook until the spinach is wilted, 5 minutes longer.

4. DIVIDE the brown rice between 2 small serving bowls and pour the lentil mixture on top. Garnish with the cilantro, if desired, and serve.

MAKES 2 SERVINGS ||| Prep time: 20 minutes ||| **Total time: 55 minutes**

Lettuce

Most greens live up to their superfood reputations, packing a good dose of potassium, vitamin K, folate, an array of antioxidants, and even calcium. But to be sure you're getting max nutrients per leaf—and avoiding pesticides in the process—opt for organic and locally grown whenever possible.

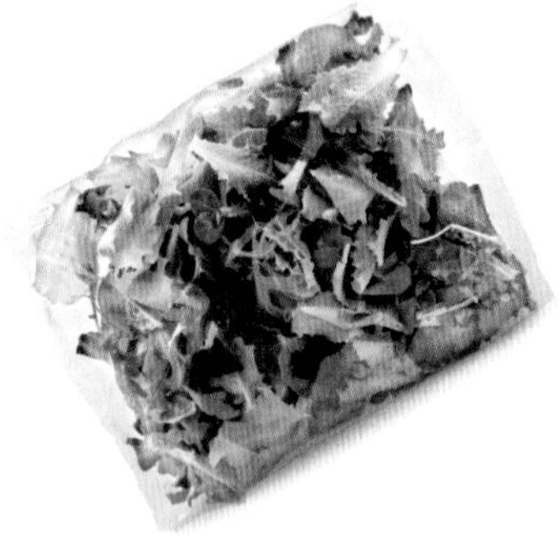

*

NOT CLEAN

REGULAR BAGGED GREENS

Conventional bagged greens are often washed with a mix of chlorine and water—not exactly appetizing. And like organic bagged greens, they're more likely to have fewer nutrients and make you sick. But perhaps worst of all is that they're grown with, and contain residues of, pesticides and fertilizers that no amount of washing can remove completely.

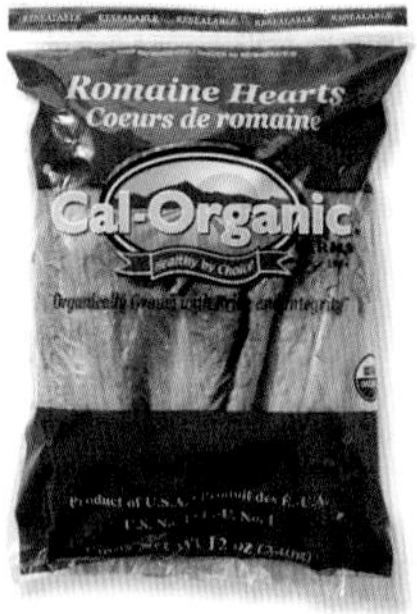

**

CLEAN

ORGANIC BAGGED GREENS

Because they're free of pesticides and funky chemicals, bagged greens are a good backup plan. But greens of any kind—even organic—can be up to 2 weeks old by the time you get them home. Meaning: fewer nutrients. Even more important, a recent investigation of 16 brands of prewashed greens found that many contained coliforms and *Enterococcus*, bacteria linked to foodborne illnesses.

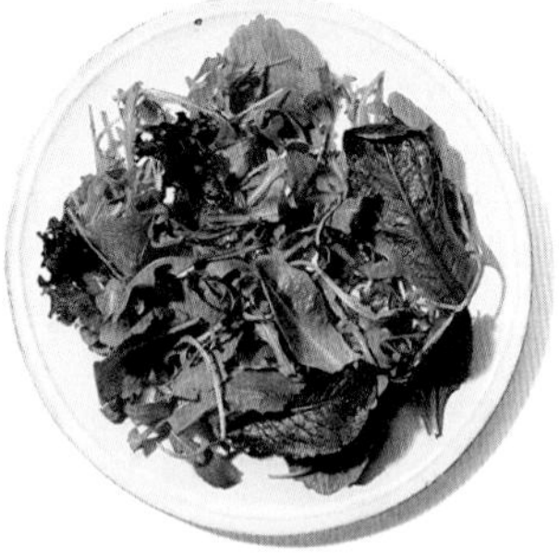

***

CLEANEST

ORGANIC LOCALLY GROWN GREENS

To get the most nutritional bang for your leafy green buck, buy locally grown organic greens that aren't prebagged. These can pack four times as many antioxidants as precut, washed, and bagged varieties, which lose more nutrients the longer they're in transit. And no bag means they're less likely to encourage the growth of dangerous pathogens that can make you sick.

KALE PESTO

- ½ cup sliced almonds
- ½ cup salted roasted sunflower seeds
- 1 cup loosely packed fresh basil leaves
- 1 cup roughly chopped and stemmed fresh kale
- ½ cup grated Parmesan
- ¾ cup extra virgin olive oil

COMBINE the almonds and sunflower seeds in a blender or food processor. Pulse to make small, even crumb-size pieces. Add the basil, kale, and Parmesan and pulse until evenly combined into the nuts. With the machine running, drizzle in the olive oil and ¼ cup water. Blend until the texture is uniform and the color is light green. Store in an airtight container in the refrigerator for up to 1 week.

MAKES 4 SERVINGS ||| Prep time: 10 minutes ||| **Total time: 10 minutes**

GREEN SMOOTHIE

- 1 Granny Smith apple, quartered
- 1½ cups spinach
- 2 inches fresh ginger, peeled
- Juice of 1 lime
- ½ cup 2% plain Greek yogurt
- 1 banana (optional: frozen banana)

COMBINE all the ingredients in a blender and process until smooth. Drink immediately.

MAKES 2 SERVINGS ||| Prep time: 5 minutes ||| **Total time: 5 minutes**

ARUGULA SALAD WITH ZUCCHINI RIBBONS

- 4 cups arugula
- 1 small zucchini (or ½ large)
- ⅓ cup salted roasted sunflower seeds
- ⅔ cup (2 ounces) pecan halves (optional: toasted)
- 1 ounce Parmesan, shaved
- 1 lemon, halved
- Grated zest of 1 small orange
- ¼ cup extra virgin olive oil

1. **PLACE** the arugula in a large bowl. Using a vegetable peeler, begin to shave the zucchini on one side over and over to make ribbons, turning every few strokes to evenly distribute peel. Stop when you reach the seedy core (and no more ribbons can be sliced). Gently distribute the ribbons on top of the arugula.

2. **SPRINKLE** on the sunflower seeds, pecans, and Parmesan shavings. Squeeze the lemon juice all around the top of the salad. Sprinkle on the orange zest and drizzle on the olive oil. Serve immediately.

MAKES 2 SERVINGS ||| Prep time: 15 minutes ||| **Total time: 15 minutes**

HEALTHY HACK

It's time to ditch your fat-free dressing: Recent research shows that a little fat can go a long way in helping you absorb more nutrients from your greens and other veggies, specifically boosting your absorption of carotenoids—antioxidants that have been linked to a reduced risk of cancer, heart disease, and macular degeneration. To get the most out of your next salad, dress your greens in olive oil and lemon juice or vinegar.

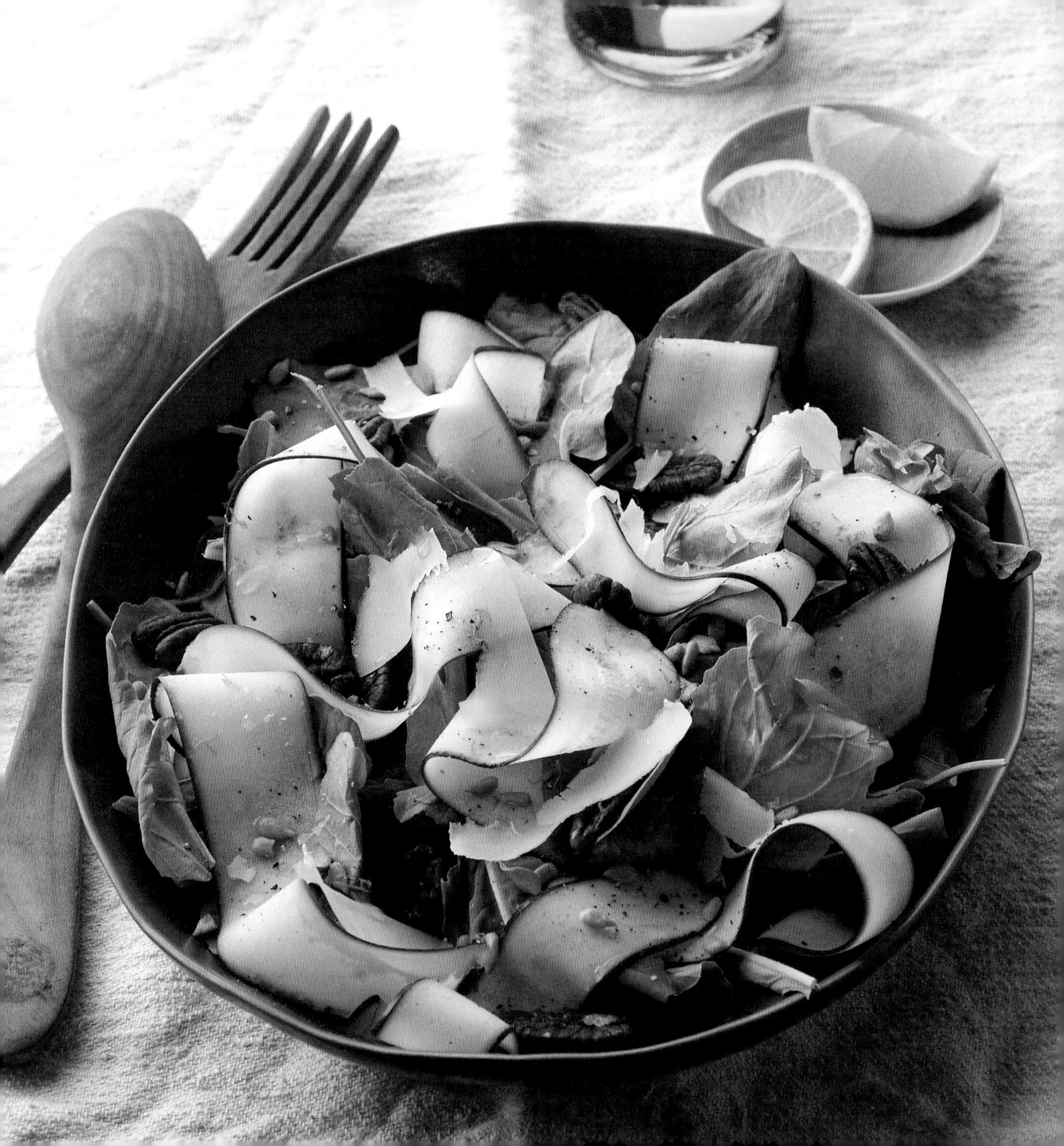

Beef

Ground beef and steak are some of the most important

foods to buy clean, given the dire state of factory farms and overuse of antibiotics and hormones—but they also have some of the most confusing label terminology out there. Your safest and most nutritious bet will always be 100% grass-fed and organic. No question.

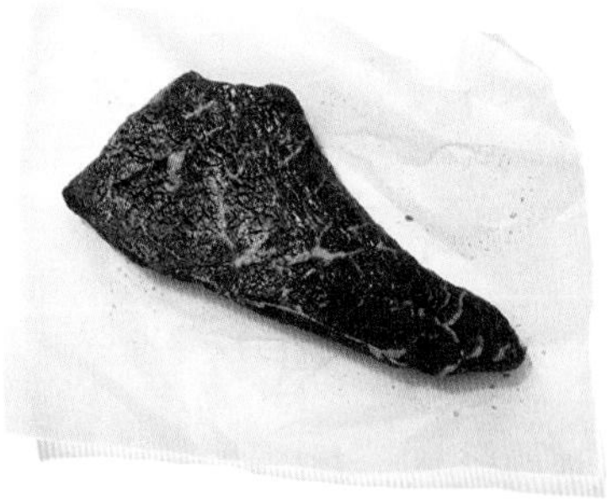

✷

NOT CLEAN

CONVENTIONAL BEEF

These animals spend much of their lives in cramped feedlots where they're fattened up on a diet of nonorganic grains, and often given growth hormones and antibiotics. Conventional beef contains far fewer omega-3s and more cholesterol and saturated fat than grass-fed and organic.

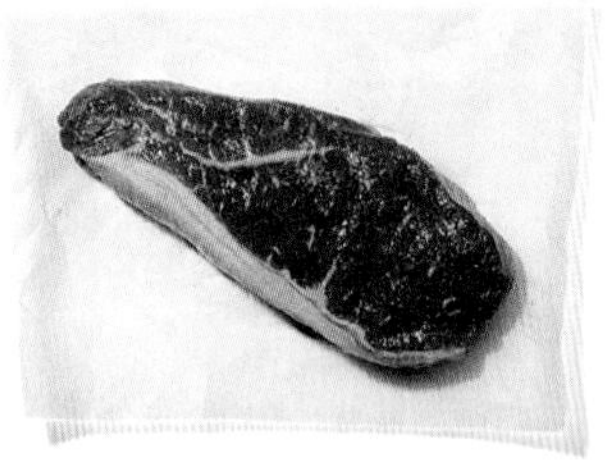

✷✷

CLEAN

ORGANIC BEEF

Organically raised cattle start on pasture. Then, to increase weight before slaughter, most cattle are fed a diet of organic grain, which diminishes the nutritional profile of their meat compared to that from 100% grass-fed cattle. On the plus side, they're never given hormones or antibiotics, and they have outdoor access throughout their lives.

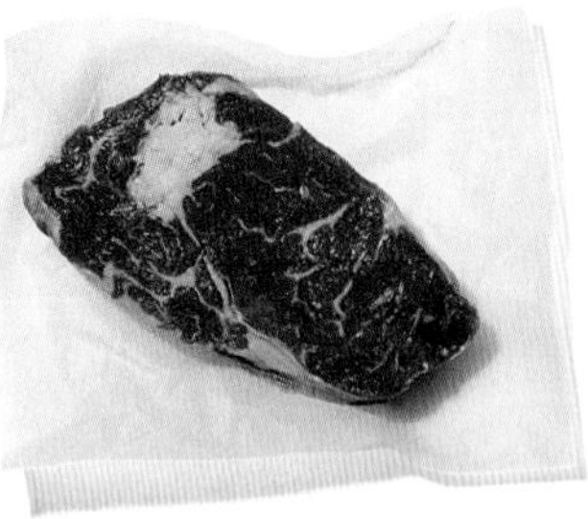

✷✷✷

CLEANEST

100% GRASS-FED BEEF

Grass-fed cattle are never injected with hormones and antibiotics, and they've grazed on pasture their entire lives—no grains allowed. The meat from grass-fed animals contains more omega-3s, conjugated linoleic acid (CLA)—a fat that may reduce risk of heart disease, cancer, and even promote weight loss—and other nutrients like beta-carotene than conventional beef.

GROUND BEEF RAGU OVER BARLEY

- 1 **tablespoon olive oil**
- 2 **tablespoons finely chopped yellow onion**
- ½ **red bell pepper, chopped**
- ½ **yellow bell pepper, chopped**
- 1 **cup chopped cremini mushrooms**
- 1 **clove garlic, minced**
- ½ **pound lean ground beef**
- ¼ **teaspoon dried basil**
- ¼ **teaspoon dried oregano**
- ¼ **teaspoon dried rosemary**
- ¼ **teaspoon dried thyme**
- ¼ **teaspoon red-pepper flakes**
- ¼ **teaspoon coarse sea salt**
- 1 **cup canned crushed tomatoes**
- 2 **tablespoons tomato paste**
- ½ **cup hulled barley**

1. HEAT the oil in a large saucepan over medium heat. Add the onion, red pepper, yellow pepper, and mushrooms and cook until soft, about 10 minutes. Add the garlic and cook, stirring constantly, for another minute.

2. PUSH the veggies to the edges of the pan and place the ground beef in the center. Break the ground beef apart and continue to cook until browned and broken into small pieces, about 5 minutes.

3. ADD the dried herbs, pepper flakes, and salt. Stir the veggies and seasonings into the beef and cook for another minute. Add the tomatoes and tomato paste. Cover and simmer until the mixture thickens and most excess liquid is gone, about 10 minutes.

4. COMBINE the barley and 1½ cups water in a medium saucepan. Bring to a boil, reduce to a low simmer, cover, and cook until the barley is tender, about 35 minutes.

5. DRAIN any excess water from the barley and serve topped with the beef ragu.

MAKES 2 SERVINGS ||| Prep time: 25 minutes ||| **Total time: 40 minutes**

SLOW-COOKED SHREDDED BEEF TACOS

- **6 ounces beef shoulder**
- **1 large tomato, roughly chopped**
- **½ yellow onion, roughly chopped**
- **1 clove garlic**
- **3 cups beef broth**
- **1 tablespoon apple cider vinegar**
- **½ teaspoon chipotle powder**
- **½ teaspoon ground cumin**
- **⅛ to ¼ teaspoon cayenne, to taste (optional)**
- **Pinch of coarse sea salt**
- **Pinch of black pepper**
- **4 corn tortillas**
- **¼ cup thinly sliced cabbage**
- **¼ cup mashed avocado**
- **4 lime wedges**

1. COMBINE the beef, tomato, onion, garlic, broth, vinegar, spices, salt, and pepper in a medium saucepan. Bring to a simmer, cover, and cook until so tender it can be pulled apart with a fork, about 2 hours 30 minutes, adding more broth as needed.

2. UNCOVER and cook until the remaining liquid reduces to form a thick sauce.

3. PULL the beef, still in the pot, into shreds using 2 forks.

4. PLACE one-fourth of shredded beef onto the center of each corn tortilla and top with 1 tablespoon cabbage, 1 tablespoon avocado, and a squeeze of lime.

MAKES 2 SERVINGS (2 TACOS EACH) ||| Prep time: 15 minutes ||| **Total time: 45 minutes**

LABEL, DECODED!

If "grass-fed" is the gold standard, then "grass-fed, grain-finished" sure sounds like a close second. But nutritionally, it's nothing more than a trick of words. Basically, anything you buy that's not 100% grass-fed is grass-fed, grain-finished. Most calves actually start out on pasture but then get shipped to feedlots to fatten up on grain, and within weeks, the nutritional perks of grass feeding are lost.

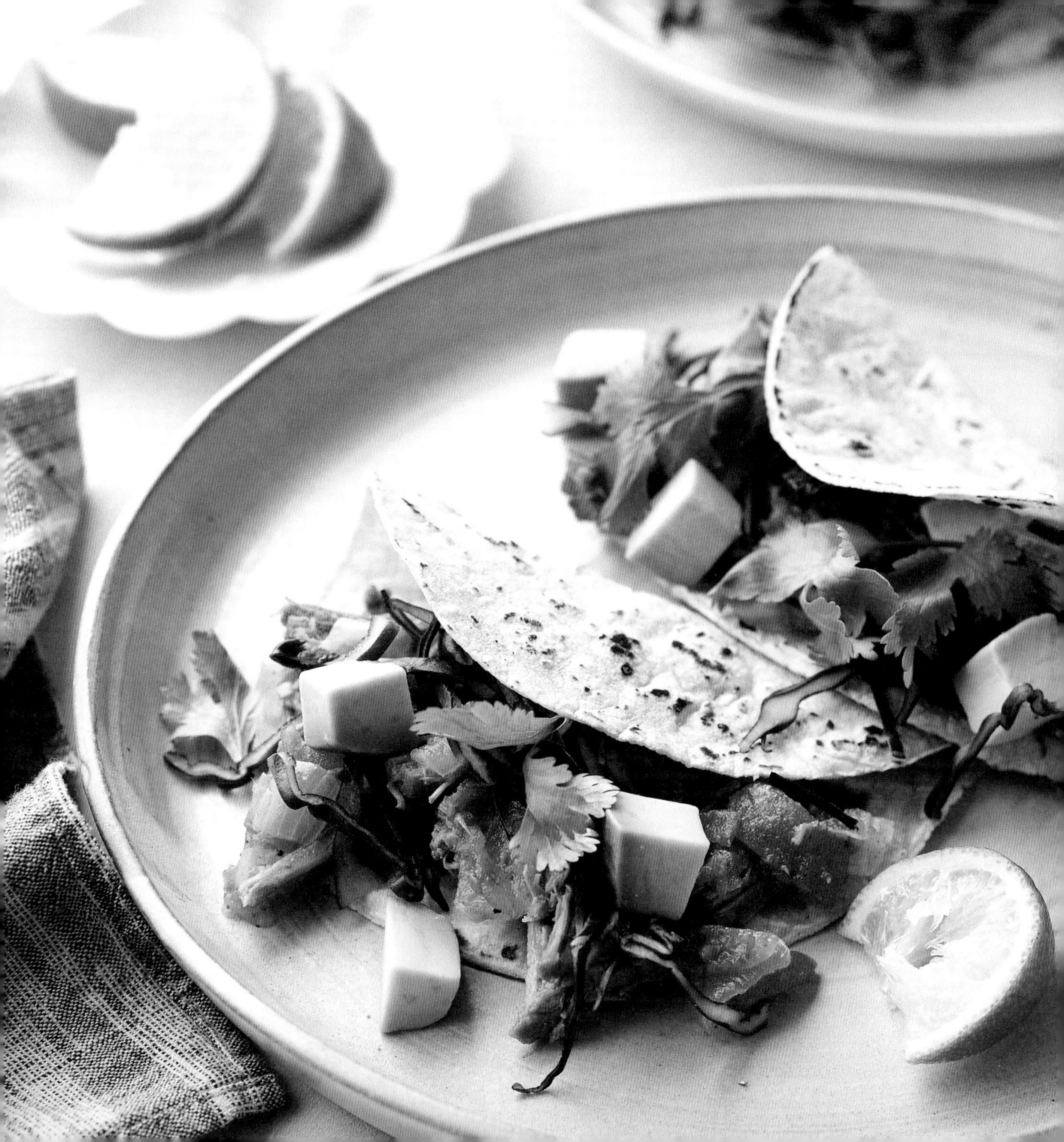

BEEF & SWEET POTATO STEW

- **1 tablespoon olive oil**
- **1 rib celery, chopped**
- **1 carrot, chopped**
- **¼ yellow onion, chopped**
- **½ large sweet potato, chopped**
- **½ cup cubed (¾-inch) lean beef, such as bottom or top round**
- **½ cup chopped cremini mushrooms**
- **2 cloves garlic, minced**
- **1 cup beef broth**
- **¼ cup stout beer**
- **1 bay leaf**
- **2 teaspoons tomato paste**

1. **HEAT** the oil in a medium saucepan over medium heat. Add the celery, carrot, onion, and sweet potato and cook until the onions become translucent, about 10 minutes.

2. **ADD** the beef and mushrooms and cook, stirring frequently, until the beef is browned and the mushrooms are softened, about 10 minutes longer. Add the garlic and stir for 1 minute.

3. **POUR** in the broth, stout, and 1 cup water. Add the bay leaf and tomato paste. Bring the mixture to a boil. Reduce to a simmer, cover, and cook for 1 hour.

MAKES 2 SERVINGS ||| Prep time: 25 minutes ||| **Total time: 1 hour 25 minutes**

Turkey

Who doesn't love turkey? It's lean, versatile, and just one serving delivers nearly half a day's worth of protein, plus a healthy dose of selenium and B vitamins. But to make sure you're getting all the good stuff, and none of the funky flavorings or antibiotics, opt for fresh and organic.

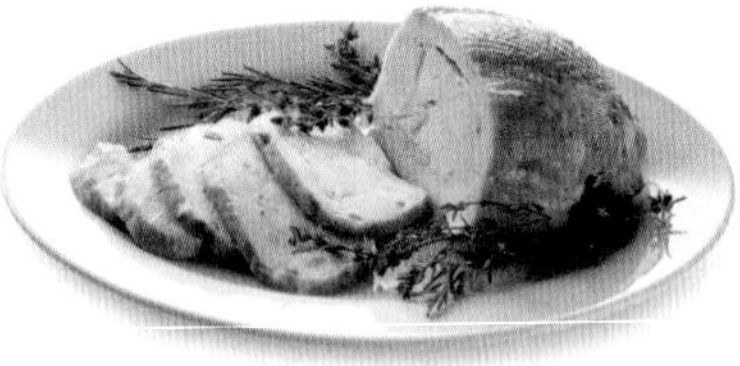

*

NOT CLEAN

CONVENTIONAL FROZEN TURKEY INJECTED WITH SODIUM OR FLAVOR

Many store-bought frozen turkeys have been injected with a solution that contains preservatives, sodium, coloring ingredients, or artificial flavors. This solution can negatively impact blood pressure.

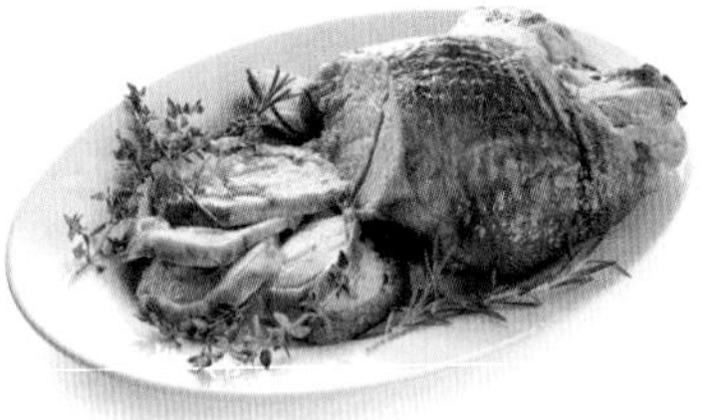

**

CLEAN

CONVENTIONAL NATURAL TURKEY

No added sodium or flavorings here, but these birds were still most likely given antibiotics; fed a diet of nonorganic, potentially pesticide-riddled feed; and raised in cramped indoor cages.

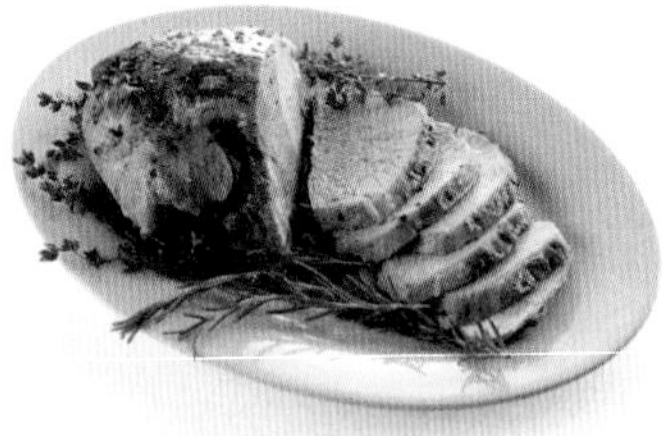

***

CLEANEST

ORGANIC NATURAL TURKEY

Buying organic means avoiding antibiotics and pesticides (from the nonorganic feed the turkeys consumed); while natural, according to the USDA, means your turkey hasn't been injected with sodium or flavorings. Pastured turkeys—ones that have been allowed to roam outdoors in their natural environment—are an added plus, but may be hard to find.

THAI TURKEY SALAD

DRESSING

- 2 tablespoons sesame oil
- Juice of 1 lemon
- 3 tablespoons water
- 2 tablespoons wheat-free tamari
- 1 inch fresh ginger, grated
- 1 small clove garlic, peeled
- 2 teaspoons creamy peanut butter
- 2 teaspoons sugar

TURKEY

- 2 tablespoons coconut oil
- ½ pound ground turkey breast
- 6 inches lemongrass, finely sliced into coins
- 1 clove garlic, grated
- 1 inch fresh ginger, grated
- Juice of 2 limes
- 1 tablespoon rice vinegar
- 2 tablespoons tahini
- Cayenne (optional)

SALAD

- 2 cups chopped spinach
- 1 red bell pepper, cut into matchsticks
- ¼ small head red cabbage, thinly sliced
- 2 ounces snow peas
- 4 or 5 large fresh basil leaves, julienned, plus small sprigs for garnish
- ¼ cup chopped salted roasted peanuts

1. MAKE the dressing: Combine the dressing ingredients in a blender and puree until smooth.

2. PREPARE the turkey: Heat the coconut oil in a medium skillet over medium-high heat. Add the turkey and chop roughly with a wooden spatula to break it up. Add the lemongrass, garlic, ginger, lime juice, vinegar, tahini, and a dash of cayenne (if using). Cook, stirring, until no pink remains. Remove from the heat and cover.

3. ASSEMBLE the salad: Layer the spinach, bell pepper, cabbage, and snow peas on 2 plates. Stir the basil into the hot turkey and fold to wilt. Divide into 2 portions and top each salad with half the dressing, or to taste. Garnish with the basil sprigs and peanuts.

MAKES 2 SERVINGS ||| Prep time: 20 minutes ||| **Total time: 30 minutes**

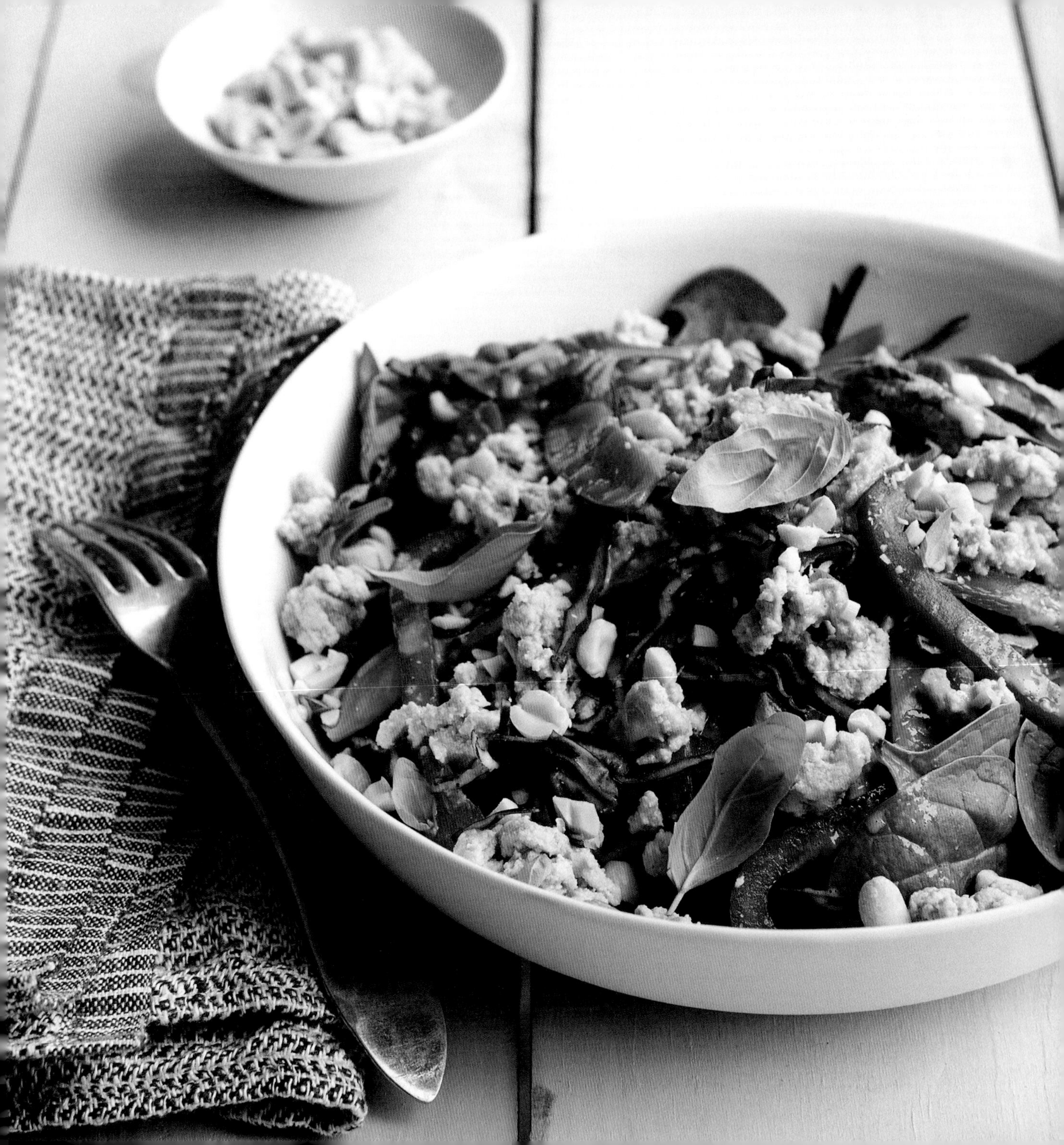

HERBED ROAST TURKEY BREAST

- ½ **teaspoon dried thyme**
- ½ **teaspoon dried savory**
- ½ **teaspoon dried marjoram**
- ½ **teaspoon dried rosemary**
- ¼ **teaspoon fine sea salt**
- ¼ **teaspoon black pepper**
- ½ **teaspoon grated lemon zest**
- 1 **bone-in turkey breast half (about 3 pounds)**
- 1 **tablespoon butter, at room temperature**

1. HEAT the oven to 400°F.

2. COMBINE the herbs, salt, pepper, and lemon zest in a small bowl.

3. PAT the turkey dry and place on an easily cleanable surface. Gently separate the skin from the meat, creating a pocket to rub the herbs and butter into. Rub the butter onto the turkey underneath and over the skin. Rub the herb mix under and over the skin.

4. PLACE on a rimmed baking sheet and roast until the internal temperature reaches 160°F, 45 to 55 minutes. Remove from the oven and let sit at room temperature for 10 minutes before slicing.

MAKES 2 SERVINGS ||| Prep time: 10 minutes ||| **Total time: 1 hour 15 minutes**

Clean Shopping Tip

Organic fresh turkeys can be hard to find, but your local butcher or a specialty food market should have the 411 on where to get the best birds and can often place an order for you. Just be sure to order a few weeks in advance around the holidays.

TURKEY TETRAZZINI WITH CREAMY CAULIFLOWER SAUCE

- ½ pound whole-grain spaghetti (or other long noodle), broken in half
- 1 small head cauliflower, broken into florets
- 1 cup water
- ¼ cup 2% plain Greek yogurt
- 2 tablespoons extra virgin olive oil
- 2 cloves garlic, minced
- 1 pound cremini mushrooms, sliced
- ½ teaspoon fine sea salt
- ½ cup dry white wine
- ¼ cup all-purpose flour
- 2 cups turkey broth or vegetable broth
- 1 pound cooked turkey, diced or shredded
- 1 cup frozen green peas
- 1½ cups frozen chopped kale
- ½ cup shredded part-skim mozzarella
- ½ cup grated Parmesan
- Salt and black pepper

1. HEAT the oven to 350°F.

2. PREPARE the pasta per package directions, cooking it 1 or 2 minutes shy of the times listed. Drain and rinse.

3. POUR 1 cup water into a separate saucepan and add the cauliflower. Simmer until fork-tender, about 8 minutes. Transfer the cauliflower and the water it cooked in to a blender. Add the yogurt and puree until smooth.

4. HEAT the olive oil in a large pot over medium-high heat. Add the garlic and sauté until just fragrant, about 1 minute. Add the mushrooms and salt, cover, and cook for 5 minutes, until reduced in size by about half. Pour in the wine and simmer uncovered for 5 minutes. Sprinkle in the flour and stir to combine, then add the broth and bring to a simmer. Stir in the cauliflower puree. Add the turkey, peas, kale, mozzarella, and ¼ cup of the Parmesan and fold to combine. Add the drained pasta and stir to coat.

5. POUR the mixture into a 9 x 9-inch baking pan and top with the remaining ¼ cup Parmesan. Bake until golden brown, 15 to 20 minutes. Let stand for 15 minutes before serving.

MAKES 4 SERVINGS ||| Prep time: 15 minutes ||| **Total time: 1 hour 15 minutes**

Deli Meat

Sure, cold cuts are a quick and easy source of protein, but they're also a speedy delivery system for not-so-delicious synthetic nitrites, excess sodium, and fillers. To ensure you're loading your organic whole-grain bread or lettuce wrap with only the good stuff, go for organic and uncured.

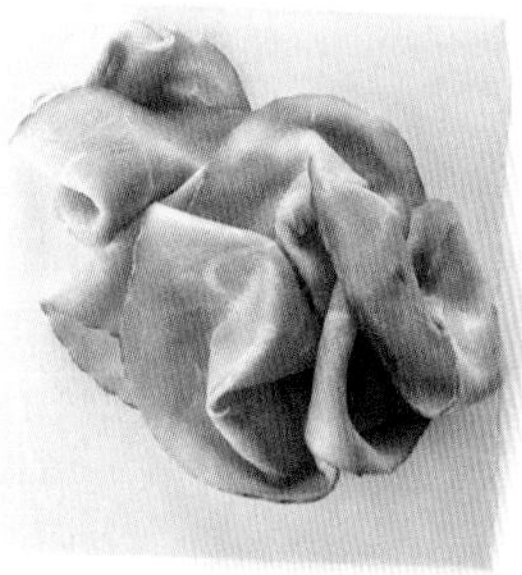

*

NOT CLEAN

TRADITIONAL CURED MEAT (WITH SYNTHETIC NITRITES)

Traditionally cured deli meats are just kind of gross—they can contain synthetic nitrites, loads of fillers, and excessive sodium, which can lead to high blood pressure. Studies suggest that sodium may increase your risk of heart disease, diabetes, and cancer.

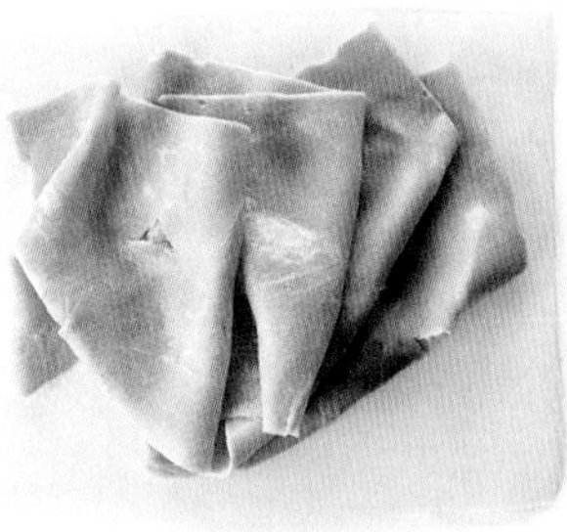

**

CLEAN

CONVENTIONAL UNCURED MEAT

These won't deliver the organic benefits—animals were likely given antibiotics and hormones—but they'll still be free of synthetic nitrites. To maintain freshness and kill pathogens, uncured meats do often contain celery powder or salt, a naturally occurring *nitrate* that's considered safer than its lab-produced counterpart. These might also contain fillers for texture such as corn syrup and carrageenan—a seaweed extract that's been linked to gut inflammation.

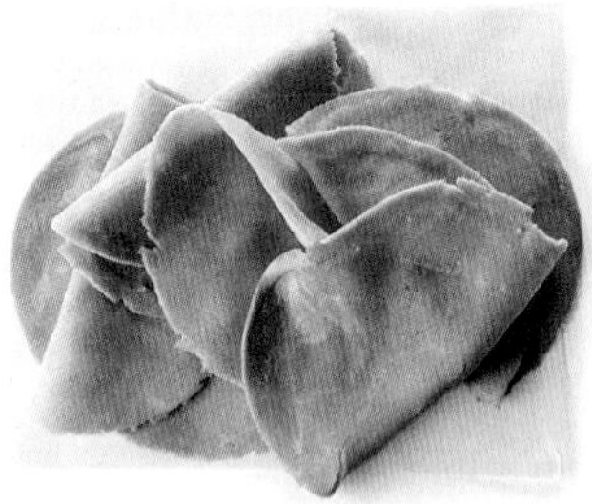

***

CLEANEST

ORGANIC UNCURED MEAT

The animals used to produce these meats were fed a cleaner diet of organic feed and not given antibiotics or hormones; and these meats weren't pumped with synthetic sodium nitrite either. All deli meat, however, can be high in sodium, so always be mindful of how much you eat. You can find presliced brands like Applegate at most markets and the deli counter at most natural food stores should have this option.

SMOKED TURKEY PANINI WITH QUICK-PICKLED ASPARAGUS

- **1 bunch asparagus (about 1 pound), tough ends trimmed**
- **1 cup rice vinegar (or other white vinegar)**
- **2 tablespoons sugar**
- **1 tablespoon fine sea salt**
- **¼ cup diced onion**
- **1 inch fresh ginger, cut into 4 pieces**
- **2 tablespoons mayonnaise**
- **2 whole wheat ciabatta rolls, split**
- **6 ounces sliced uncured smoked turkey**
- **2 ounces sliced Havarti cheese**
- **8 fresh basil leaves**
- **1 tablespoon extra virgin olive oil**

1. CUT the asparagus into 2- to 3-inch pieces and place in a heatproof bowl with room for 2 cups of additional liquid.

2. COMBINE 1 cup water, the vinegar, sugar, salt, onion, and ginger in a medium saucepan and bring to a boil. Pour the boiling mixture over the asparagus. Cover the bowl with plastic wrap or foil and let cool for 30 minutes at room temperature. Transfer to the refrigerator to chill for 1 hour. (The pickled asparagus can be made well ahead; they will keep for up to 1 week.)

3. ASSEMBLE the panini: Spread 1 tablespoon mayo on the cut sides of each roll. Divide the turkey, cheese, and basil between the rolls. Add 10 to 12 pieces of asparagus per sandwich and close the rolls. Brush the outside of the rolls with the olive oil.

4. HEAT a panini press. Add the sandwiches and cook until the outside is golden brown and crisp, while the inside stays soft and warm. (If you're not using a panini press, heat a medium skillet over medium-high heat. Add the sandwiches and weight down with a heavy-bottomed pan to press the sandwich during cooking.)

MAKES 2 SERVINGS ||| Prep time: 10 minutes ||| **Total time: 20 minutes + 1 hour chilling time**

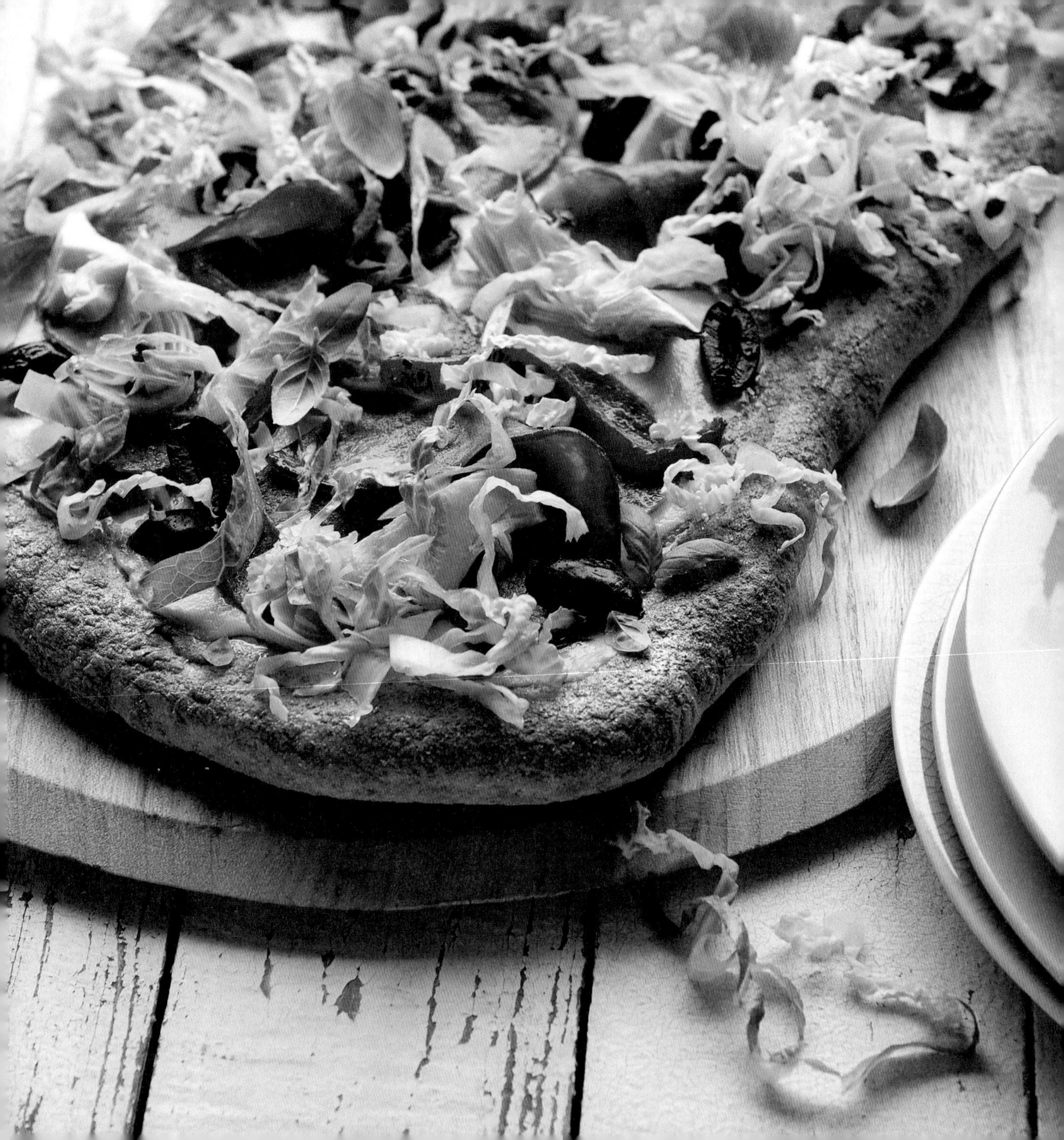

SALAMI & HAM FLATBREAD

DOUGH

- **1 envelope (2¼ teaspoons) rapid rise yeast**
- **1½ cups whole wheat flour**
- **1 teaspoon dried oregano**
- **1 tablespoon sugar**
- **½ teaspoon fine sea salt**
- **½ cup warm (not hot) water**

TOPPINGS

- **2 ounces uncured salami, sliced**
- **2 ounces uncured sliced ham, rolled into straws**
- **⅓ cup kalamata olives**
- **1 large roasted red pepper, thinly sliced**
- **¾ cup water-packed canned artichoke hearts, drained**
- **2 ounces sliced mozzarella**
- **1 cup chopped romaine lettuce**
- **3 tablespoons fresh basil leaves, roughly chopped**
- **3 tablespoons fresh mint leaves, roughly chopped**
- **2 tablespoons extra virgin olive oil**

1. HEAT the oven to 425°F.

2. MAKE the dough: Combine the yeast, 1 cup of the flour, the oregano, sugar, and salt in a bowl, stirring to mix evenly. Pour in the warm water and stir gently until evenly mixed (the dough will be wet). Spread the remaining ½ cup flour on a clean, flat surface and turn the dough out onto it. Knead in enough additional flour so the dough is not sticky, then knead for 3 to 4 minutes to develop gluten. Place in a warm place to sit for 5 minutes to allow the yeast to work.

3. PREPARE the toppings while the dough rests.

4. STRETCH the dough into a rough 14-inch square on a baking sheet. Brush or drizzle with the olive oil and bake for 10 minutes. Reduce the oven temperature to 375°F. Remove from the oven and layer on the meats, olives, roasted pepper, artichokes, and cheese. Bake for 10 minutes longer, just to warm the ingredients.

5. GARNISH with the lettuce and fresh herbs. Cut into squares to serve.

MAKES 2 SERVINGS ||| Prep time: 15 minutes ||| **Total time: 35 minutes**

MEDITERRANEAN CHICKEN WRAPS

- ½ **small cucumber**
- 4 **tablespoons olive hummus**
- 2 **whole wheat tortillas (8-inch diameter)**
- ¼ **cup crumbled feta cheese (1 ounce)**
- 4 **ounces deli sliced chicken breast**
- 1 **small tomato, sliced**
- 1 **ounce uncured salami, sliced**
- 1 **cup fresh spinach**
- 2 **sprigs fresh dill**

1. PEEL the cucumber into ribbons with a vegetable peeler, turning to shave ribbons from each of 4 sides.

2. SPREAD 2 tablespoons of hummus over each tortilla. Sprinkle each with half the feta. Divide the cucumber, chicken, tomato, salami, spinach, and dill between the two. Fold the wrap up and use a toothpick to secure if not eating immediately.

MAKES 2 SERVINGS ||| Prep time: 5 minutes ||| **Total time: 5 minutes**

Did You Know?

Synthetic nitrites, which are used to preserve meat, have gotten a bad rap since scientists discovered that the compounds may convert to potential carcinogens under high temperatures. Yet there are also *natural* nitrites, a byproduct produced when we eat fruits and veggies rich in naturally occurring dietary *nitrates*, like beets and leafy greens. Natural sources seem to pose no harm: Two new studies suggest they reduce risk for blood clots, stroke, and heart attack. Some food manufacturers now cure meat with natural nitrate sources, like celery extract, in place of synthetic nitrites.

Salmon

Salmon may be everyone's favorite superfood of the sea—

it's got loads of heart-healthy omega-3s, filling protein, and pretty much tastes incredible however you prep it. But if you want to avoid seriously scary pollutants and antibiotics, go wild.

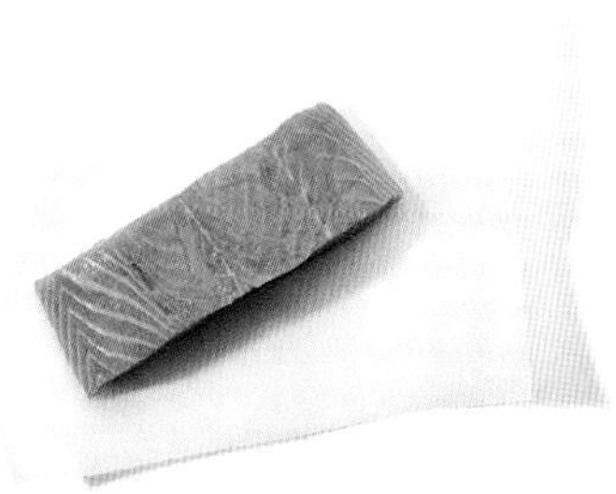

✱

NOT CLEAN

FARM-RAISED SALMON

Farm-raised salmon are far more likely to be exposed to persistent organic pollutants (POPs) than fish that have lived their lives in a natural environment.

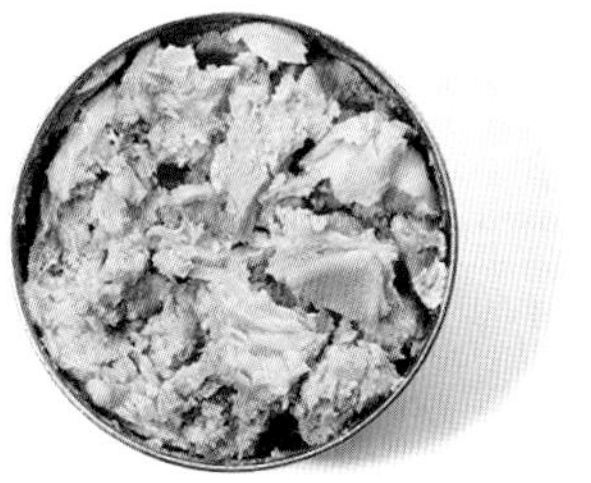

✱✱

CLEAN

CANNED WILD SALMON

Seems strange, but if you can't get fresh wild salmon, go for canned instead of fresh farmed salmon. Canned salmon will still give you a helping of omega-3 fatty acids, essential nutrients that your body cannot produce on its own. These fats help promote healthy joints and skin, and reduce your risk of heart disease.

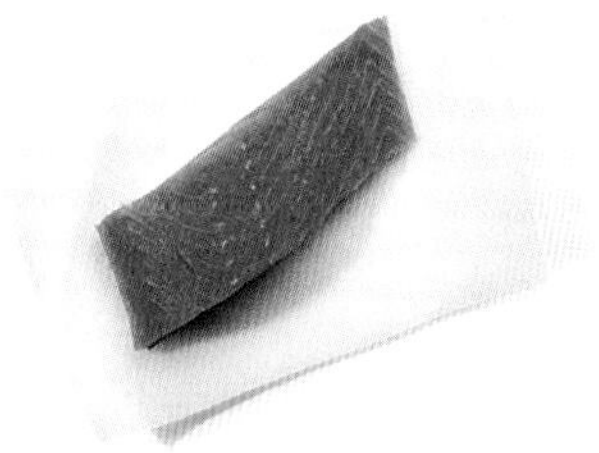

✱✱✱

CLEANEST

FRESH WILD OR ALASKAN SALMON

Wild salmon is both more nutritious and safer than farmed salmon—it has fewer calories and a significantly lower fat content than farmed salmon, but still packs a good dose of heart-healthy omega-3s. Eating wild also means you're avoiding POPs, which have been associated with obesity, diabetes, and cancer.

CITRUS WILD SALMON WITH MANGO RED PEPPER SALSA

SALSA

- **2 tablespoons fresh lime juice**
- **1 tablespoon fresh lemon juice**
- **2 teaspoons honey**
- **Pinch of black pepper**
- **1 cup diced mango**
- **1 cup diced red bell pepper**
- **2 tablespoons finely chopped red onion**
- **2 tablespoons chopped cilantro**

SALMON

- **3 tablespoons orange juice**
- **2 tablespoons lemon juice**
- **¼ cup vegetable broth**
- **1 tablespoon olive oil**
- **1 tablespoon tamari**
- **1 teaspoon honey**
- **Pinch each of salt and black pepper**
- **1 teaspoon minced garlic**
- **1 teaspoon minced fresh ginger**
- **2 skin-on wild salmon fillets (6 ounces each)**

1. MAKE the salsa: Combine the lime juice, lemon juice, honey, and black pepper in a medium bowl. Gently stir in the mango, bell pepper, red onion, and cilantro until coated evenly. Cover and chill in the refrigerator until serving time.

2. PREPARE the salmon: Combine the orange juice, lemon juice, broth, olive oil, tamari, honey, salt, pepper, garlic, and ginger in a large zip-top plastic bag (or a shallow nonporous dish). Add the salmon, seal the bag, and turn to coat (or carefully flip the salmon over with a spatula). Let marinate in the refrigerator for at least 15 and up to 30 minutes.

3. HEAT a grill or grill pan to medium-high. Lightly oil the grill surface when ready to cook.

4. REMOVE the salmon from the marinade (discard the marinade). Carefully place the salmon skin side down on the grill surface. Grill for 3 to 4 minutes per side. The salmon is done when the fish is no longer translucent in the center and it easily pulls into flakes. Serve topped with the salsa.

MAKES 2 SERVINGS ||| Prep time: 15 minutes ||| **Total time: 15 minutes + 15–30 minutes marinating time**

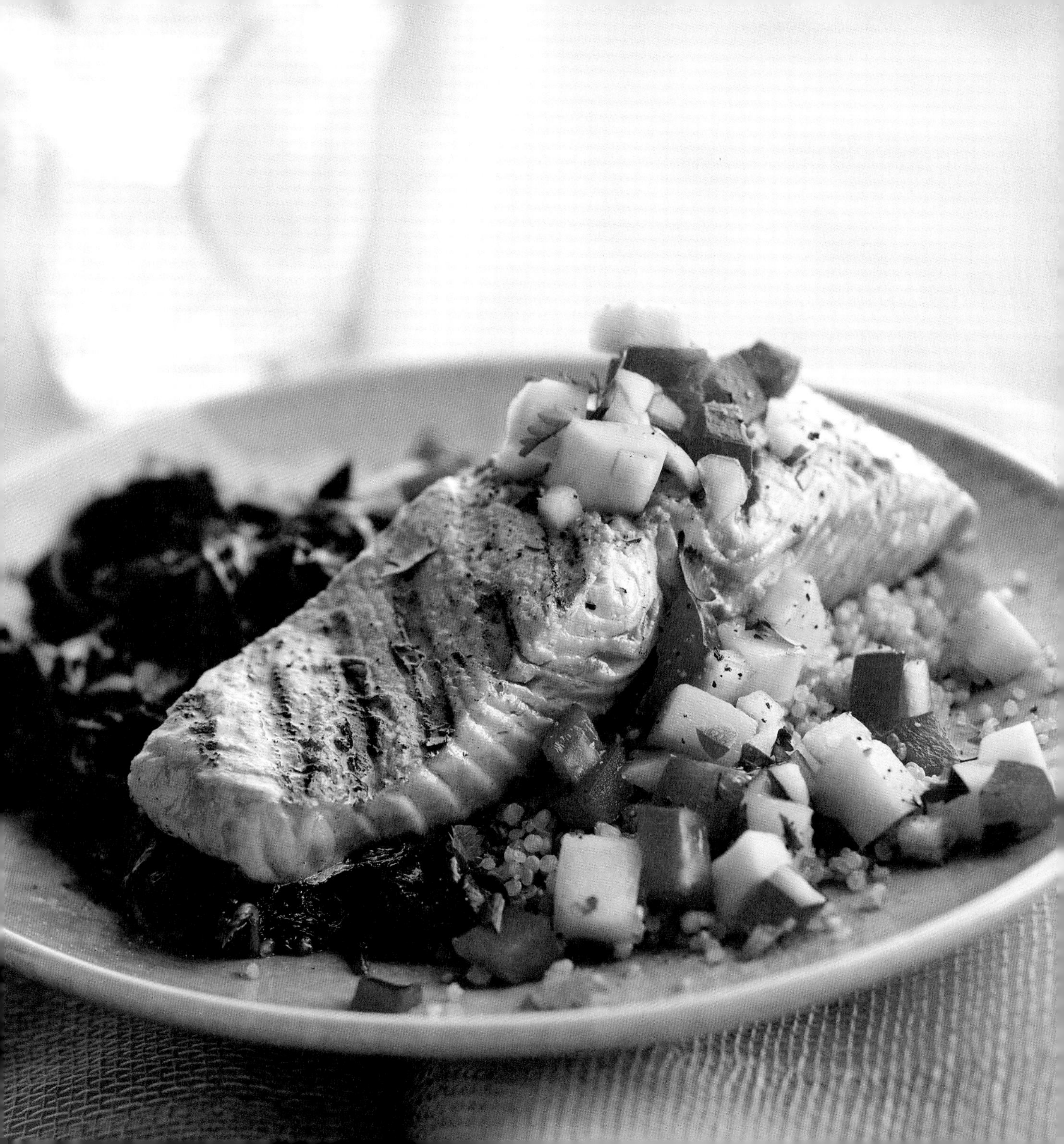

ALASKA SALMON & SWEET POTATO CUMIN CAKES

- **2 medium sweet potatoes, skin on**
- **3 ounces skin-on Alaska salmon fillet**
- **1 teaspoon olive oil**
- **Black pepper**
- **2 teaspoons cilantro**
- **1 tablespoon tahini**
- **1 tablespoon fresh lime juice**
- **1 large egg**
- **1 teaspoon finely minced garlic**
- **1½ teaspoons ground cumin**
- **1 teaspoon chili powder**
- **3 tablespoons plus ⅓ cup whole wheat flour**
- **1 tablespoon plus 1 teaspoon grapeseed oil**

1. HEAT the oven to 400°F. Line a baking sheet with foil.

2. PIERCE the sweet potatoes with a fork 5 or 6 times. Place on the baking sheet (but leave a little room for the salmon, which will be added in) and bake for 30 minutes.

3. BRUSH the salmon with the olive oil and season lightly with pepper. When the sweet potatoes have been in the oven 30 minutes, add the salmon skin side down to the baking sheet and bake for 12 to 15 minutes longer, until the salmon is cooked through and flaky and the sweet potatoes are tender.

4. SCOOP the sweet potato flesh into a medium bowl and lightly mash. Chop the salmon and add to the bowl. Add the cilantro, tahini, lime juice, egg, garlic, cumin, chili powder, and 3 tablespoons of the flour and stir well.

5. PLACE the remaining ⅓ cup flour in a shallow bowl. Form the salmon-sweet potato mixture into 6 patties. Lightly coat the cakes in the flour and set aside on a cutting board.

6. LINE a plate with paper towels and set by the stove. Heat 1 tablespoon of the grapeseed oil in a large skillet over -medium-high heat. Place half of the patties in the skillet and cook until browned on the bottom, about 3 minutes. Flip and cook until browned on the other side, about 3 minutes longer. Transfer to the lined plate. Repeat with the remaining 1 teaspoon oil and patties. Serve hot.

MAKES 2 SERVINGS ||| Prep time: 5 minutes ||| **Total time: 20 minutes**

CURRY-SPICED SALMON OVER CILANTRO-SUNCHOKE PUREE

- **1½ tablespoons reduced-sodium wheat-free tamari**
- **1 teaspoon curry powder**
- **1 teaspoon grated lemon zest**
- **2 teaspoons fresh lemon juice**
- **⅛ teaspoon black pepper**
- **3 teaspoons grapeseed oil**
- **2 skin-on wild salmon fillets (4 ounces each)**
- **¼ pound Yukon Gold potatoes, cubed**
- **½ pound sunchokes, peeled and cubed**
- **Fine sea salt**
- **½ tablespoon unsalted butter**
- **¼ teaspoon minced fresh ginger**
- **¼ teaspoon minced garlic**
- **½ teaspoon ground coriander**
- **⅛ teaspoon ground cumin**
- **¼ cup chopped cilantro**

1. COMBINE the tamari, curry powder, lemon zest, lemon juice, black pepper, and 1 teaspoon of the grapeseed oil in a large zip-top plastic bag (or a shallow nonporous dish). Add the salmon and seal the bag and turn to coat (or carefully flip the salmon over with a spatula). Marinate in the refrigerator for 15 to 30 minutes.

2. COMBINE the potatoes, sunchokes, ⅛ teaspoon salt, and water to cover in a medium saucepan. Bring to a boil, then reduce the heat to medium and cook until the potatoes and sunchokes are tender, about 10 minutes. Drain and transfer to a food processor.

3. ADD the butter, ginger, garlic, coriander, cumin, and cilantro. Puree until smooth. Season to taste with salt. Set aside and cover to keep warm.

4. HEAT the remaining 2 teaspoons oil in a medium skillet over medium heat. Drain the salmon (discard the marinade). Increase the heat to high and carefully place the salmon skin side down in the skillet. Cook until the fish is no longer translucent in the center and it pulls easily into flakes, 3 to 4 minutes per side.

5. SERVE the salmon on a bed of the sunchoke puree.

MAKES 2 SERVINGS ||| Prep time: 15 minutes ||| **Total time: 50 minutes**

Canned Fish

Canned fish is an easy and convenient way to get a dose of protein and omega-3s in your diet without all the prep work of fresh. But fear about toxins is warranted when it comes to this convenience food, so minimize your exposure by choosing the sagest seafood.

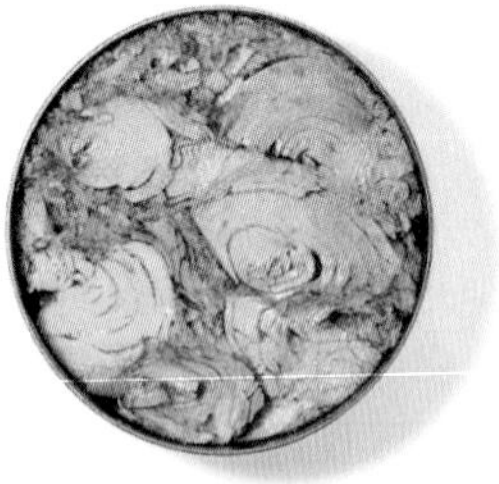

*

NOT CLEAN

WHITE OR ALBACORE TUNA

Mercury levels in canned white or albacore tuna can be up to three times that of light tuna! Even worse, most conventionally processed brands on the market are lower in omega-3s than both light tuna and canned salmon.

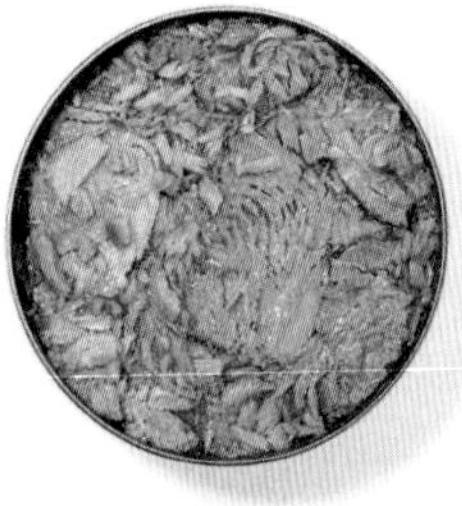

**

CLEAN

LIGHT TUNA

If you can't give up your tuna salad, opt for light tuna over white or albacore. Light tuna, made from lower-mercury skipjack tuna, not only contains fewer calories than white or albacore, but has less sodium, and more selenium, vitamin B_{12}, and iron.

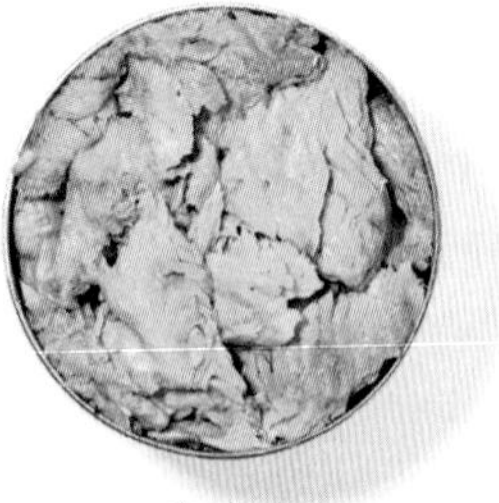

***

CLEANEST

CANNED SALMON

Canned salmon provides more omega-3s in the form of DHA and EPA– two fatty acids that are essential for a healthy brain–than other canned fish (about 500 milligrams in an 8-ounce serving). Bonus: Because salmon is lower on the food chain (typically feeding on microscopic plankton), it's likely to contain fewer toxins like mercury than tuna.

SALMON CROQUETTES

- **1 can (14 ounces) wild salmon, drained**
- **1 large egg**
- **½ cup frozen spinach, thawed, drained of excess water, and chopped**
- **2 tablespoons chopped garlic or 1 teaspoon garlic powder**
- **1 teaspoon onion powder**
- **Juice of ½ lemon**
- **¾ cup whole wheat bread crumbs**

1. HEAT the oven to 350°F. Line a baking sheet with parchment paper.

2. MIX together the salmon, egg, spinach, garlic, onion powder, lemon juice, and ½ cup of the bread crumbs in a bowl until all the ingredients are evenly distributed.

3. PLACE the remaining ¼ cup bread crumbs in a small bowl. Shape the salmon mixture into spheres the size of a golf ball, then roll in the bread crumbs. Place on the baking sheet and bake until lightly browned on the outside, about 30 minutes. Serve warm.

MAKES 2 SERVINGS (6 CROQUETTES EACH) ||| Prep time: 10 minutes ||| **Total time: 45 minutes**

Clean Shopping Tip

A couple of smaller brands like Wild Planet and Safe Catch are leading the charge in canning low-mercury, high-omega-3 products. Wild Planet purposefully selects smaller, younger tuna that have had less time to accumulate mercury, while Safe Catch actually tests each and every fish to make sure its mercury levels are safe. Bonus: Both brands use a "once-cooked" method that preserves the maximum amount of omega-3s, fatty acids that may actually help counteract mercury's damaging effects.

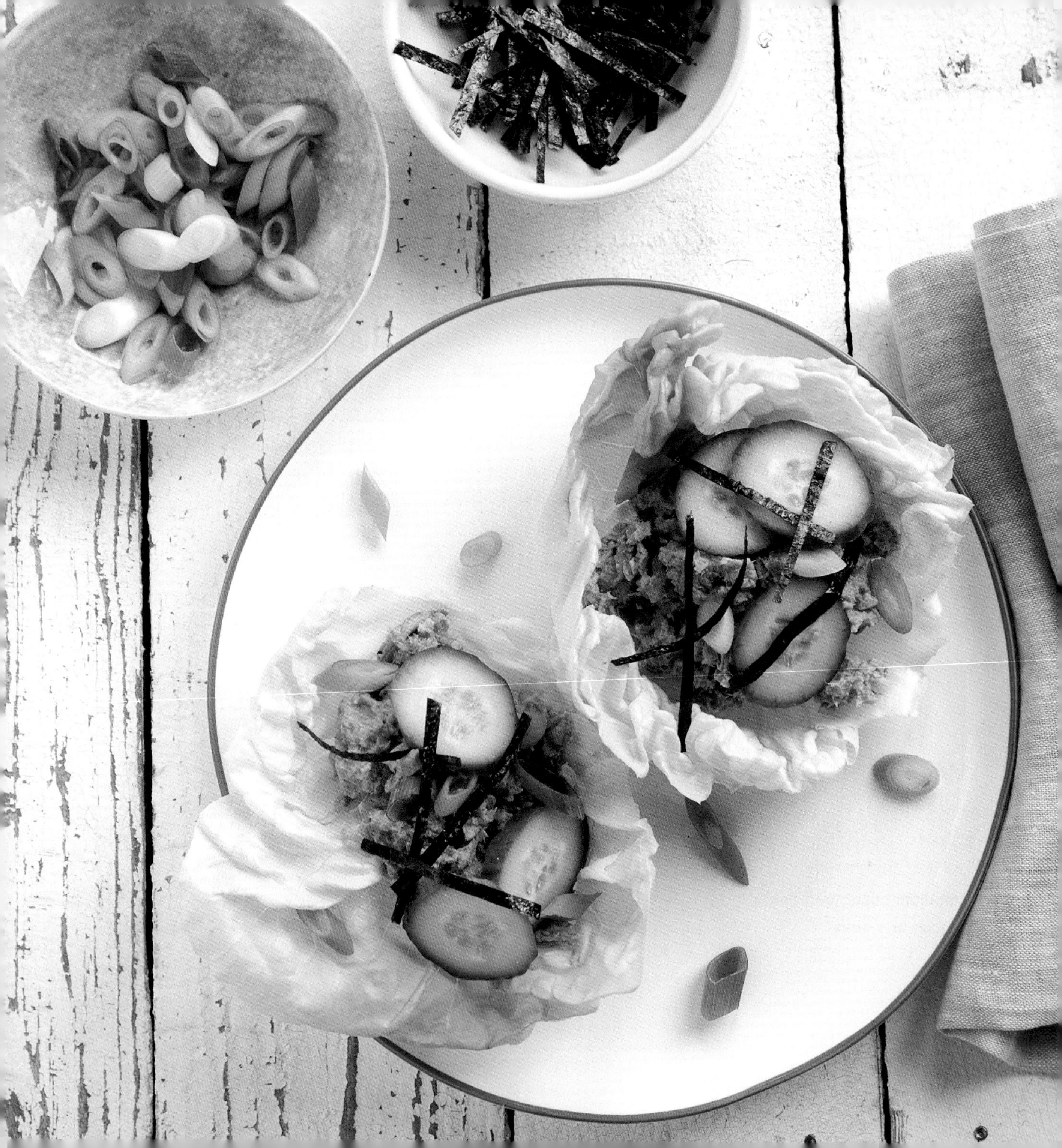

SALMON SALAD LETTUCE WRAPS

ASIAN DRESSING

- **3 tablespoons 2% plain Greek yogurt**
- **1 tablespoon reduced-sodium wheat-free tamari**
- **1 tablespoon rice vinegar**
- **¼ teaspoon ground ginger**
- **¼ teaspoon garlic powder**
- **¼ teaspoon onion powder**
- **Cayenne, to taste**

SALAD

- **2 cans (5 ounces each) wild salmon, drained**
- **3 tablespoons finely chopped celery**
- **2 tablespoons shredded carrot**
- **2 tablespoons chopped cashews**
- **1 tablespoon chopped scallion**
- **Seaweed snacks or ribbons of nori, for garnish**
- **½ medium cucumber, thinly sliced into coins**
- **6 large bibb or butterhead lettuce leaves**

1. MAKE the dressing: Puree all the ingredients together in a small food processor or blend with a whisk.

2. ASSEMBLE the salad: Toss together the salmon, celery, carrot, and cashews in a medium bowl. Add the dressing, stirring and folding until evenly coated. Transfer to a serving bowl and garnish with the scallion and seaweed.

3. DIVIDE the cucumber slices among the lettuce leaves. Add a few spoonfuls of salmon salad to each leaf.

MAKES 2 SERVINGS ||| Prep time: 15 minutes ||| **Total time: 15 minutes**

HEALTHY HACK

The easiest way to figure out which seafood is safest (and which to avoid) is to download the Monterey Bay Aquarium Seafood Watch guide at seafoodwatch.org. The easy-to-read chart provides convenient color-coded info on "Best Choices," "Good Alternatives," and fish to "Avoid," based on the region of the country that you live in. Print it out and tuck it in a reusable shopping bag or purse so you always have it at the store. You can also download an app for your phone at the same site.

SALMON NIÇOISE

DRESSING

- 1 can (2 ounces) oil-packed anchovy fillets
- 1 tablespoon mayonnaise
- 1 tablespoon 2% plain Greek yogurt
- 1 lemon
- 1 tablespoon rice vinegar
- 1 small clove garlic
- Dash each of salt and black pepper

SALAD

- 6 small red potatoes, quartered
- Fine sea salt
- ½ pound green beans
- 2 cups baby spinach
- ¼ cup fresh basil leaves
- 3 hard-boiled eggs, peeled and quartered
- 4 ounces canned wild salmon, drained
- 1 medium tomato, cut into bite-size wedges
- ½ cup kalamata olives

1. MAKE the dressing: Puree all the dressing ingredients in a blender or food processor.

2. PREPARE the salad ingredients: Place the potatoes in a microwaveable bowl and cover with a lid or wax paper. Microwave until fork-tender, 5 to 7 minutes. Sprinkle with salt.

3. SET up a bowl of ice and water. Blanch the green beans in a small pot of boiling water for 2 to 3 minutes. Drain and plunge into the ice water, to stop the cooking.

4. SPREAD the spinach and basil on 2 plates. Divide the potatoes, green beans, eggs, salmon, tomato, and olives between the plates, placing them each in a small section of the plate. Drizzle the dressing over the salads. Or divide between 2 small bowls for dipping.

MAKES 2 SERVINGS ||| Prep time: 10 minutes ||| **Total time: 15 minutes**

Eggs

Scrambled eggs can be the perfect quick and clean breakfast, packed with nutrients like choline, which is essential for healthy liver function. But all the different labels applied to eggs are enough to make your head spin. In reality, there's only one variety you can truly feel good about eating: organic and pasture-raised.

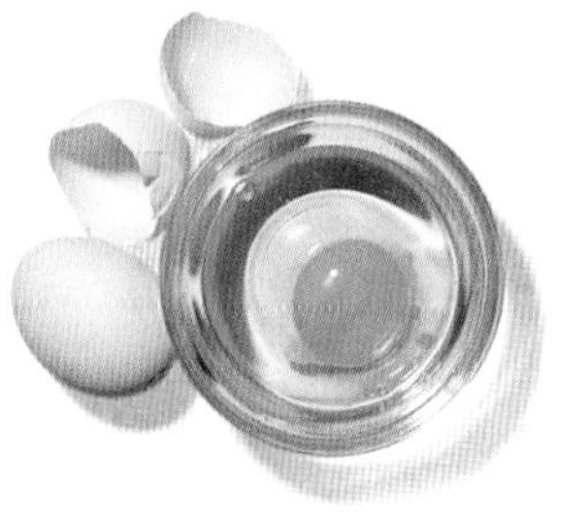

*

NOT CLEAN

CONVENTIONAL EGGS

Conventional eggs are best avoided. Not only are they less nutritious than pasture-raised eggs, but studies show that they have higher levels of salmonella than eggs from organic and cage-free hens. This is in large part because cramped quarters and lots of cages generate more fecal matter, attract more disease-carrying insects and rodents, are difficult to disinfect, and stress out hens, which may lower their natural immunity. Sounds pretty darn horrific, doesn't it?

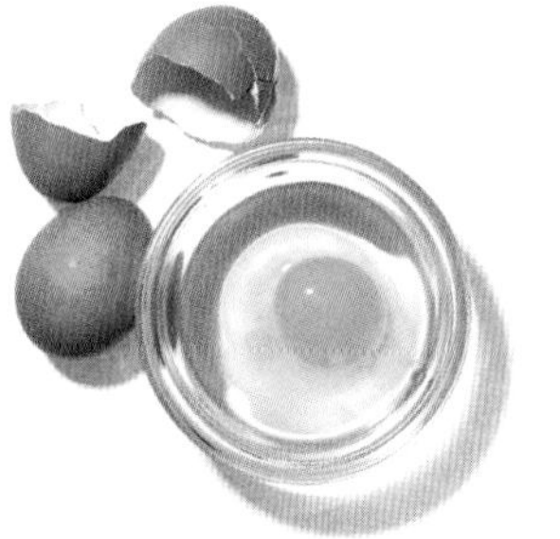

**

CLEAN

CAGE-FREE EGGS

Cage-free eggs come from hens not confined to cages, but they could still be in close quarters. They can spread their wings and lay eggs in nest boxes. It's also easier to maintain sanitary conditions. But unless they're raised organic, cage-free hens are fed grains made from crops heavily treated with chemical pesticides. There's no mandatory third-party auditing for the term "cage-free," so look for the term along with a seal such as "Certified Humane" or "Animal Welfare Approved."

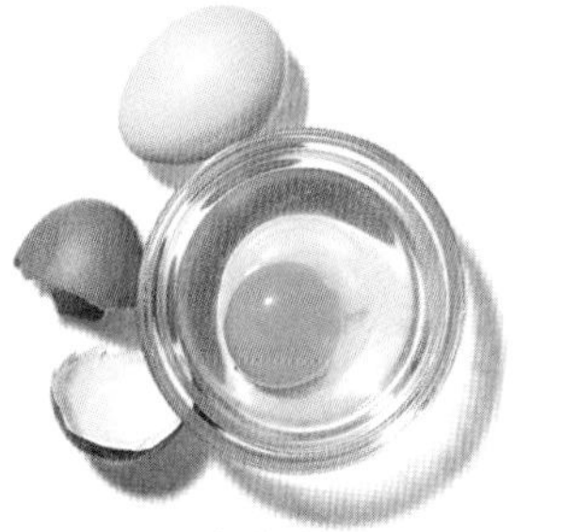

***

CLEANEST

ORGANIC PASTURE-RAISED EGGS

Pasture-raised hens hunt and peck for grass and insects, and their diets may be supplemented with organic feed. These eggs can contain two and a half times the amount of omega-3s and twice as much vitamin E as conventional. There's no mandatory third-party auditing for the term "pasture-raised," however, so seek these eggs out from a farmer you trust or from a brand that's been pasture-raised certified ("Certified Humane" or "American Humane Certified") such as Vital Farms Alfresco Eggs.

SOUTHWEST SKILLET EGGS

- **2 tablespoons canola oil**
- **½ large onion, diced**
- **1 clove garlic, minced**
- **1 can (14.5 ounces) diced tomatoes**
- **⅔ cup cooked or canned black beans**
- **½ cup brown rice**
- **1 tablespoon smoked paprika**
- **1 teaspoon ground cumin**
- **½ teaspoon fine sea salt**
- **½ teaspoon black pepper**
- **Cayenne**
- **4 ounces baby spinach, roughly chopped**
- **4 large eggs**
- **½ cup chopped cilantro**
- **½ cup 2% plain Greek yogurt**
- **½ avocado, sliced**

1. HEAT the oil in a large (12 to 16 inches) shallow, lidded pan over medium-high heat. Add the onion and garlic and cook until the onion is translucent, 2 to 3 minutes. Add the tomatoes (with juice), beans, rice, 1 cup water, the paprika, cumin, salt, black pepper, and cayenne to taste. Reduce to a simmer, cover, and cook until the rice is tender, about 40 minutes. Add the spinach and gently wilt, about 3 minutes.

2. CRACK an egg into each quarter of the pan. Cover again and cook until the eggs are opaque, 3 to 5 minutes. Uncover and garnish with the cilantro, yogurt, and avocado. Serve from the pan.

MAKES 2 SERVINGS ||| Prep time: 5 minutes ||| **Total time: 55 minutes**

HEALTHY HACK

You can actually use eggs to increase the nutrient value of the other foods you eat. A recent study found that topping your salad with a hard-boiled egg can help you absorb a whopping 500% more beta-carotene from your veggies. This antioxidant is essential for healthy eyes, skin, and immune function.

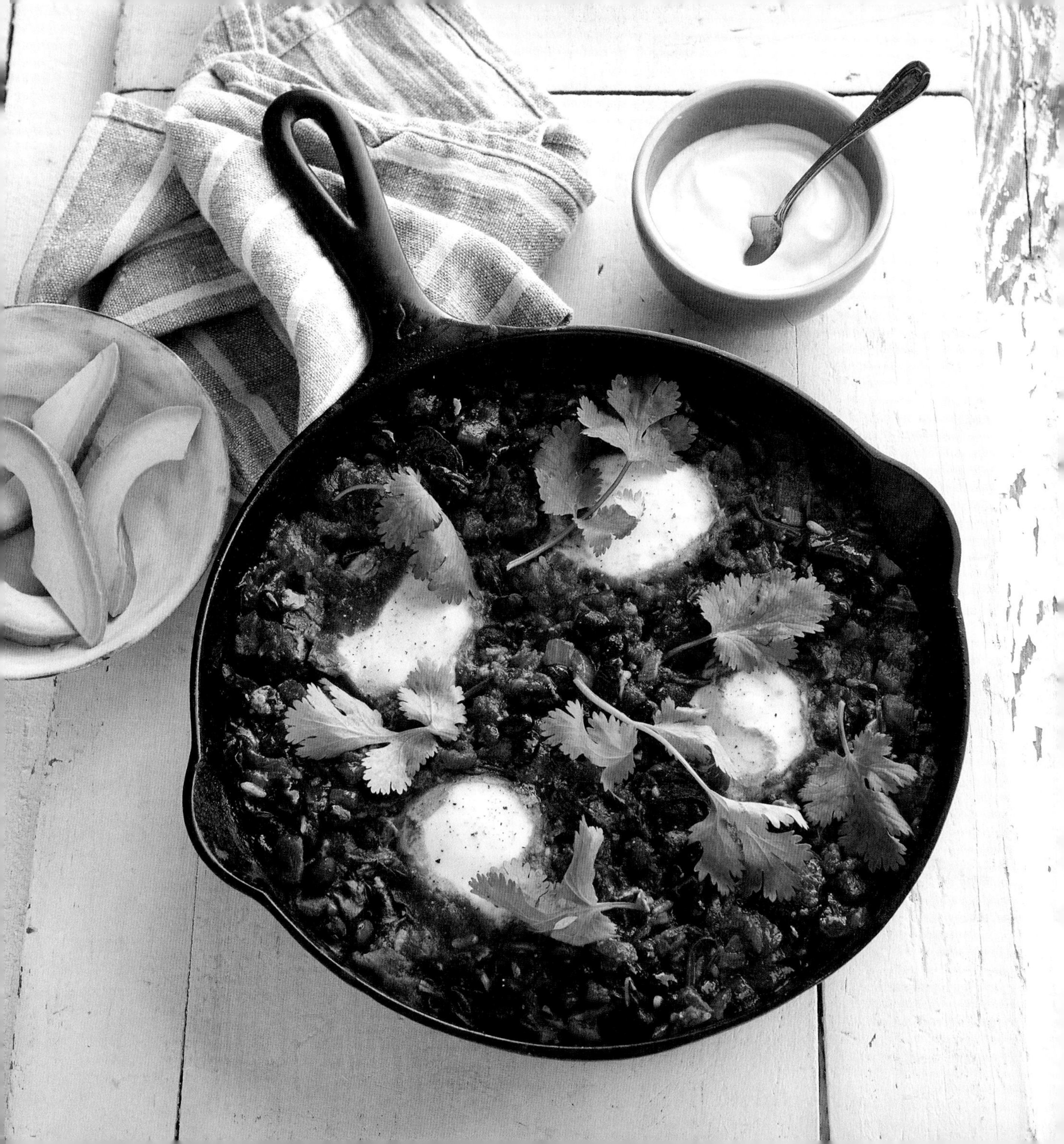

CREMINI EGG DROP SOUP

- 1 **tablespoon coconut oil**
- 1 **inch fresh ginger, grated**
- ¾ **cup sliced cremini mushrooms**
- 3 **tablespoons sliced scallion whites**
- ¼ **teaspoon garlic powder**
- 4 **cups vegetable broth**
- 1 **tablespoon wheat-free tamari**
- 2 **large eggs**
- 2 **cups spinach leaves**
- 6 **tablespoons sliced scallion greens**
- **Salt (optional)**

1. HEAT the oil in a soup pot over medium heat. Add the ginger, mushrooms, and scallion whites and cook until the vegetables soften and the ginger is fragrant, about 3 minutes. Sprinkle on the garlic powder, then add the vegetable broth and tamari and bring to a boil.

2. WHISK together the eggs and few tablespoons water in a container with a spout.

3. REMOVE the boiling broth from the heat and stir to set up a whirlpool. As the broth is swirling, drizzle in the whisked eggs so that thin strands form (try to avoid letting chunks of eggs form in any one place). Add the spinach and stir gently until wilted. Stir in the scallions greens. Taste and add salt if needed.

MAKES 2 TO 4 SERVINGS ||| Prep time: 10 minutes ||| **Total time: 15 minutes**

HASH BROWN FRITTATA

- **1 large russet (baking) potato**
- **2 tablespoons extra virgin olive oil**
- **Fine sea salt**
- **1 small onion, diced**
- **1 red bell pepper, diced**
- **2 cups kale leaves (tough ribs removed)**
- **4 large eggs**
- **½ cup 1% milk**
- **½ teaspoon garlic powder**
- **½ teaspoon onion powder**
- **½ cup shredded part-skim mozzarella (2 ounces)**
- **1 cup cilantro, roughly chopped**
- **1 lime, halved**
- **½ avocado, pitted, peeled, and sliced**

1. SHRED the unpeeled potato on the large holes of a box grater.

2. HEAT 1 tablespoon of the oil in an ovenproof 9-inch non-stick skillet over medium-high heat. Add the potato and a dash of salt and cook, stirring, until lightly browned. Spread the potato evenly in the pan and gently press to form a base layer. Remove from the heat.

3. HEAT the remaining 1 tablespoon oil in a separate skillet over medium-high heat. Add the onion, bell pepper, and kale and cook until the volume is reduced by about half, 5 to 6 minutes. Spread the vegetables evenly over the potato base.

4. WHISK together the eggs, milk, garlic powder, and onion powder in a bowl. Whisk in the mozzarella.

5. POSITION an oven rack 6 inches from the heating element and heat the broiler.

6. PUT the pan with the potatoes and vegetables back over medium-high heat and pour the egg mixture over. Cook until the eggs are set on the bottom, 2 to 3 minutes. Place the pan under the broiler until golden brown on top and cooked through in the middle (test with a knife), 8 to 10 minutes.

7. CUT into wedges and serve topped with cilantro, a squeeze of lime, and the avocado.

MAKES 2 SERVINGS ||| Prep time: 10 minutes ||| **Total time: 30 minutes**

Beans

Think of beans as a superfood for your heart. Their high fiber, potassium, and magnesium contents work together to help keep blood pressure in check. Bonus: Just 1 cup packs 15 grams of vegetarian-friendly protein. But packaging and added ingredients can make certain brands clean-diet killers.

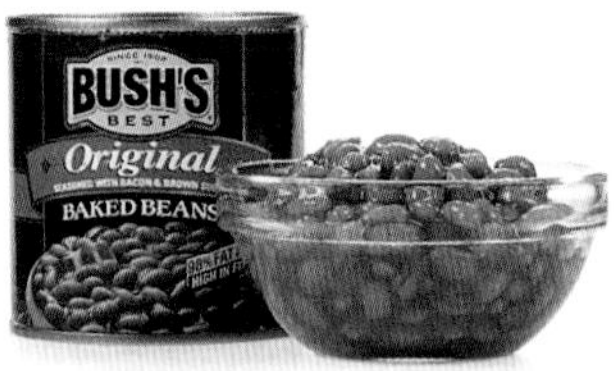

✱

NOT CLEAN

BAKED BEANS

Sure, they're delicious and may be okay for that once-in-a-while cookout, but in general, pass on the baked beans. They contain added sugar (some packing 12 grams in just ½ cup), salt, fat, and preservatives.

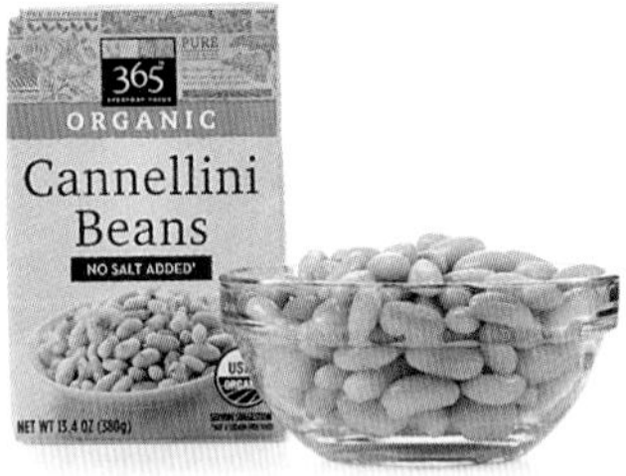

✱✱

CLEAN

UNFLAVORED PACKAGED BEANS

Regular packaged beans will still provide beneficial nutrients like protein and fiber, but you'll often end up consuming quite a bit of sodium, and, in the case of canned varieties, exposing yourself to dangerous BPA. Some canned beans—usually the organic brands, like Eden Foods—use BPA-free lined cans, so opt for those; or choose beans that come in cardboard Tetra Pak packaging such as Whole Foods' 365 Organic brand, which are always BPA-free.

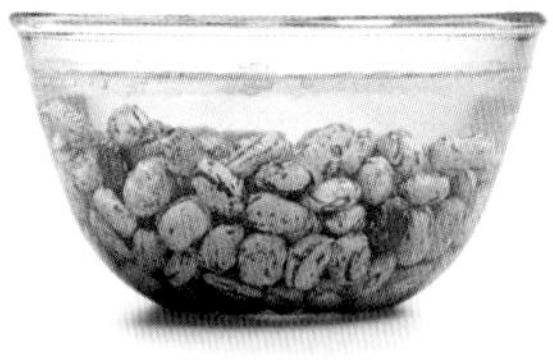

✱✱✱

CLEANEST

DRIED BEANS

Buying dried beans, rather than in a can, will ensure that they're free of added salt and BPA—a chemical linked to a slew of health problems, including breast cancer. Recent research shows that avoiding BPA-containing packaging can immediately reduce BPA levels in the body. Soak them overnight to cut down on cooking time the next day.

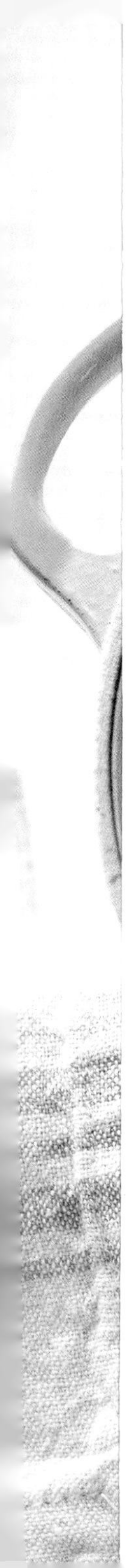

GASLESS BEANS

- **1 cup dried pinto beans**
- **1 tablespoon finely chopped yellow onion**
- **1 teaspoon ground cumin**
- **½ teaspoon black pepper**
- **½ teaspoon fine sea salt**
- **1 teaspoon minced garlic**

1. COMBINE the beans and water to cover by 1 inch in a medium saucepan. Bring to a boil. Boil for 5 minutes and then turn the heat off. Cover and let soak 8 hours or overnight.

2. DRAIN the beans in a colander and rinse with water. Return to the saucepan and add water to cover by 1 inch. Bring to a boil, then reduce to a simmer. Add the onion, cumin, pepper, salt, and garlic and simmer until tender, about 45 minutes.

3. LET cool before freezing in 1- to 2-cup containers to use in place of canned beans.

MAKES 3 CUPS ||| Prep time: 5 minutes |||
Total time: 50 minutes+ 8 hours or overnight soaking

HEALTHY HACK

Beans aren't just for savory meals. Instantly up the health cred of your favorite boxed brownie mix or homemade recipe by substituting pureed black beans for the oil and eggs. Use one 15-ounce can of undrained black beans, pureed, in place of one egg plus ⅓ to ½ cup oil. The result will be perfectly fudgy brownies (that don't taste like beans) with far fewer calories and lots of plant-based protein and fiber.

LOADED REFRIED BEANS

- **3 cups cooked pinto beans**
- **½ to 1 cup reduced-sodium vegetable broth**
- **2 tablespoons olive oil**
- **½ yellow onion, chopped**
- **2 cloves garlic, minced**
- **2 large tomatoes, chopped**

1. COMBINE the beans and ½ cup broth in a blender and pulse until some of the beans are smooth and some are still chunky, adding additional broth if needed to blend into the right consistency.

2. HEAT the oil in a medium skillet over medium heat. Add the onion and cook until soft, about 5 minutes.

3. ADD the garlic and tomatoes and cook until most of the water from the tomatoes is gone, about 8 minutes.

4. STIR in the beans and cook, stirring, until thickened and hot throughout.

MAKES 3 CUPS ||| Prep time: 15 minutes ||| **Total time: 20 minutes**

Soy

Soy sure is controversial: Allergies to this legume are on the rise, 90% of soy is genetically modified, and researchers keep going back and forth on whether soy isoflavones are good or bad. But for the majority of people, high-quality soy products consumed in moderation are likely safe and healthy. Stick to organic, though, if you want to avoid GMOs.

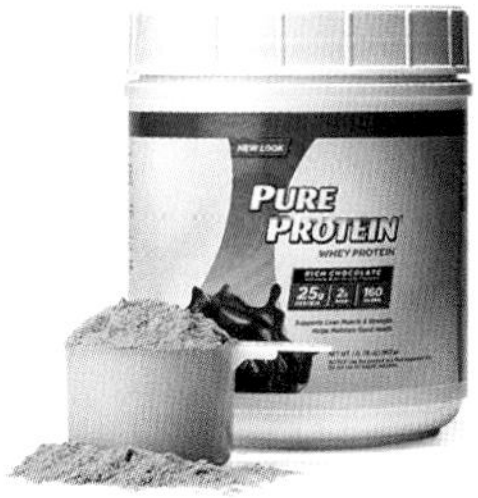

*

NOT CLEAN

SOY PROTEIN

Soy protein, ubiquitous in protein bars and other packaged foods, is not your friend. The process of isolating protein from soy often requires the use of the harsh chemical solvent hexane, which has unknown effects on the body. Getting your hands on organic varieties is also difficult.

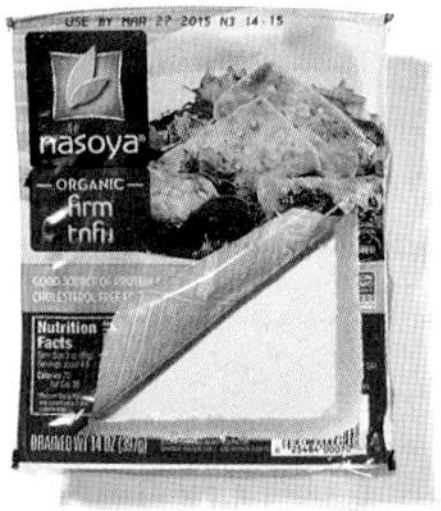

**

CLEAN

TOFU

Tofu contains less fiber than tempeh and none of the benefits of fermentation. It does, however, make a convenient source of quality protein for vegans. Like all soy, it contains all essential amino acids, so it's a complete source of protein.

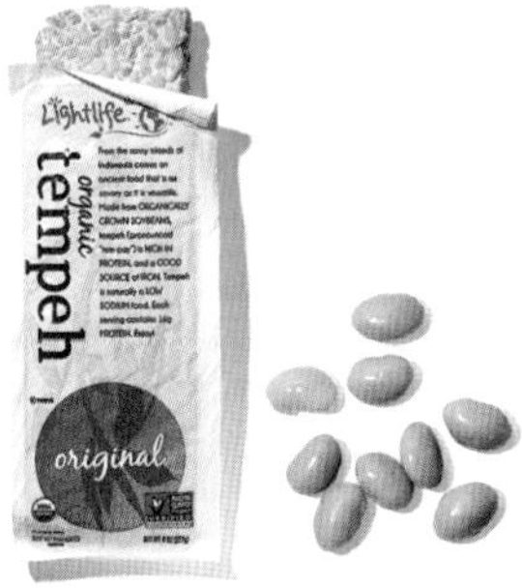

***

CLEANEST

TEMPEH OR FRESH EDAMAME

Tempeh, tofu's nutty-tasting, more texturized cousin is made of soybeans that have been fermented with a fungus starter, which makes it easier to digest and helps you absorb nutrients more readily than with other soy products. Whole edamame also makes a great clean appetizer alternative to typical fried and cheesy restaurant fare.

SLOW-COOKER TEMPEH CURRY WITH CAULIFLOWER

- **1 cup coconut milk**
- **1 can (15 ounces) unsweetened pumpkin puree**
- **2 cups vegetable broth**
- **1 inch fresh ginger, peeled and grated**
- **2 tablespoons curry powder**
- **½ cup chopped onion**
- **1 large russet (baking) potato, diced with skin on**
- **½ head cauliflower, broken into florets**
- **1 package (8 ounces) tempeh, cut into ½-inch squares**
- **2 cups green peas, thawed**
- **1 cup cooked rice**
- **Fresh basil leaves (optional)**

COMBINE the coconut milk, pumpkin puree, broth, ginger, curry powder, and onion in a large slow cooker, stirring to mix. Add the potato, cauliflower, and tempeh, stirring to coat in the sauce. Cover and cook on low for 7 hours. Fold in the peas and serve over rice. Garnish with basil leaves, if desired.

MAKES 2 LARGE SERVINGS ||| Prep time: 10 minutes ||| **Total time: 7 hours 10 minutes**

Clean Shopping Tip

If soy protein is a no-go for you, there are oodles of other plant-based options in protein powders and protein-fortified foods. Your best bet: A blend of plant proteins like pea, rice, and hemp to make sure you're getting a complete protein. All are unlikely to be genetically modified or processed with hexane, but be sure to stick to no-sugar-added and flavor-free varieties. Good choices include NOW Foods non-GMO Pea Protein and Nutriva Organic Hemp Protein.

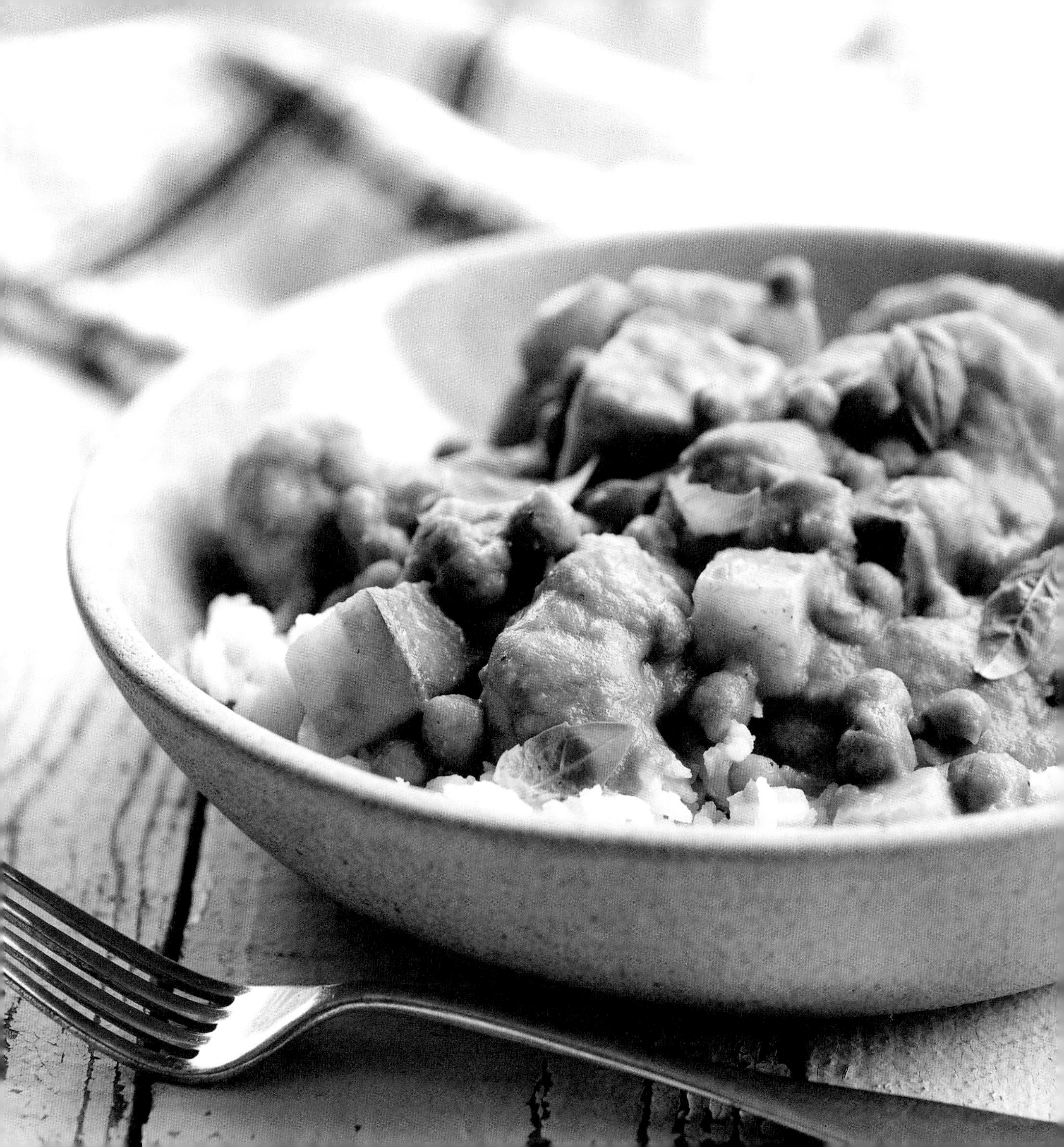

TEMPEH BOLOGNESE SAUCE WITH PAPPARDELLE

- **2 tablespoons extra virgin olive oil**
- **1 small onion, diced**
- **1 clove garlic**
- **1 piece tempeh (8 ounces), roughly chopped into tiny pieces**
- **5 ounces mushrooms, roughly chopped into tiny pieces**
- **1 tablespoon tomato paste**
- **½ cup dry red wine**
- **2 teaspoons vegetable broth concentrate (or bouillon paste)**
- **1 can (15 ounces) tomato sauce**
- **1 tablespoon wheat-free tamari**
- **½ teaspoon fine sea salt**
- **Black pepper**
- **4 ounces pappardelle pasta**

1. HEAT the oil in a large saucepan over medium-high heat. Add the onion and garlic and cook until translucent, about 5 minutes. Add the tempeh and mushrooms and cook, stirring, until the mushrooms are soft and tender, about 5 minutes.

2. STIR in the tomato paste and cook, allowing the heat to brown the red color. Pour in the wine and simmer until absorbed, then add the broth, tomato sauce, tamari, salt, and a dash of pepper. Reduce to a simmer, stir to combine, cover, and cook for 15 to 20 minutes to blend the flavors.

3. PREPARE the pappardelle per package directions. Drain and place in 2 pasta bowls, then divide the sauce between the bowls.

MAKES 2 SERVINGS ||| Prep time: 10 minutes ||| **Total time: 50 minutes**

DRY-RUB TEMPEH

- ¼ **cup wheat-free tamari**
- **2 tablespoons distilled white vinegar**
- **1 teaspoon garlic powder**
- **1 teaspoon onion powder**
- **1 8-ounce package tempeh**
- **1 teaspoon smoked paprika**
- **1 teaspoon dried rosemary**
- ½ **teaspoon ground cumin**
- ¼ **teaspoon fine sea salt**

1. COMBINE 1 cup water, tamari, vinegar, and ½ teaspoon each of the garlic powder and onion powder in a pot large enough to hold the tempeh in a single layer. Bring to a boil. Poke the tempeh with a fork on both sides so that the surface has small holes, about 1 inch apart. Add to the pot, cover, and simmer for 5 minutes to allow the flavors of the sauce to cook into the tempeh.

2. STIR together the paprika, rosemary, cumin, salt, and remaining ½ teaspoon each garlic and onion powders in a small bowl.

3. REMOVE the tempeh from the marinating liquid and rub the spice mixture on both sides.

4. GRILL or broil until the spices are toasted and the tempeh is warm, about 4 minutes on each side. Slice into inch-wide pieces to add to a wrap, or chop into cubes to add to a salad.

MAKES 2 SERVINGS ||| Prep time: 10 minutes ||| **Total time: 20 minutes**

Veggie Burgers

Veggie burgers can be a healthy alternative to a typical burger, and they're great for vegetarians and carnivores alike. As with most foods, the cleanest option is one that you make at home, so you can control what goes into it.

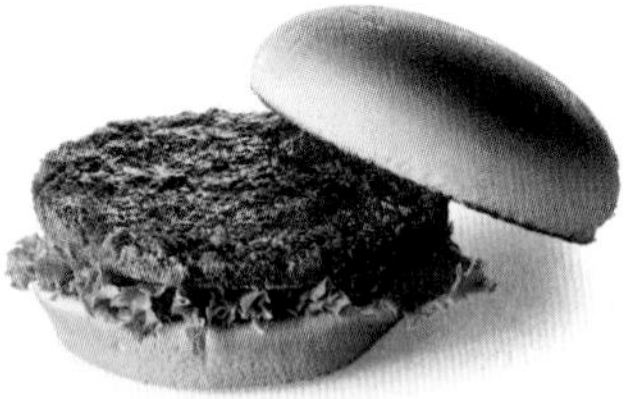

*

NOT CLEAN

PATTIES WITH SYNTHETIC INGREDIENTS

Be on the lookout for store-bought veggie burgers containing soy protein isolate, textured vegetable protein, or synthetic fillers. These are overly processed, likely to contain loads of sodium, and often contain genetically modified ingredients.

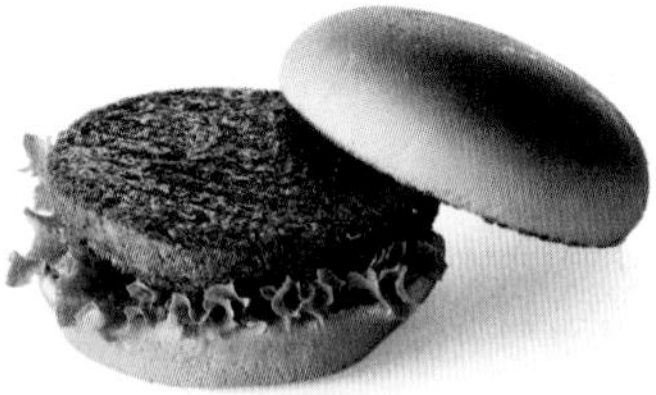

**

CLEAN

ORGANIC FROZEN PATTIES MADE FROM WHOLE-FOOD INGREDIENTS

If you opt for a store-bought veggie burger, be sure to choose one that's organic or non-GMO and made from only whole-food ingredients. The shorter the ingredient list, the better.

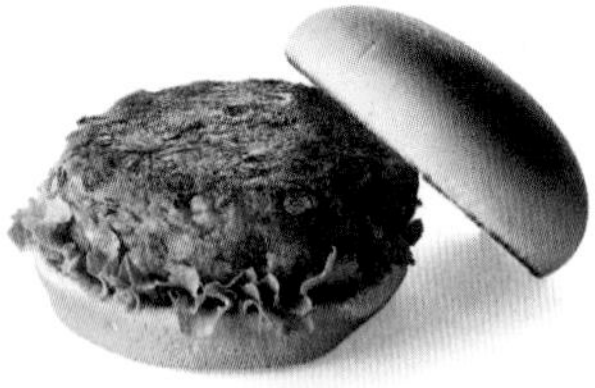

***

CLEANEST

HOMEMADE

A nutritious veggie burger can be made with your favorite beans, vegetables, whole grains, eggs, and spices. Make a few and freeze them the next time you have some leftover rice or quinoa sitting in the fridge. Keep things interesting with one of the delicious veggie burger recipes starting on the opposite page.

BLACK BEAN & MUSHROOM BURGERS

- **8 ounces mushrooms**
- **½ cup cilantro leaves**
- **2 scallions**
- **1 can (15 ounces) black beans, rinsed and drained**
- **Juice of 1 lime**
- **½ cup bread crumbs**
- **Fine sea salt**

1. POSITION a rack 6 inches from the heating element and heat the broiler. Line a baking sheet with parchment paper.

2. MINCE the mushrooms, cilantro, and scallions (or do this by pulsing in a food processor). Place in a bowl and add half the black beans, mashing to combine. Add the remaining beans, lime juice, bread crumbs, and a dash of salt. Shape into 4 patties.

3. ARRANGE the patties a few inches apart on the baking sheet and broil until browned and crisp on the outside, 6 to 8 minutes per side.

Note: If you want to grill the burgers, be sure to use a grill topper, because the patties will not hold their shape if placed directly on a grill grate.

MAKES 2 SERVINGS (2 BURGERS EACH) ||| Prep time: 10 minutes ||| **Total time: 25 minutes**

HEALTHY HACK

Instantly boost the nutrition and flavor profile of your best veggie burger by topping it with slices of avocado or a dollop of guac. You'll not only add a delicious richness, but the healthy monounsaturated fats in this fruit (yep, it's technically a large berry) actually help you absorb more nutrients from your vegetables.

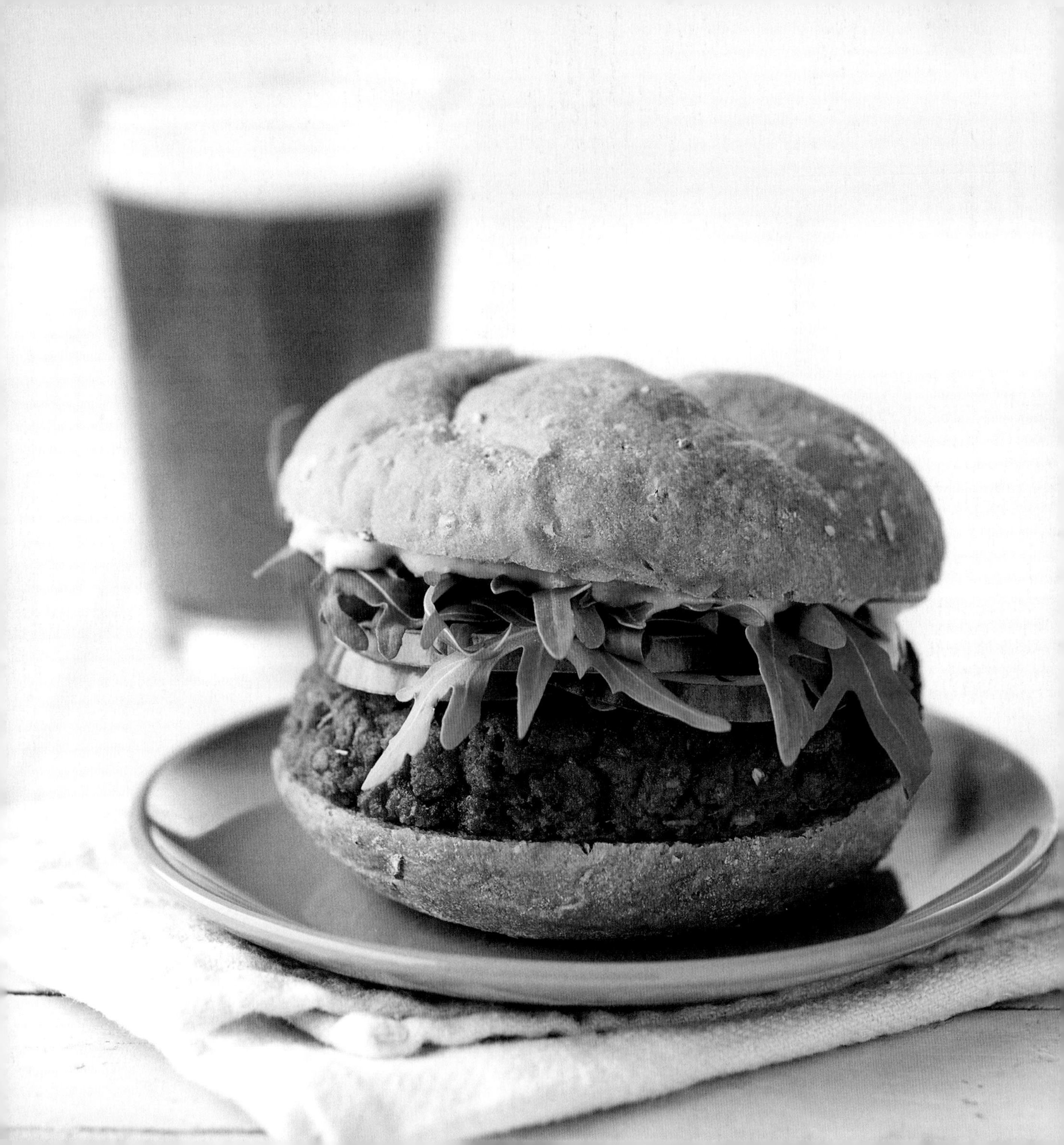

SWEET POTATO LENTIL BURGERS

- ½ **cup red lentils**
- **1 cup vegetable broth**
- **1 medium sweet potato, skin on, diced**
- **1 tablespoon smoked paprika**
- **1 teaspoon ground cumin**
- **2 tablespoons minced onion**
- ⅓ **cup bread crumbs**
- **2 roasted red peppers, diced**
- **Fine sea salt**
- **3 tablespoons extra virgin olive oil**

1. COOK the lentils in the broth, covered, in a small saucepan until softened but still firm.

2. PLACE the sweet potato in a microwaveable bowl, cover, and microwave on high for 6 to 7 minutes, until soft enough to mash easily.

3. POSITION a rack in the top third of the oven and heat the broiler. Line a baking sheet with parchment or foil.

4. COMBINE the drained lentils and sweet potato (still warm), paprika, cumin, and onion in a medium bowl. Mash with a potato masher or fork until the mixture becomes sticky. Fold in the bread crumbs and roasted peppers. Form into 4 patties ½ inch thick.

5. ARRANGE the patties on the baking sheet and sprinkle with a dash of salt, then drizzle on the olive oil. Broil for 3 to 5 minutes per side, until golden brown and crisp on the outside. Let cool for 7 to 10 minutes before serving on a roll or as part of a salad.

MAKES 2 SERVINGS (2 BURGERS EACH) ||| Prep time: 10 minutes |||
Total time: 50 minutes

FALAFEL BURGERS

- **2 tablespoons olive oil**
- **1 small eggplant, cut into ½-inch cubes, skin on**
- **Salt and black pepper**
- **1 can (15 ounces) chickpeas, drained**
- **⅓ cup chopped fresh parsley**
- **1 tablespoon chopped scallion**
- **½ teaspoon garlic powder**
- **½ teaspoon ground cumin**
- **Juice of ½ lemon**
- **1½ tablespoons tahini**
- **½ cup bread crumbs**

1. HEAT 1 tablespoon of the oil in a skillet over medium-high heat. Add the eggplant and sprinkle with a dash of salt and pepper. Cook until all sides are browned, about 5 minutes. Continue cooking until reduced in size by about half, about 10 minutes.

2. COMBINE the chickpeas, parsley, scallion, garlic powder, cumin, lemon juice, tahini, and bread crumbs.

3. SCRAPE the eggplant into the bowl with the chickpeas and roughly mash until the mixture becomes sticky. Form into 4 patties.

4. HEAT the remaining 1 tablespoon oil in a nonstick skillet over medium heat. Add the patties and cook until golden brown, 6 to 8 minutes on each side.

MAKES 4 SERVINGS ||| Prep time: 15 minutes ||| **Total time: 40 minutes**

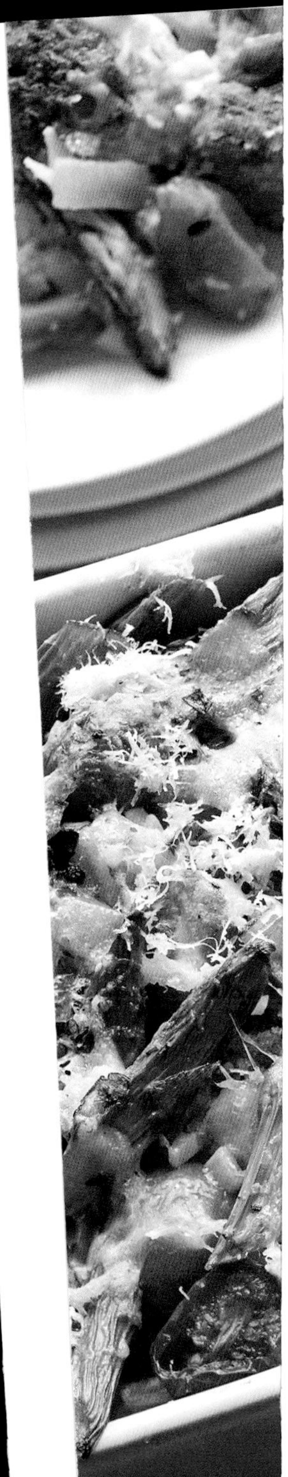

Bread

Ditching white bread for whole wheat is a no brainer, but you shouldn't stop there. For max nutrition per slice, minimal funky additives, and fewer refined carb–induced cravings, your best bet is organic whole wheat bread.

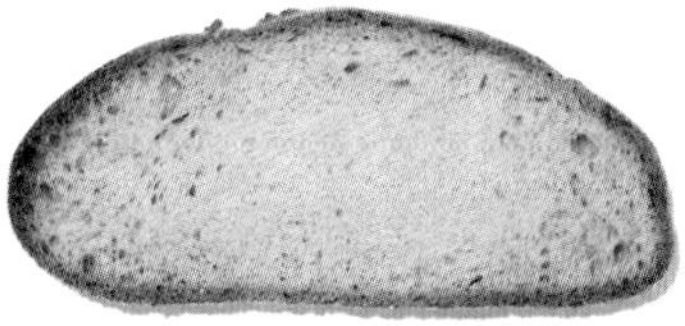

✱

NOT CLEAN

WHEAT OR WHITE BREAD

Bread made with refined flour should be skipped altogether. Most of the naturally occurring nutrients from the wheat kernels have been stripped away, and you're missing out on some of that blood sugar–stabilizing fiber and protein.

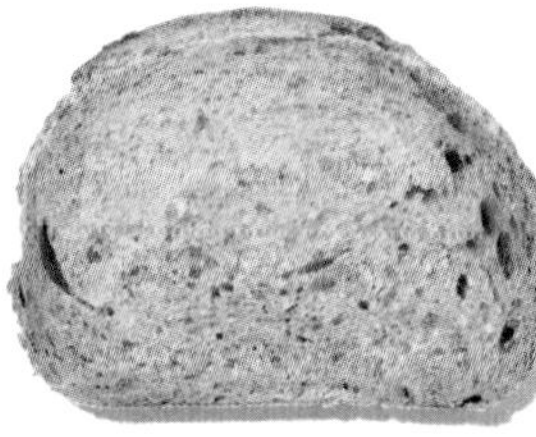

✱✱

CLEAN

WHOLE WHEAT OR WHOLE-GRAIN BREAD

The grains used in nonorganic whole wheat or whole-grain bread have likely been treated with pesticides called organophosphates—linked to lower IQ and ADHD in children, with unknown effects on adults. Nonorganic breads have also been found to have more preservatives, thickeners, and refined flours.

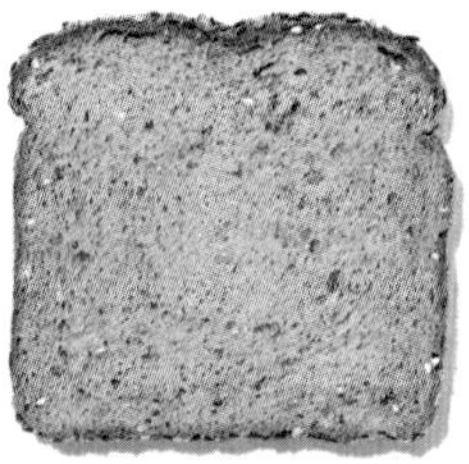

✱✱✱

CLEANEST

ORGANIC WHOLE WHEAT OR WHOLE-GRAIN BREAD

Whole wheat bread contains the original kernel (bran, germ, and endosperm), leaving fiber and protein intact. Bread made with other grains is also a good choice, as long as the word "whole" appears before them on the ingredient list. Studies have shown that consuming whole grains helps promote a healthy weight. Buy organic whenever possible to avoid pesticides.

Rice

Don't know about you, but the last time we looked at the varieties of rice in the grocery store, we were a tad overwhelmed. It's not just a matter of white versus brown anymore—jasmine, basmati, Arborio, black, red, and wild are all options. Next time you need a base for your stir-fry, pick the one that packs the most nutrients: wild.

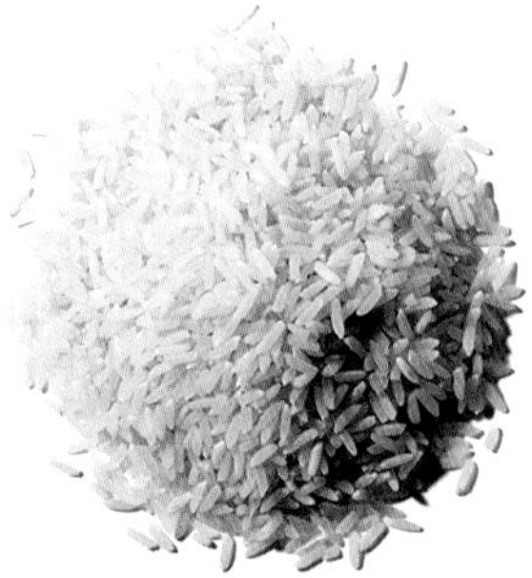

✷

NOT CLEAN

WHITE RICE

Your typical white rice isn't necessarily unhealthy, but its nutritional value simply doesn't begin to measure up to wild or brown rice.

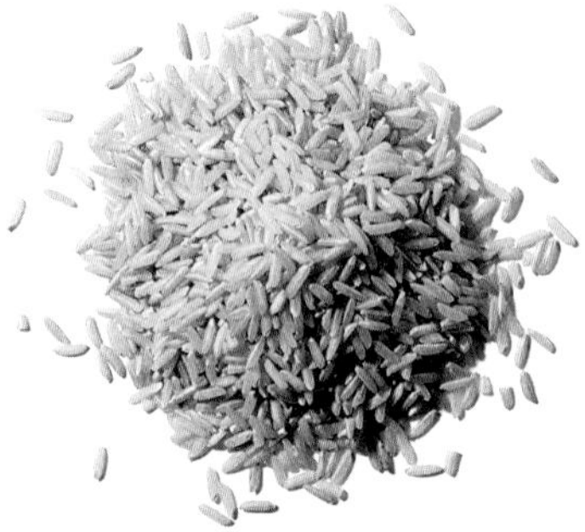

✷✷

CLEAN

BROWN RICE

Mild and nutty brown rice still beats white. It's considered a whole grain because, unlike white, it still contains the bran and the germ, which provide you with a dose of fiber, making it less likely to contribute to blood sugar spikes and drops.

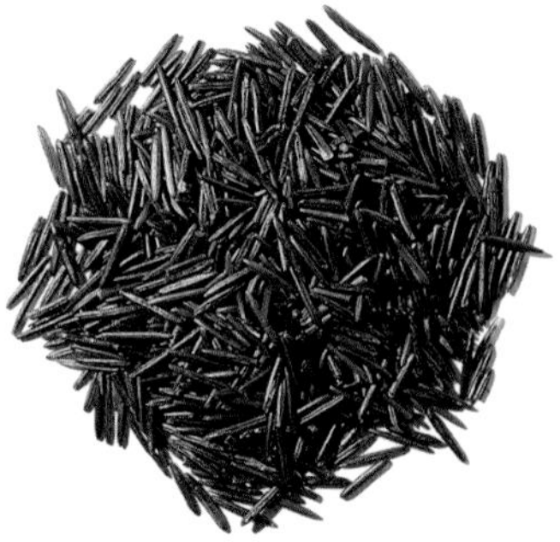

✷✷✷

CLEANEST

WILD RICE

Wild rice is actually the seed of a marsh grass found near the Great Lakes. It contains protein, fiber, folate, manganese, zinc, magnesium, phosphorus, niacin, and iron—making it more nutrient-dense (and lower in carbs!) than even our beloved brown rice.

WILD RICE WITH CARROTS & PORTOBELLOS

- 1 cup wild rice
- 3 cups broth (vegetable or meat)
- 1 tablespoon olive oil
- 3 large carrots, cut into ¼-inch-thick coins
- 2 large portobello mushrooms, cut into ½-inch dice
- 2 cloves garlic, finely diced
- ½ teaspoon fine sea salt
- 1 teaspoon dried rosemary

1. COOK the wild rice in the broth per package directions.

2. HEAT the oil in a skillet over medium-high heat. Add the carrots, mushrooms, and garlic and cook, stirring frequently, until the carrots are fork-tender, 10 to 15 minutes. Season with the salt and rosemary.

3. ADD the cooked wild rice to the vegetables and stir until well combined. Serve warm.

MAKES 2 SERVINGS ||| Prep time: 10 minutes ||| **Total time: 1 hour 10 minutes**

HEALTHY HACK

It's true, your favorite starchy staple can contain unwanted arsenic, a known human carcinogen. But there's an effortless way to slash arsenic in rice by 30 to 40%. Simply rinse 1 cup of brown rice thoroughly, boil it in approximately 4 to 6 cups of water for 30 to 45 minutes or until tender, and drain like you would pasta.

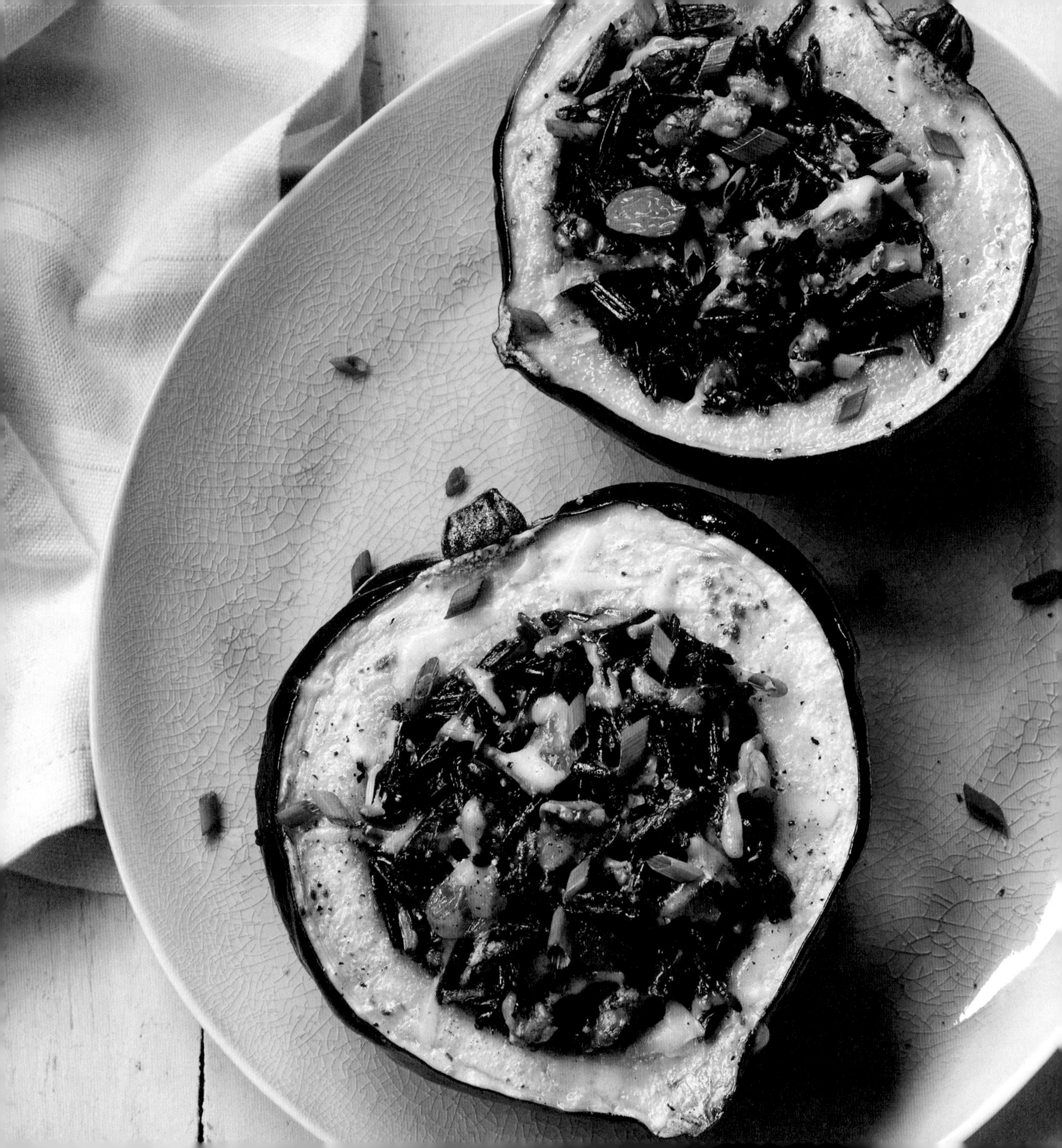

SQUASH STUFFED WITH WILD RICE & GOLDEN RAISINS

- **½ cup wild rice**
- **2 small dumpling or acorn squash**
- **4 ounces mushrooms, finely diced**
- **2 tablespoons golden raisins**
- **½ cup shredded Gruyère cheese (2 ounces)**
- **3 tablespoons roughly chopped walnuts**
- **1 egg**

1. **COOK** the wild rice in 1½ cups lightly salted water in a small pot until the rice is tender, 45 to 50 minutes.

2. **HEAT** the oven to 350°F.

3. **CUT** each squash in half, lengthwise, and scoop the seeds out with a spoon.

4. **PLACE** the squash halves on a baking sheet, cut side up, and bake until just tender but still firm, about 30 minutes.

5. **FOLD** the warm rice into the mushrooms, raisins, cheese, and walnuts in a small bowl. Stir in the egg to coat all ingredients. Divide the stuffing between the parcooked squash halves.

6. **RETURN** the stuffed squash to the oven and bake until the filling is heated through and the squash is fork-tender, about 15 minutes longer.

MAKES 2 SERVINGS ||| Prep time: 10 minutes ||| **Total time: 1 hour 10 minutes**

WILD RICE CASSEROLE

1 cup wild rice

1 cup brown rice

8 cups vegetable or chicken broth

2 large onions

2 cups baby spinach

1 cup shredded Cheddar (4 ounces)

1 cup fresh whole wheat bread crumbs

2 large eggs, beaten

1 tablespoon olive oil

½ cup grated Parmesan

1. ADD the wild and brown rice to 6 cups of the broth. Bring to a boil and then turn down the heat. Simmer, covered, until the liquid is absorbed, about 45 minutes. Transfer to a large bowl.

2. HEAT the oven to 350°F. Grease a 9 x 13-inch baking dish.

3. DICE 1 of the onions and cut the other into rings or half-moons.

4. ADD the diced onion, spinach, Cheddar, bread crumbs, and eggs to the rice mixture, gently mixing until evenly combined. Spread the mixture in the baking dish. Sprinkle with the remaining 2 cups broth and cover the baking dish. Bake for 20 minutes.

5. HEAT the oil in a skillet over medium-high heat. Add the onion rings and cook until translucent, about 5 minutes. Reduce the heat to medium-low and cook, stirring occasionally, until the onions are caramelized and brown, 15 to 20 minutes longer.

6. UNCOVER the baking dish, spread on the caramelized onions, and sprinkle on the Parmesan. Bake uncovered until the cheese is golden, 15 to 20 minutes longer. Let stand for 15 minutes before serving.

MAKES 4 SERVINGS ||| Prep time: 15 minutes ||| **Total time: 1 hour 50 minutes**

Pasta

Yes, pasta can still be a part of your clean diet, but you're going to have to replace the traditional white stuff with 100% whole-grain pasta for maximum nutrition. Oh, and you know, avoid covering it with cheese.

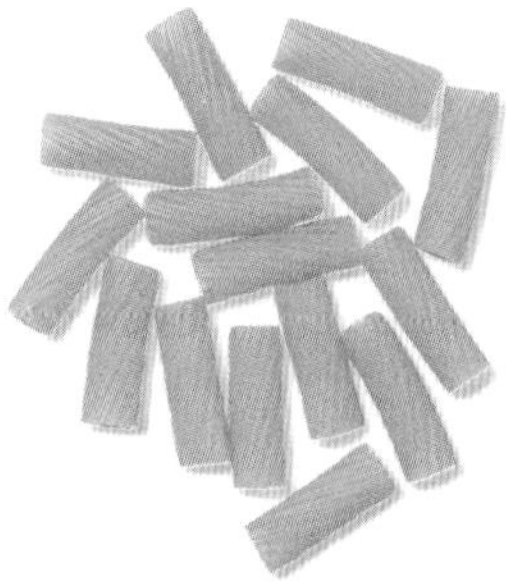

✱

NOT CLEAN

TRADITIONAL PASTA

White pasta made from enriched wheat flour is refined and starchy, and these kinds of carbs can induce cravings—thanks to a rapid spike and then drop in blood sugar—and thus promote weight gain.

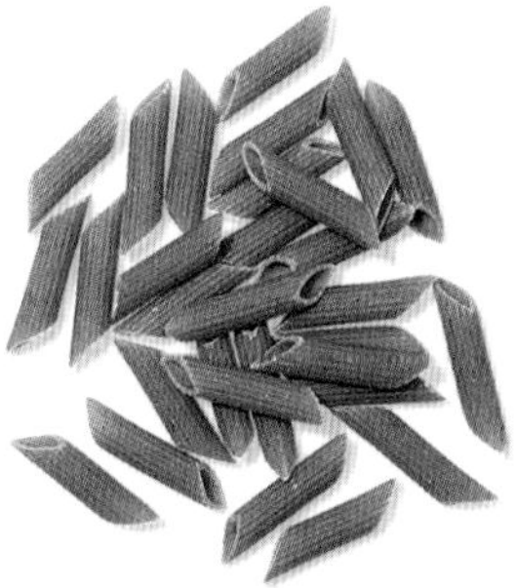

✱✱

CLEAN

WHOLE-GRAIN PASTA THAT INCLUDES REFINED FLOURS

Be on the lookout for whole-grain pastas that are made with other refined flours—you're not going to get the same protein, fiber, and micronutrient benefits as you would from 100% whole grain.

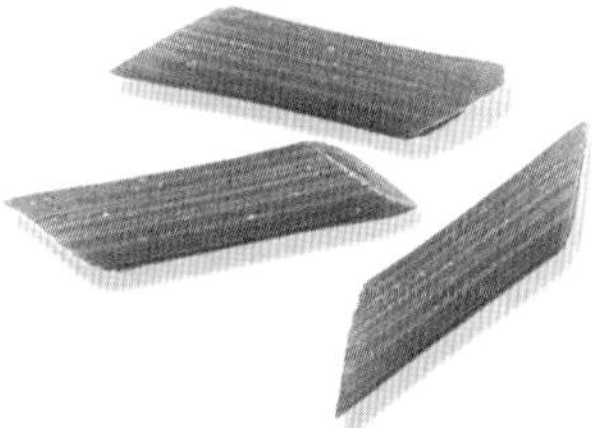

✱✱✱

CLEANEST

100% WHOLE WHEAT PASTA

Because 100% whole grain pasta is made from all three parts of the grain—bran, germ, and endosperm—it contains more fiber and protein than other varieties and is digested more slowly, keeping energy levels stable. It also contains a variety of minerals important for things like blood sugar regulation and nerve function. True whole grain pasta will always say 100% whole grain or 100% whole wheat on the package.

SPICY GREEN COCONUT SHRIMP CURRY RAMEN

- 1½ tablespoons coconut oil
- ½ red onion, thinly sliced
- ½ cup thinly sliced red bell pepper
- 1 jalapeño or 2 small Thai chiles
- 2 teaspoons grated fresh ginger
- 2 cloves garlic, minced
- 2 teaspoons green curry paste
- ¾ cup coconut milk
- 1 kaffir lime leaf (optional)
- 1 cup thinly sliced carrot coins
- ½ cup green beans, halved crosswise
- 1 teaspoon light brown sugar
- 1 tablespoon fresh lime juice
- ½ pound peeled cooked large shrimp
- 1 package (3 ounces) ramen noodles (no seasoning packet)
- 2 tablespoons thinly sliced radish
- 1 tablespoon roughly chopped cilantro
- 1 tablespoon chopped Thai basil (optional)

1. HEAT the oil in a large pot over medium-high heat. Add the onion, bell pepper, and jalapeño and cook until slightly soft, about 2 minutes. Add the ginger, garlic, and green curry paste and cook until fragrant, about 2 minutes longer.

2. ADD the coconut milk, ½ cup water, kaffir lime leaf (if using), carrots, and green beans. Bring to a slow boil, then reduce to a simmer and cook for 5 minutes. Stir in the brown sugar, lime juice, and shrimp and simmer 5 minutes longer.

3. PREPARE the ramen per package directions.

4. ADD the ramen to the curry pot and stir to combine. Serve topped with radish, cilantro, and Thai basil (if using).

MAKES 2 SERVINGS ||| Prep time: 10 minutes ||| **Total time: 30 minutes**

Cereal

The problem with most cereal today is that it's actually dessert in disguise. Let's be real, Reese's Puffs are anything but wholesome. Healthy options do exist, but you have to be a savvy shopper and keep sugar, fiber, and protein top of mind.

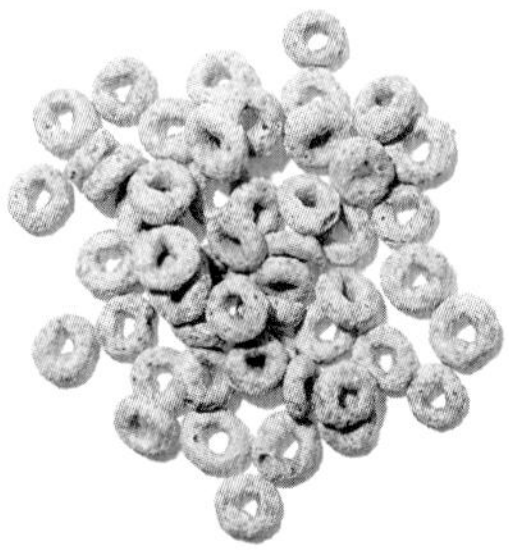

✱

NOT CLEAN

MOST STORE-BOUGHT CEREAL

Be careful with the majority of store-bought cereals—they're often made with refined grains, processed sugars, a slew of preservatives, and artificial colors, derived from petroleum, that have been linked to behavior problems in children.

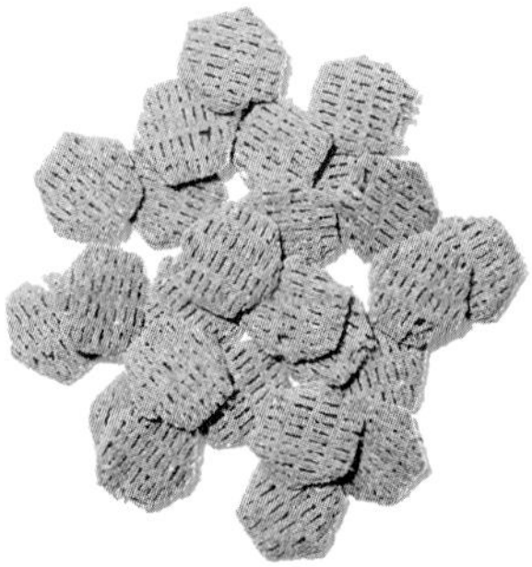

✱✱

CLEAN

WHOLE-GRAIN CEREAL WITH LESS THAN 10 GRAMS SUGAR

If you're having a hard time finding a cereal that meets all of our clean criteria, the most important factor to consider is sugar—keep it under 10 grams per serving to avoid crazy spikes in blood sugar, which put you at risk for overeating later.

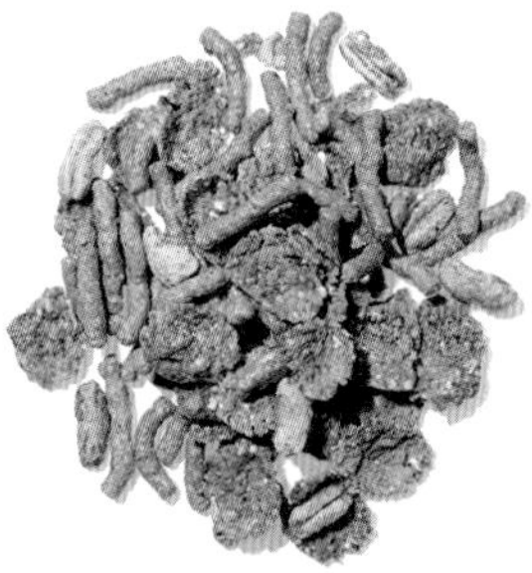

✱✱✱

CLEANEST

ORGANIC WHOLE-GRAIN CEREAL LOW IN SUGAR AND HIGH IN PROTEIN OR FIBER

To feel satisfied and energized, choose an organic whole-grain cereal with less than 10 grams of sugar and at least 5 grams of fiber and/or protein per serving. And be wary of what that serving size is—you might find an option that fits the bill only to discover that the serving is a measly ¾ cup, putting you at risk of overdoing it on sugar if you pour a full bowl.

CRANBERRY-WALNUT HERITAGE FLAKE MUFFINS

- **1¼ cups whole wheat flour**
- **2 tablespoons granulated sugar**
- **2 tablespoons light brown sugar**
- **¾ teaspoon baking soda**
- **½ teaspoon cinnamon**
- **¼ teaspoon fine sea salt**
- **2½ cups Nature's Path Heritage Flake cereal (or any 100% whole grain flake cereal)**
- **1 large egg**
- **1½ cups buttermilk**
- **2 tablespoons coconut oil, melted**
- **½ teaspoon vanilla extract**
- **½ cup dried cranberries**
- **⅓ cup chopped walnuts**

1. HEAT the oven to 375°F. Coat 12 cups of a muffin tin with cooking spray or line with paper liners.

2. WHISK together the flour, sugars, baking soda, cinnamon, and salt in a large bowl. Stir in the cereal. Whisk together the egg, buttermilk, coconut oil, and vanilla in a medium bowl.

3. POUR the wet ingredients over the dry ingredients, and fold in until completely combined, being careful not to overmix. Stir in the cranberries and walnuts.

4. LET the batter stand at room temperature for at least 45 minutes, or in the refrigerator in an airtight container for up to 3 days. This allows the cereal flakes to soften.

5. POUR the batter into the prepared muffin tin and bake until a skewer inserted into the center comes out clean, about 25 minutes. Remove from the muffin tin and allow to cool on a wire rack.

MAKES 12 MUFFINS ||| Prep time: 10 minutes ||| **Total time: 80 minutes**

Did You Know?

Breakfast can actually boost brainpower and help you fight disease all day long. Years of research shows that a morning meal—regardless of its effect on weight loss—hones cognitive performance, supplies extra energy for exercise (no matter what time of day you work out), and can help stave off type 2 diabetes, high cholesterol, and even heart disease.

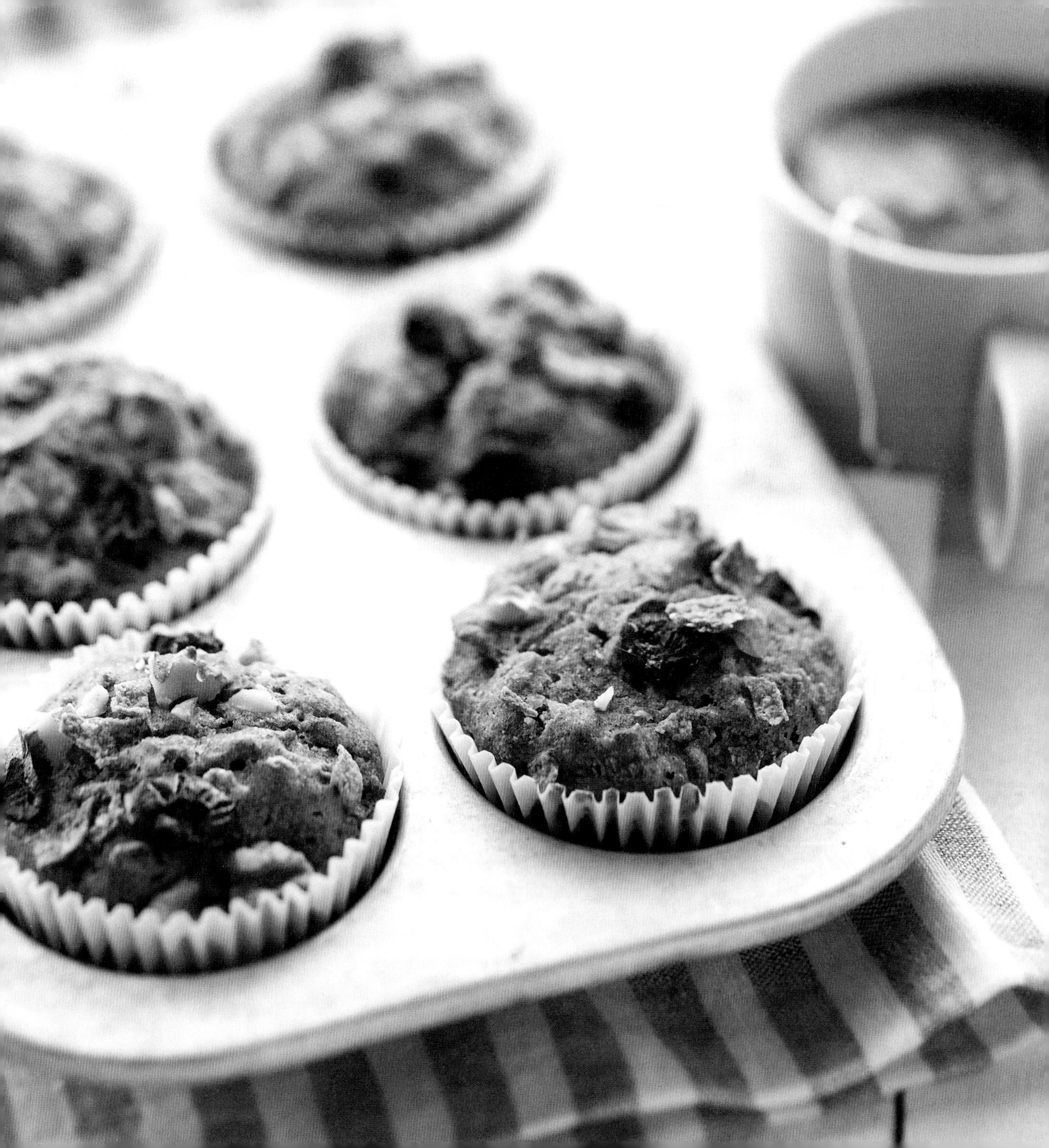

PEANUT BUTTER WHOLE-GRAIN O BARS

- **¼ cup creamy peanut butter**
- **2 tablespoons honey**
- **1 tablespoon maple syrup**
- **Dash of cinnamon**
- **1½ cups whole-grain O's cereal**

1. LINE an 8 x 8-inch baking pan with parchment paper.

2. COMBINE the peanut butter, honey, maple syrup, and cinnamon in a large saucepan. Heat over medium heat, stirring until well combined, about 3 minutes. Remove from the heat and add the cereal, gently combining until the cereal is well coated.

3. SPREAD the mixture out in the pan. Use your hands to even out the top.

4. CHILL in the refrigerator for at least 1 hour before cutting into 4 bars. Store in an airtight container.

MAKES 4 BARS ||| Prep time: 5 minutes ||| **Total time: 10 minutes + chilling time**

PECAN & HERITAGE FLAKE FISH FINGERS

- **1 cup Nature's Path Heritage Flake cereal (or any 100% whole grain flake cereal)**
- **2 tablespoons chopped pecans**
- **1 tablespoon chopped fresh curly parsley**
- **1 tablespoon chopped fresh basil**
- **¼ teaspoon dried oregano**
- **¼ teaspoon garlic powder**
- **2 tablespoons buttermilk**
- **¼ teaspoon fine sea salt**
- **¼ teaspoon black pepper**
- **2 tilapia fish fillets (4 ounces each)**

1. HEAT the oven to 425°F. Set a wire rack over a baking sheet and coat with olive oil cooking spray.

2. COMBINE the cereal, pecans, parsley, basil oregano, and garlic powder in a blender. (Make sure the herbs are fully dried first if they were just washed.) Pulse until the mixture resembles bread crumbs. Transfer to a shallow bowl.

3. WHISK together the buttermilk, salt, and pepper in a second shallow bowl.

4. DIP each tilapia filet in the buttermilk mixture, shaking off the excess. Then dredge each fillet in the cereal crumbs to evenly coat. Arrange on the rack over the baking sheet.

5. BAKE for 15 minutes, or until the coating is crispy and the fish is cooked through.

MAKES 2 SERVINGS ||| Prep time: 10 minutes ||| **Total time: 25 minutes**

Granola

This versatile, satisfying snack can certainly have a place

in a clean kitchen. But store-bought varieties are often loaded with sugar and overly processed vegetable oils—not a good thing when you eat it by the handful! Your best bet: Make it yourself! We promise, it's easy. Try one of our favorite recipes starting on the opposite page.

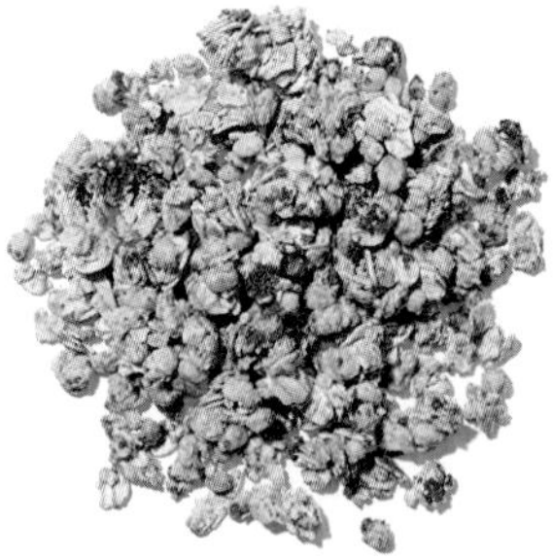

*

NOT CLEAN

CONVENTIONAL STORE-BOUGHT

If a granola has added sugars, unnatural ingredients, fillers, or corn syrup, it's best to pass, as all that junk isn't worth what few nutrients you'll get.

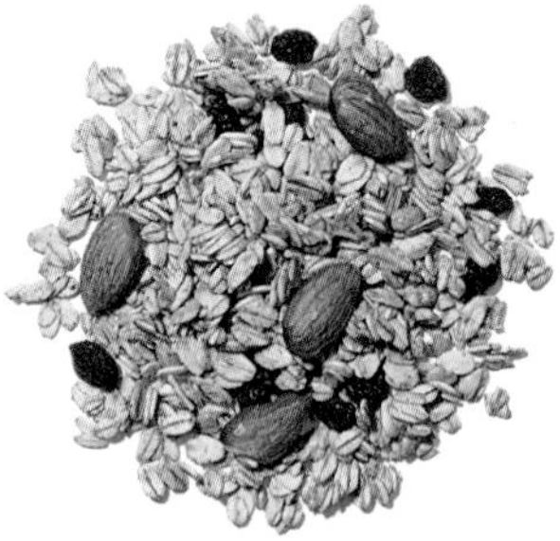

**

CLEAN

ORGANIC STORE-BOUGHT

If you're buying granola, read the ingredients carefully. You want less than 10 grams of sugar and a short ingredient list–granola should generally only contain things like oats, nuts, seeds, coconut, oil, and dried fruit.

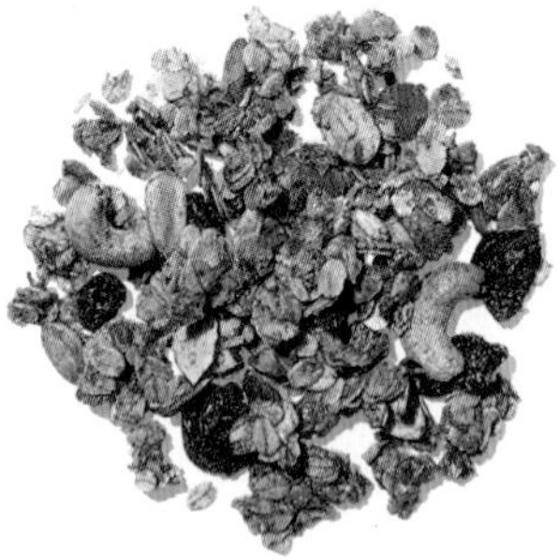

***

CLEANEST

HOMEMADE GRANOLA

Tailor granola to your personal taste–and keep sugar low–by making it with your favorite grains, nuts, seeds, and dried fruits. Oats are high in fiber, keep you full, and can help lower cholesterol; nuts and seeds contain heart-healthy fats and protein; and dried fruit delivers a dose of antioxidants and even more fiber.

COCOA OAT & DATE GRANOLA

- 1 pound chopped pitted Medjool dates
- 2 tablespoons maple syrup
- 1 tablespoon vanilla extract
- ½ cup unsweetened cocoa powder
- ½ teaspoon cinnamon
- ¼ teaspoon fine sea salt
- 4 cups rolled oats

1. HEAT the oven to 325°F. Line 2 baking sheets with parchment paper.

2. PLACE half of the dates, ⅔ cup water, the maple syrup, vanilla, cocoa, cinnamon, and salt in a food processor or blender. Blend until smooth, about 10 minutes. Scrape down the sides every few minutes. Pour the date mixture into a medium bowl. Add the oats and stir until coated.

3. SPREAD the granola mixture evenly on the prepared baking sheets. Bake until the granola is dry to the touch and somewhat crisp, 40 to 50 minutes. Remove from the oven and stir in the remaining chopped dates. The granola will become crunchy once it is cooled. Store in an airtight container at room temperature.

MAKES 8 SERVINGS (½ CUP EACH) ||| Prep time: 15 minutes ||| Total time: 55 minutes

HEALTHY HACK

Granola can actually be made grain-free–a great option for Paleo dieters and low-carb eaters. Simply toss some chopped nuts, unsweetened coconut flakes, seeds, and dried fruit together with olive oil or melted coconut oil, spread on a parchment-lined baking sheet, and bake until crunchy.

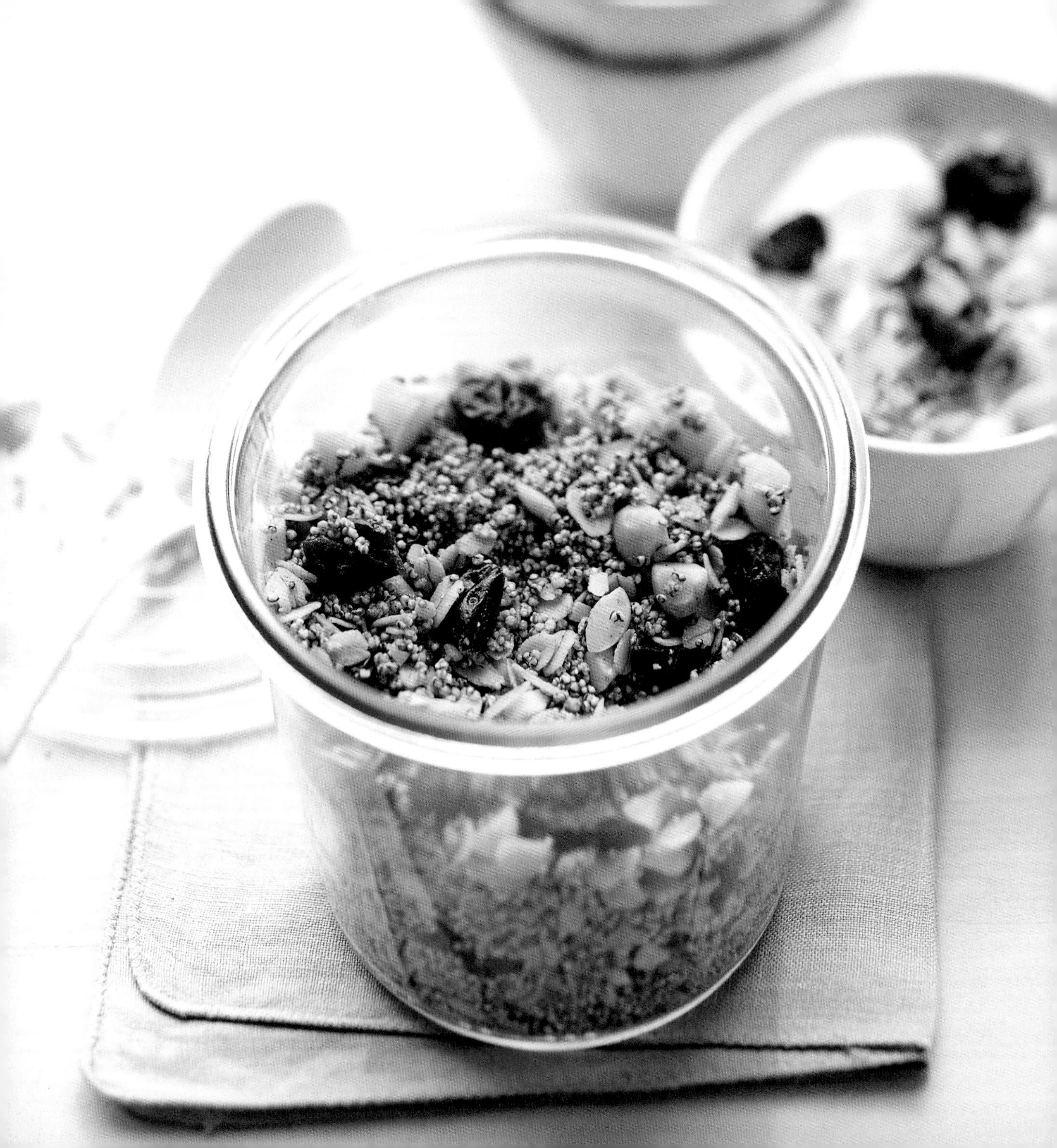

CINNAMON-VANILLA POPPED AMARANTH, DRIED CHERRY & MACADAMIA GRANOLA

- ½ **cup amaranth grain**
- 1 **cup rolled oats**
- 1 **cup roughly chopped macadamia nuts**
- 1 **teaspoon cinnamon**
- ¼ **teaspoon fine sea salt**
- ⅓ **cup pure maple syrup**
- ¼ **cup coconut oil**
- 1 **teaspoon vanilla extract**
- ¾ **cup dried cherries, chopped**

1. HEAT the oven to 275°F. Line a baking sheet with parchment paper.

2. PLACE a dry heavy-bottomed medium saucepan with a tight-fitting lid over medium-high heat. Check if the pan is hot enough by sprinkling a drop of water on the pan. If the water vaporizes immediately, it is ready. Pop the amaranth by placing 1 tablespoon of grain in the pan at a time, stirring constantly until the seeds pop. They should be done popping within 10 or 15 seconds. Once the first tablespoon is popped, transfer to a large bowl. Add the next tablespoon of amaranth to thc pan. Repeat until you have popped all of the amaranth.

3. ADD the oats, macadamia nuts, cinnamon, and salt to the bowl of popped amaranth and stir to mix.

4. COMBINE the maple syrup and coconut oil in a small saucepan and bring to a boil over medium heat. Remove from the heat and stir in the vanilla.

5. POUR the liquid mixture over the granola mixture and stir carefully to coat. Spread evenly on the prepared baking sheet. Bake for 35 to 40 minutes, stirring halfway.

6. REMOVE the granola from the oven and stir in the dried cherries. Cool completely and store in an airtight container.

MAKES 8 SERVINGS (½ CUP EACH) ||| Prep time: 15 minutes ||| **Total time: 50 minutes**

GINGERBREAD-SPICED BUCKWHEAT & QUINOA GRANOLA

- **1 cup buckwheat groats**
- **1 cup quinoa**
- **½ cup chopped walnuts or pecans**
- **¼ cup unsweetened applesauce**
- **2 tablespoons molasses**
- **2 tablespoons pure maple syrup**
- **2 tablespoons coconut oil, melted**
- **1 teaspoon vanilla extract**
- **1 teaspoon ground ginger**
- **½ teaspoon cinnamon**
- **¼ teaspoon fine sea salt**

1. HEAT the oven to 300°F. Line 2 baking sheets with parchment paper.

2. COMBINE the buckwheat, quinoa, and nuts in a large bowl.

3. STIR together the applesauce, molasses, maple syrup, coconut oil, vanilla, ginger, cinnamon, and salt in a small bowl. Drizzle over the buckwheat/quinoa mixture and stir to combine.

4. SPREAD out evenly on the baking sheets. Bake for 30 minutes. Remove from the oven and gently stir, being careful not to break clusters. Return to the oven and bake until the granola is dry to the touch, 20 to 30 minutes longer. The granola will become crunchy once it is cooled. Store in an airtight container at room temperature.

MAKES 8 SERVINGS (½ CUP EACH) ||| Prep time: 10 minutes ||| **Total time: 1 hour**

Oatmeal

Wholesome, filling, fiber-packed oatmeal: Well, that's what it should be anyway. But not all oatmeal is created equal. Your best choice is the one that's least messed-around-with: steel-cut.

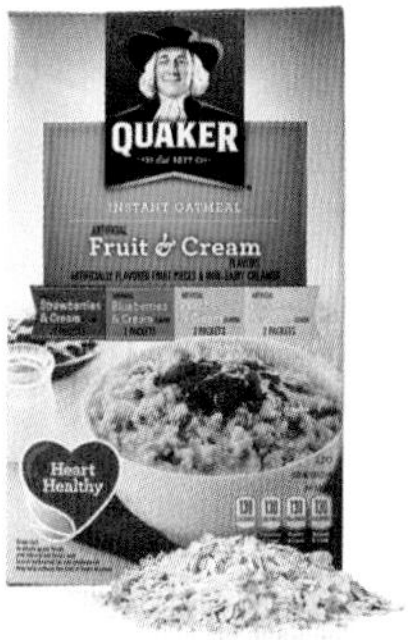

✱

NOT CLEAN

FLAVORED INSTANT OATMEAL

Pass on packets of flavored instant oatmeal. The oats have been highly processed, and the packet contains artificial flavors, excessive sugar, and preservatives. If you want convenience, toss some quick-cooking oats in a plastic baggy to take to the office or to have on hand throughout the week.

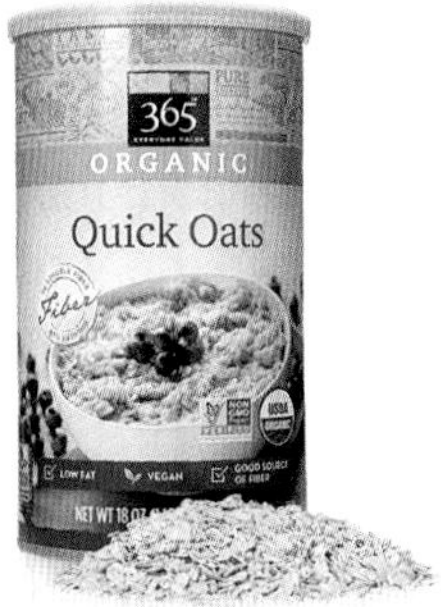

✱✱

CLEAN

PLAIN ROLLED OR QUICK-COOKING OATS

While rolled oats also help lower cholesterol, the way they're processed—they're steamed, rolled, steamed again, and toasted—gives them a higher glycemic index, meaning your blood sugar will experience more of a spike. But these are still a great option for the time-strapped.

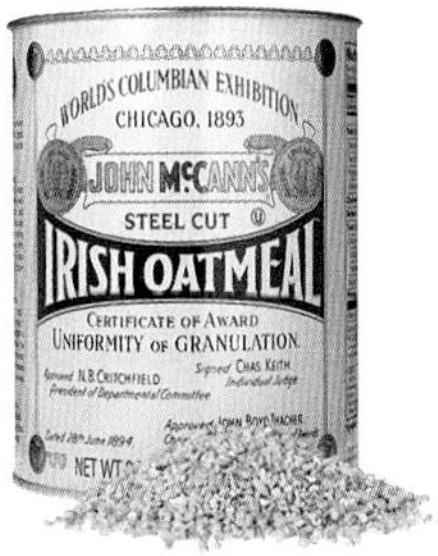

✱✱✱

CLEANEST

STEEL-CUT OATS

Steel-cut oats are simply whole oat groats that have been cut into neat little pieces on a mill. Because they're the least processed, they are also lowest on the glycemic index of all oat varieties, meaning it takes more time for the body to convert them into glucose for energy, keeping your blood sugar levels stable.

SIMPLE OVERNIGHT STEEL-CUT OATS

- **1⅔ cups 1% milk or unsweetened milk alternative**
- **⅔ cup steel-cut oats**
- **2 Medjool dates, chopped**
- **¼ teaspoon cinnamon**
- **1 tablespoon almond butter**
- **2 tablespoons chopped walnuts**

COMBINE the milk, oats, dates, cinnamon, and almond butter in a blender and blend until the dates are nearly pureed. Some small pieces might remain. Pour the mixture into a container, cover, and refrigerate overnight. In the morning, stir and top with the walnuts.

MAKES 2 SERVINGS ||| Prep time: 5 minutes ||| **Total time: 5 minutes + overnight soaking**

Did You Know?

Eating oatmeal for breakfast can actually help you lose weight. In a recent study, when people breakfasted on oatmeal instead of consuming its caloric equivalent in sugared cornflakes or skipping the meal altogether, they took in 31% fewer calories at their next meal.

STEEL-CUT OATS WITH CHICKEN SAUSAGE & CREMINI

- ½ cup steel-cut oats
- 1¼ cups reduced-sodium chicken broth
- ¼ teaspoon black pepper
- Pinch of cinnamon
- 1 tablespoon olive oil
- ¼ cup diced yellow onion
- 1 cup sliced cremini mushrooms
- 2 organic precooked chicken sausages (about 3 ounces each), chopped
- 1 teaspoon Dijon mustard
- 2 tablespoons balsamic vinegar
- ½ teaspoon dried thyme

1. COMBINE the oats and 1 cup of the broth in a small saucepan and bring to a boil over high heat. Reduce to a simmer, stir in the pepper and cinnamon, cover, and cook until all the liquid is gone and the mixture is thickened. Set aside to cool completely.

2. HEAT the olive oil in a medium skillet over medium-high heat. Add the onion, mushrooms, and chicken sausage and cook until the vegetables are softened and browned with no liquid or oil residue left in the bottom of the pan, about 5 minutes.

3. STIR the mustard into the vinegar in a small bowl and add to the skillet along with the remaining ¼ cup chicken broth and the thyme. Continue to cook over medium-high heat, gently scraping the bottom of the pan to release any remnants of onions or sausage. Simmer until the liquid is nearly gone. Remove from the heat.

4. SERVE the oats topped with the sausage mixture.

MAKES 2 SERVINGS ||| Prep time: 25 minutes ||| **Total time: 35 minutes**

Jams/ Jellies

Fruit spreads are a healthy way to satisfy a sweet craving

when slathered on a thick slice of whole-grain toast or as part of a classic PB&J. Just be sure to keep it real—most conventional jams and jellies are nothing more than hidden sources of high fructose corn syrup.

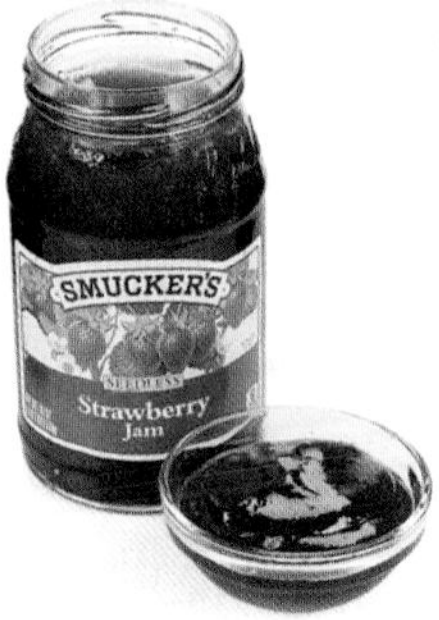

*

NOT CLEAN

SPREADS MADE FROM FRUIT AND HIGH FRUCTOSE CORN SYRUP

Skip conventional jams and jellies altogether, as they're often loaded with added colors, preservatives, and high fructose corn syrup.

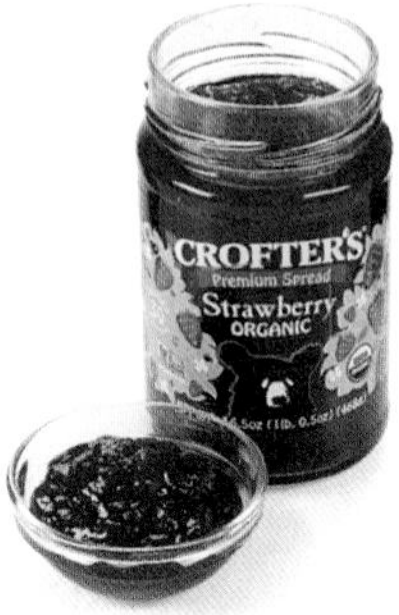

**

CLEAN

SPREADS MADE FROM FRUIT AND NATURAL SWEETENERS

A fruit spread that's sweetened should only contain natural sugars such as cane sugar or honey. And even then, pick a brand that contains 6 grams or less of sugar per serving.

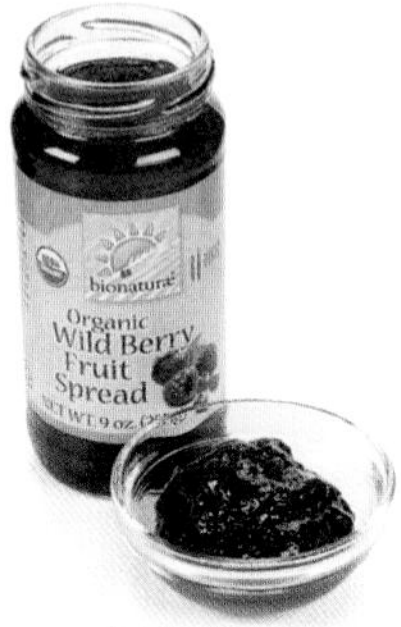

***

CLEANEST

SPREADS MADE FROM FRUIT ONLY

A 100% fruit spread made with no added sugars, preferably organic, is your healthiest bet. Bursting with flavor, natural jams and jellies that let the naturally delicious taste of strawberries, raspberries, or blackberries come through will keep you from missing any additional sugar.

RASPBERRY CHIA JAM

3 cups fresh or frozen raspberries
3 tablespoons orange juice
2 tablespoons chia seeds
½ teaspoon vanilla extract

STIR the raspberries, chia seeds, and orange juice together in a medium saucepan. Bring to a light boil, then reduce the heat to simmer and cook, uncovered, until the raspberries break down and the mixture thickens, 10 to 12 minutes. Remove from the heat and stir in the vanilla. Let cool 20 minutes. The jam will thicken more as it cools. If you prefer a smoother jam, use an immersion/hand blender to puree to the desired consistency.

MAKES 1 CUP ||| Prep time: 5 minutes ||| **Total time: 20 minutes**

Did You Know?

Since sugar acts as a preservative, spreads made from fruit only will spoil more quickly than jams and jellies that include sweeteners. Most fruit-only spreads include expiration dates on the jars and recommend using within 1 month after opening. To prevent early spoilage, keep your spreads in the back of the refrigerator where it's colder, not in the door shelf.

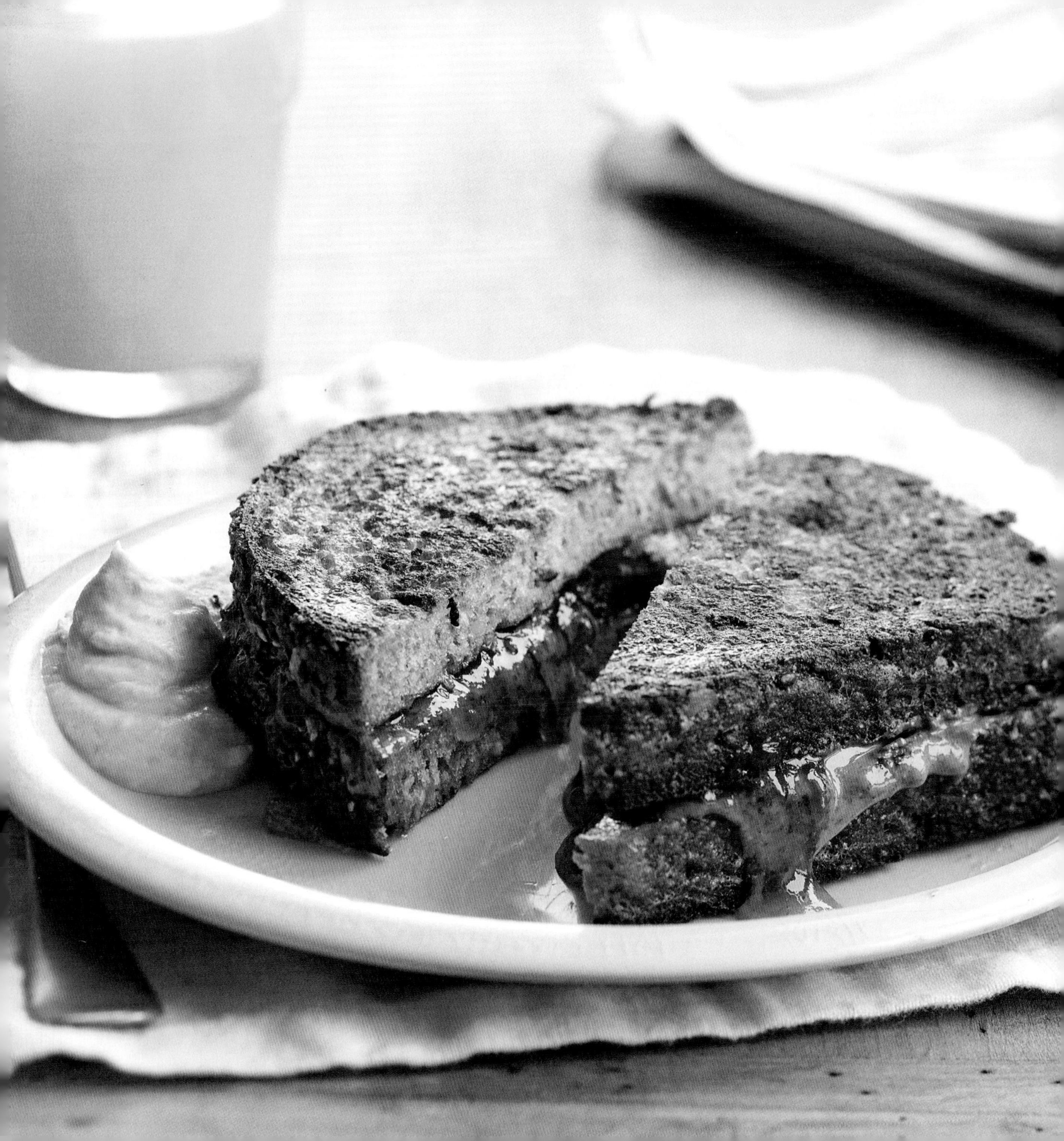

STUFFED FRENCH TOAST WITH ORANGE-COCONUT CREAM

2 tablespoons canned coconut cream (see Note)
2 teaspoons powdered sugar
1 teaspoon vanilla extract
2 teaspoons grated orange zest
1 large egg
⅓ cup unsweetened vanilla almond milk
Pinch of ground nutmeg
4 thick slices crusty whole-grain bread (preferably a day or two old)
3 teaspoons coconut oil
4 teaspoons almond butter
4 teaspoons no-sugar-added apricot preserves

1. BEAT the thickened coconut cream in a bowl with the powdered, sugar, ½ teaspoon of the vanilla, and ½ teaspoon of the orange zest until creamy, about 30 seconds.

2. WHISK the egg with the almond milk, nutmeg, and the remaining ½ teaspoon vanilla and 1½ teaspoons orange zest in a shallow bowl. Dip each side of the bread slices in the egg mixture until coated, but do not saturate.

3. HEAT the coconut oil in a skillet over medium heat. Cook the bread until lightly browned on both sides, about 3 minutes per side.

4. SPREAD half of the still-warm slices with the almond butter. Spread the other 2 slices with the apricot preserves. Create sandwiches by putting 1 jam slice and 1 almond butter slice together. Cut on a diagonal. Top each serving with coconut cream.

Note: To get coconut cream, refrigerate an unopened can of coconut milk. The thick cream will rise to the top and solidify. Scoop out the 2 tablespoons needed for the recipe. Beat while the cream is still chilled and solid.

MAKES 2 SERVINGS ||| Prep time: 10 minutes ||| **Total time: 20 minutes**

WHOLE-GRAIN THUMBPRINT COOKIES WITH RASPBERRY CHIA JAM

- **¼ cup rolled oats**
- **1¼ cups whole wheat pastry flour**
- **2 cups almond meal/flour**
- **½ teaspoon fine sea salt**
- **½ teaspoon cinnamon**
- **½ cup coconut oil, melted**
- **½ cup pure maple syrup**
- **½ cup Raspberry Chia Jam (page 141)**

1. HEAT the oven to 350°F. Line a baking sheet with parchment paper.

2. PULSE the oats in a blender or food processor until they form a coarse flour, about 30 seconds.

3. COMBINE the oats, flour, almond meal, salt, and cinnamon in a large bowl. Stir in the coconut oil and maple syrup to combine.

4. SHAPE the dough into balls using about 1 tablespoon per cookie and arrange 1½ inches apart on the baking sheet. Gently make an indentation in the center of each cookie using your thumb. Fill the indentation of each cookie with ½ to ¾ teaspoon jam.

5. BAKE until the cookies are golden brown, about 20 minutes. Allow to cool for a couple minutes on the baking sheet before moving to a wire rack to cool completely.

MAKES 24 COOKIES ||| Prep time: 10 minutes ||| **Total time: 30 minutes**

Nut Butters

Peanut, almond, and cashew butter (just to name a few)

are perfect ways to add protein and healthy fats to your diet. Research even suggests that eating more nuts, in their various forms, can reduce risk of heart disease and diabetes. Good news, but don't let pesticides and nasty packaging counter these health benefits.

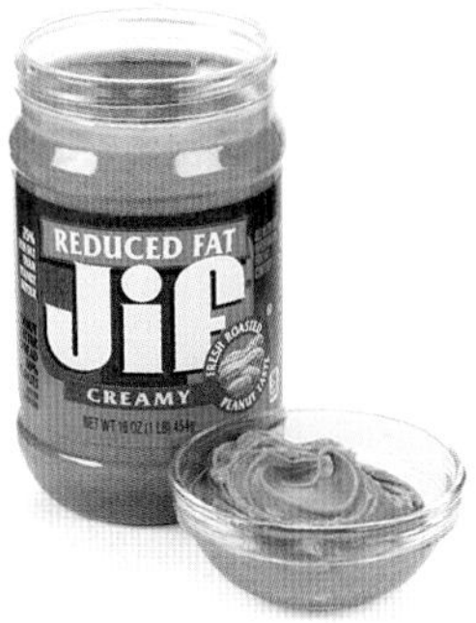

✷

NOT CLEAN

REDUCED-FAT NUT BUTTERS

Don't buy into low-fat claims on nut butter jars: While there may be less fat, there's more sugar; and the healthy monounsaturated fats in nut butters are an important part of your diet that shouldn't be stripped away.

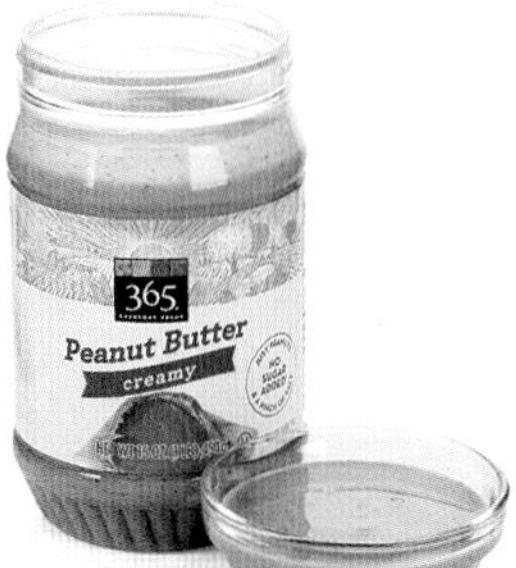

✷✷

CLEAN

CONVENTIONAL NUT BUTTERS WITHOUT ADDED SWEETENERS

Nonorganic nut butters can contain pesticides and other synthetic ingredients. Plastic nut butter jars may also contain potentially dangerous chemicals that may leach into your food.

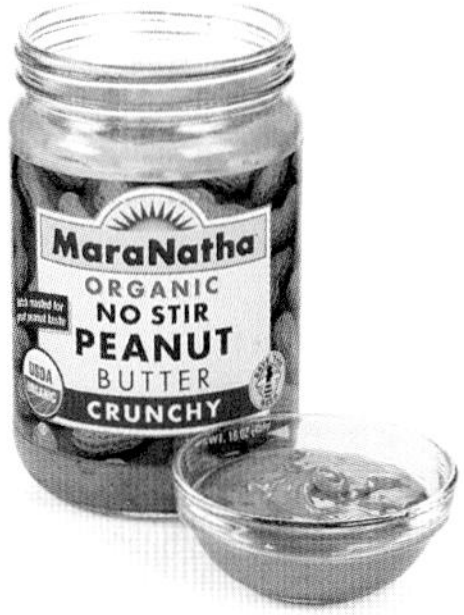

✷✷✷

CLEANEST

ORGANIC NUT BUTTERS WITHOUT ADDED SWEETENERS IN GLASS JARS

Whichever nut butter you prefer, select organic varieties sold in a glass jar. They'll be free of pesticides and potentially carcinogenic chemicals found in plastic packaging. Also, since many manufacturers add sugar to peanut butter, check the label to be sure your product pick doesn't include any sweeteners.

HOMEMADE COCOA-HAZELNUT BUTTER

1 cup unsalted dry-roasted skinned hazelnuts

1 teaspoon coconut or grapeseed oil

2 tablespoons honey

1 tablespoon vanilla extract

¼ cup plus 2 tablespoons soy or nut milk

3 tablespoons Dutch process cocoa powder

Fine sea salt

1. PLACE the hazelnuts in a food processor and grind to a fine powder, scraping down the sides every few minutes, for up to 10 minutes. With the processor running, slowly add the oil, honey, and vanilla and process for 5 minutes, frequently scraping down the sides to ensure it mixes evenly.

2. ADD the milk and process until it is smooth, 2 to 4 minutes. Add the cocoa powder and a dash of salt and process until creamy, up to 5 minutes. Store in a glass jar in the refrigerator.

MAKES ABOUT ¾ CUP ||| Prep time: 15 minutes ||| **Total time: 15 minutes**

Did You Know?

Enjoying peanut butter on your whole-grain English muffin in the morning is a great way to curb cravings throughout the day. Research has found that nut butters consumed at breakfast profoundly impact your blood sugar, keeping it stable past lunch and achieving what's called the "second meal effect."

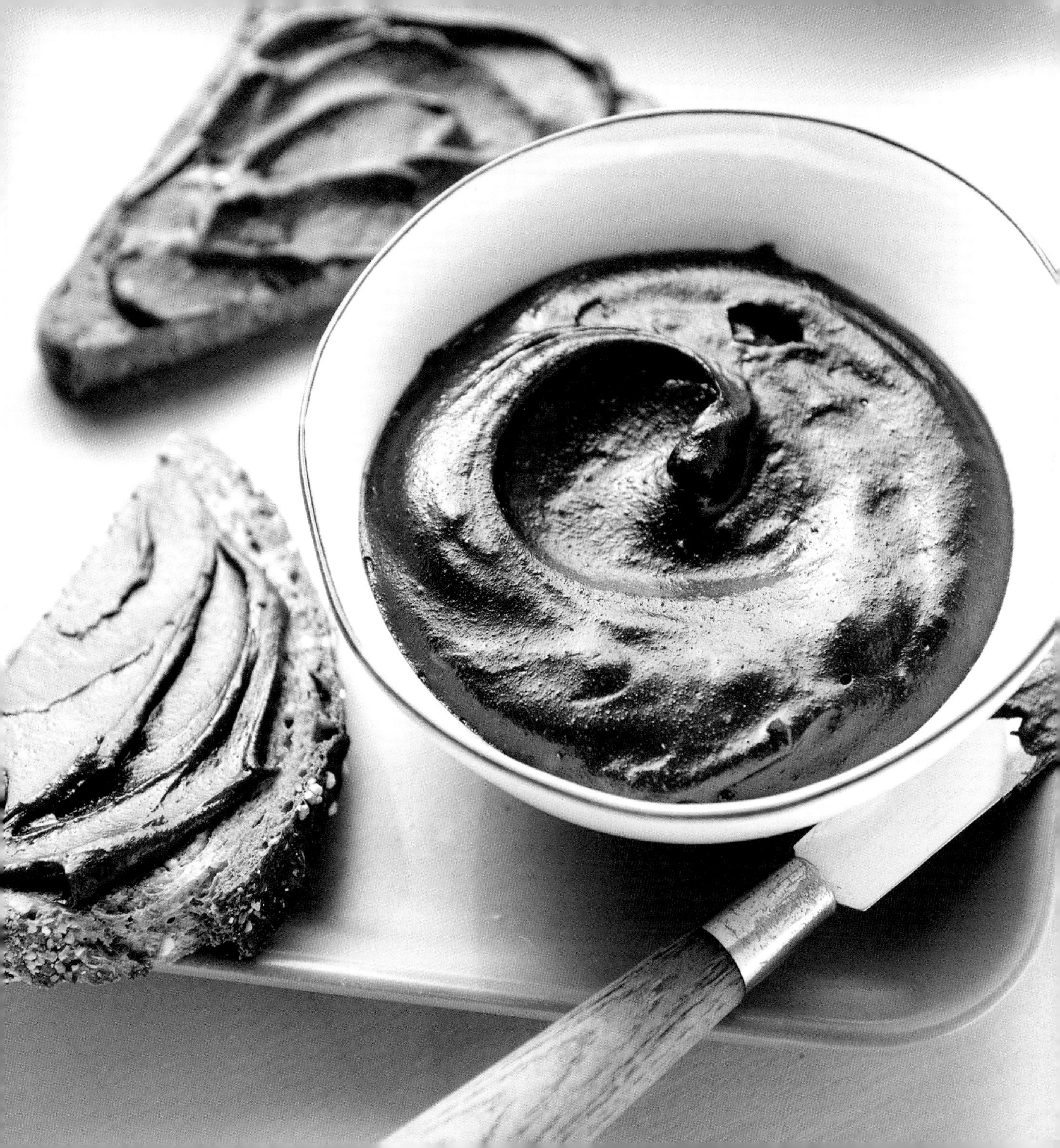

PEANUT BUTTER, DATE & OAT BALLS

- ½ **pound (1 cup packed) pitted Medjool dates**
- 1 **cup rolled oats**
- ¼ **cup plus 1 tablespoon peanut butter**
- 1 **tablespoon honey**
- 1 **tablespoon vanilla extract**
- **Dash of fine sea salt**
- **Dash of cinnamon**

1. PLACE all the ingredients in a food processor. Process until crumbly, about 3 minutes.

2. USE a 1½-tablespoon cookie scoop to pack the mixture into a ball. You may need to lightly squeeze the dough between your hands to help it stick together at first. Roll into a ball and set aside on a cutting board or piece of wax paper. Repeat with the remaining mixture. Store in an airtight container.

MAKES 12 BALLS ||| Prep time: 10 minutes ||| **Total time: 10 minutes**

SPICY GINGER-ALMOND SAUCE

- ¼ **cup almond butter**
- 3 **tablespoons canned lite coconut milk**
- 2 **tablespoons reduced-sodium wheat-free tamari**
- 1 **teaspoon honey**
- ½ **teaspoon minced fresh ginger**
- ¼ **teaspoon minced garlic**
- ¼ **teaspoon Sriracha sauce**
- ¼ **teaspoon sesame oil**

WHISK together all of the ingredients in a small bowl. Serve as a sauce, dip, or sandwich spread. Store in an airtight container in the refrigerator.

MAKES ABOUT ½ CUP ||| Prep time: 5 minutes ||| **Total time: 5 minutes**

Butter

Once thought of as a complete "diet don't," real butter is finally making a comeback, and for good reason. High-quality varieties are thought to contain more beta-carotene and a healthier fatty acid profile than lab-made margarine, which is a sneaky source of dangerous trans fats.

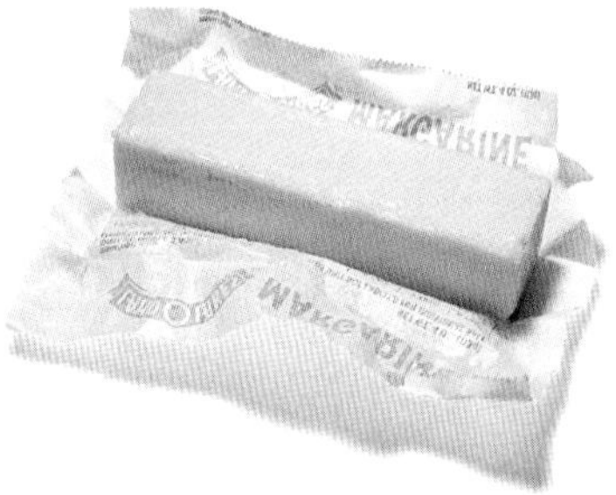

✱

NOT CLEAN

MARGARINE

Margarine and other "buttery spreads" can contain trans fats—the fat that's most strongly associated with heart disease—as well as synthetic vitamins, soy protein isolate, and other additives and preservatives. Some studies have shown that people who eat margarine are twice as likely to suffer from cardiovascular disease.

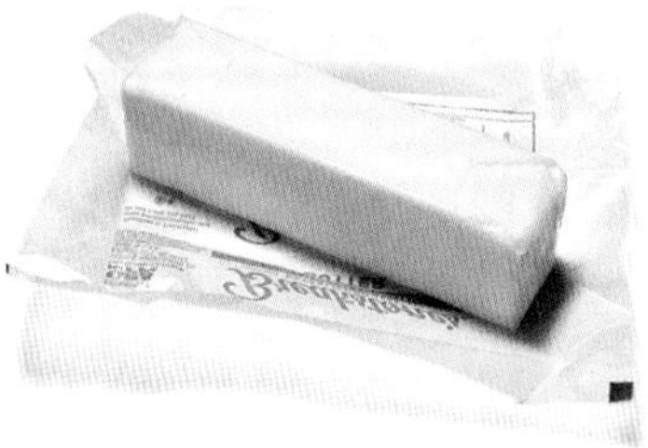

✱✱

CLEAN

CONVENTIONAL BUTTER

Think twice about conventional butter, as it's likely produced from cows that have been given antibiotics and growth hormones. That being said, it's still more natural than margarine, and any type of fat will help boost your absorption of disease-fighting nutrients from the veggies you consume.

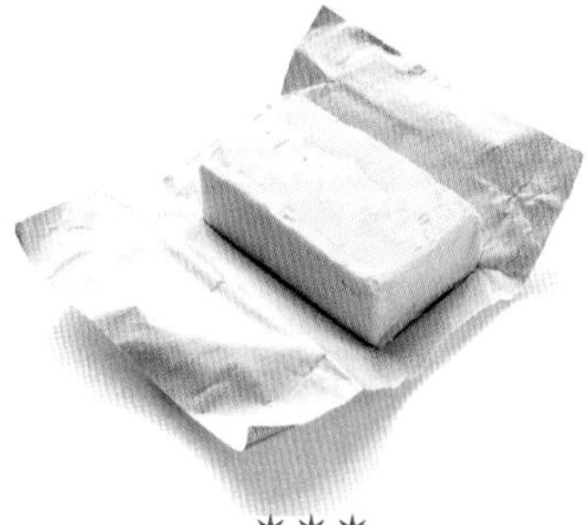

✱✱✱

CLEANEST

ORGANIC GRASS-FED BUTTER

Butter from grass-fed cows has been shown to contain healthier fats than butter from grain-fed cattle. A grass-fed diet also contributes to increased amounts of beta-carotene, which the body converts to vitamin A.

BROWN BUTTER SAUTÉED CARROTS

- **1 pound young whole carrots**
- **1½ tablespoons unsalted butter**
- **¼ teaspoon fine sea salt**
- **¼ teaspoon ground cumin**
- **¼ teaspoon ground coriander**
- **Pinch of black pepper**

1. STEAM the carrots until just tender, about 5 minutes.

2. HEAT the butter in a medium skillet over medium-low heat, swirling the pan until the butter begins to brown. When the butter begins to smell like baked goods, add the salt, cumin, coriander, and pepper and continue to swirl for another minute.

3. ADD the carrots, toss to coat, and allow to cook in the butter mixture for 3 minutes longer.

MAKES 2 SERVINGS ||| Prep time: 15 minutes ||| **Total time: 15 minutes**

Did You Know?

Dietary cholesterol found in butter, beef, and other animal-based foods isn't as bad for heart health as doctors and nutritionists have been telling us for decades. After reviewing piles of research, the group that advises the US government on dietary guidelines recently reported that it's "not a nutrient of concern for overconsumption," meaning that the cholesterol you eat isn't likely to raise your heart disease risk. Bigger culprits in heart disease seem to be sugars and trans fats.

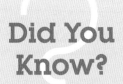

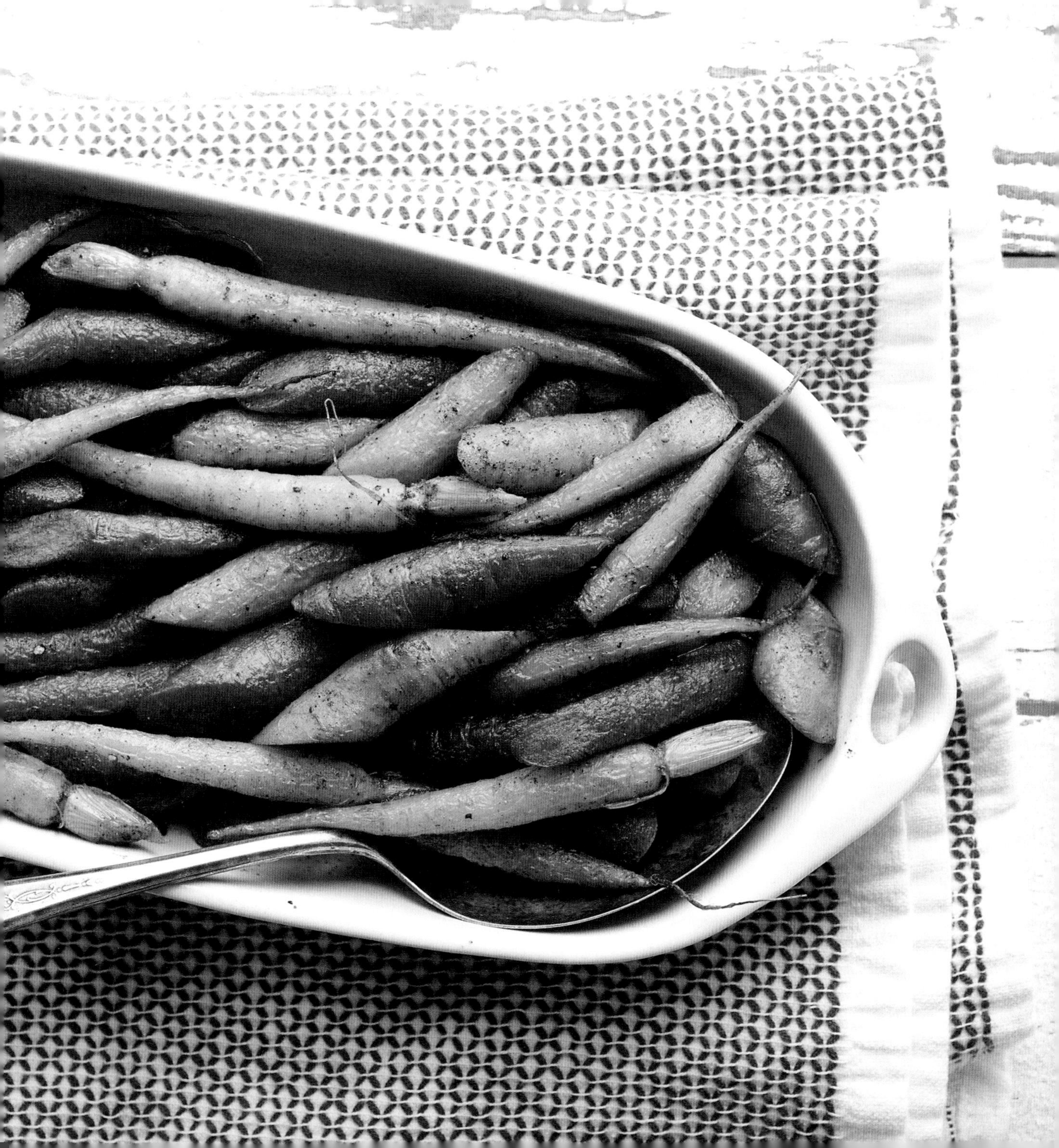

FLOURLESS BANANA BREAD

1½ cups rolled oats
½ cup almond meal/flour
1 teaspoon baking soda
1 teaspoon baking powder
2 teaspoons cinnamon
⅛ teaspoon fine sea salt
4 Medjool dates, soaked in water for 30 minutes
4 very ripe bananas
4 tablespoons unsalted butter
2 large eggs, separated
1 teaspoon vanilla extract

1. HEAT the oven to 350°F. Grease a 9 x 5-inch loaf pan very well with butter.

2. GRIND the oats in a blender until fully ground and powdery. Transfer to a bowl and stir in the almond meal, baking soda, baking powder, cinnamon, and salt.

3. DRAIN the dates and add to the blender. Add the banana, butter, and egg yolks to the blender and puree. Mix into the dry ingredients until just incorporated.

4. WHIP the egg whites in a bowl with an electric mixer until stiff peaks form. Gently fold half the egg whites into the batter until incorporated. Then fold the second half of the whites in.

5. POUR the batter into the prepared loaf pan and bake until firm in the center and browned, about 1 hour 15 minutes. Allow to cool completely in the pan before removing and slicing.

MAKES ONE 9-INCH LOAF (ABOUT 8 SLICES) ||| Prep time: 15 minutes ||| **Total time: 1 hour 30 minutes**

OMELET STUFFED WITH BUTTER-SAUTÉED MUSHROOMS

- **4 large eggs**
- **1½ tablespoons unsalted butter**
- **1½ cups thinly sliced mixed mushrooms**
- **1 clove garlic, minced**
- **¼ teaspoon dried ground sage**
- **¼ teaspoon fine sea salt**
- **2 tablespoons chopped fresh chives**

1. WHISK the eggs with 2 tablespoons water in a bowl. Set aside.

2. HEAT half of the butter in a medium skillet over medium heat and add the mushrooms. Cook until lightly browned, about 8 minutes. Add the garlic, sage, and salt and cook for 1 minute longer. Transfer the mushrooms to a plate..

3. ADD the remaining butter to the pan and melt over medium heat. Pour in the eggs and use a spatula to gently move the egg mixture from the sides to the center, allowing the liquid egg to fill in around the edges. This will help the egg cook evenly.

4. FLIP the omelet over in the pan and top one half with the mushroom mixture and chives. Fold in half to serve.

MAKES 2 SERVINGS ||| Prep time: 15 minutes ||| **Total time: 15 minutes**

Salad Dressing

Topping your lovingly prepared salads with a trans fat–loaded dressing (or even a fat-free one) should be a crime. Unfortunately, that makes up a lot of what's lining store shelves. Keep it simple and make your own—it literally takes 30 seconds! Try one of our three unique recipes starting on the opposite page.

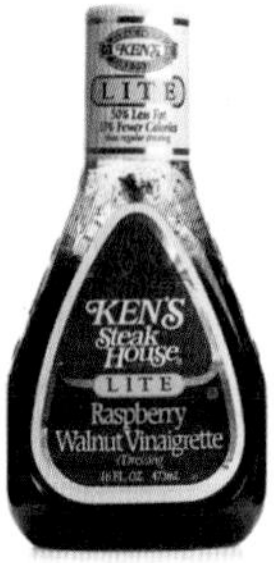

✷

NOT CLEAN

CONVENTIONAL STORE-BOUGHT DRESSINGS

Most of these are loaded with added sugar, sodium, artificial colorings, and preservatives. They may also contain trans fats in the form of partially hydrogenated vegetable oils, which are linked to heart disease.

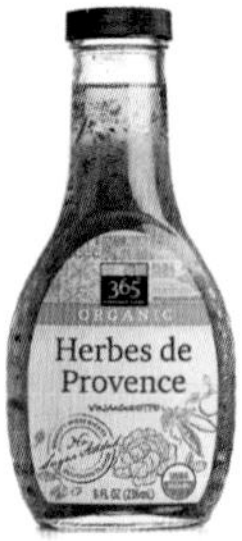

✷✷

CLEAN

ORGANIC OR NON-GMO STORE-BOUGHT DRESSINGS

If you buy bottled dressing, look for an organic or non-GMO dressing, nothing synthetic, few ingredients, and less than 5 grams of sugar per 2 tablespoons. Oh, and pick one that has some fat (at least 3 grams, although the more, the better)—it helps you absorb the nutrients in your veggies.

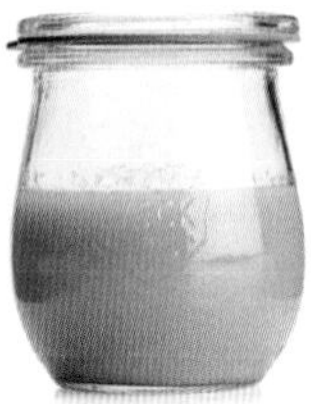

✷✷✷

CLEANEST

HOMEMADE DRESSING

A homemade vinaigrette of olive oil and vinegar will make your salad even better for you. Olive oil contains anti-inflammatory monounsaturated fats, and apple cider vinegar consumed before a carb-heavy meal can slow the rise of blood sugar (reducing cravings) and improve insulin sensitivity.

ASIAN GINGER VINAIGRETTE

- ½ cup dark sesame oil
- ¼ cup wheat-free tamari
- 1 inch fresh ginger, peeled
- 1 clove garlic, peeled
- 1 tablespoon creamy peanut butter
- 1 tablespoon tahini
- Juice of 1 lemon
- ¼ cup water
- 2 teaspoons sugar
- ¼ teaspoon cayenne (or to taste)

COMBINE the sesame oil, tamari, ginger, garlic, peanut butter, tahini, lemon juice, ¼ cup water, sugar, and cayenne in a food processor or blender. Puree until smooth. Store in the refrigerator for up to 1 week.

MAKES 4 SERVINGS ||| Prep time: 5 minutes ||| **Total time: 5 minutes**

CREAMY VEGAN RANCH DRESSING

- 1 cup cashews
- 3 tablespoons finely chopped fresh parsley
- 2 tablespoons finely chopped fresh dill
- 1 teaspoon garlic powder
- 1 teaspoon onion powder
- ½ teaspoon fine sea salt

1. **SOAK** the cashews overnight in water to cover. Drain.

2. **COMBINE** the cashews, 1 cup fresh water, parsley, dill, garlic powder, onion powder, and salt in a blender or food processor. Puree until smooth and creamy. Add water if a thinner consistency desired.

MAKES 6 SERVINGS ||| Prep time: 5 minutes ||| **Total time: 5 minutes + overnight soaking**

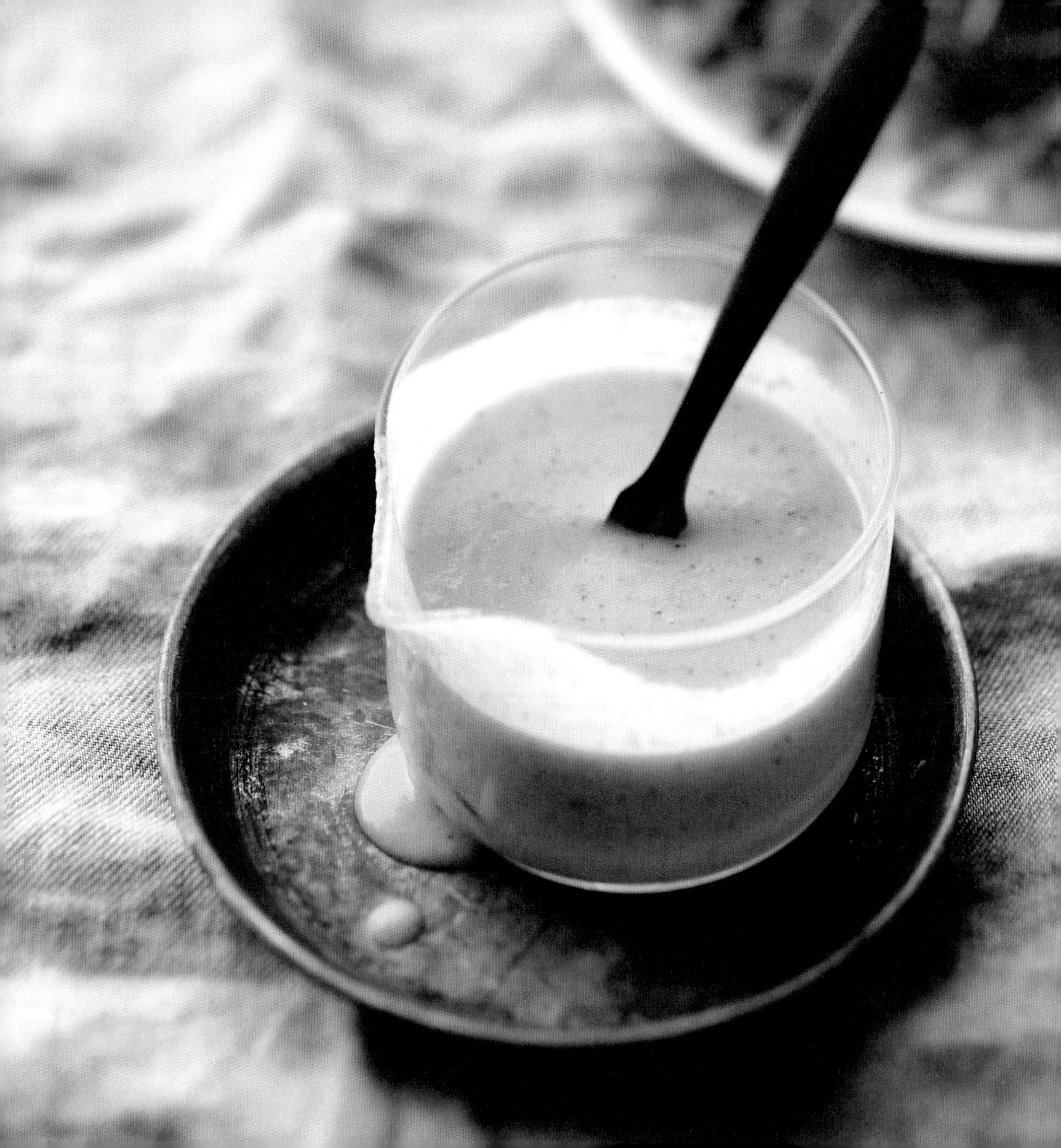

CILANTRO-PEAR VINAIGRETTE

- **½ cup cilantro leaves**
- **1 small pear, cored and quartered**
- **1 clove garlic, peeled**
- **Juice of 1 lemon**
- **2 tablespoons white wine vinegar**
- **½ cup extra virgin olive oil**

PUREE the cilantro, pear, garlic, lemon juice, and vinegar in a blender until smooth. On low speed, drizzle in the olive oil and blend to emulsify. Serve immediately or store covered in the refrigerator for up to 4 days. Shake to redistribute if settling occurs.

MAKES 4 SERVINGS ||| Prep time: 5 minutes ||| **Total time: 5 minutes**

HEALTHY HACK

Stuck in a repetitive rut and always reach for olive oil any time you make a dressing or marinade? One of the simplest ways to mix up the flavor and nutrition profile of any dressing is by switching up the oils. Some of the most flavorful (and healthiest) options include avocado, walnut, flax, and safflower.

Pasta Sauce

Topping whole wheat pasta, veggies, and a lean protein with a little marinara is an easy and nutritious meal. But don't ruin it all with the wrong sauce. Pick something that will enhance your meal's nutrition, not detract from it.

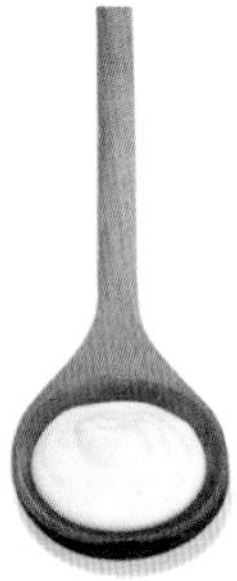

*

NOT CLEAN

STORE-BOUGHT CREAM SAUCE

Just say no to dairy-based cream sauces. They're full of unhealthy fats, sodium, and preservatives—and you definitely don't get the antioxidant benefits of tomatoes. If you ever indulge in a cream sauce, make it yourself and use quality ingredients.

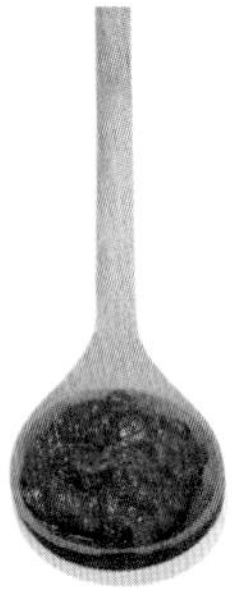

**

CLEAN

REGULAR TOMATO SAUCE

Standard store-bought tomato sauce can contain as many as 12 grams of sugar per ½ cup, and this may come in the form of high fructose corn syrup—not to mention the excess sodium, preservatives, and traces of pesticides.

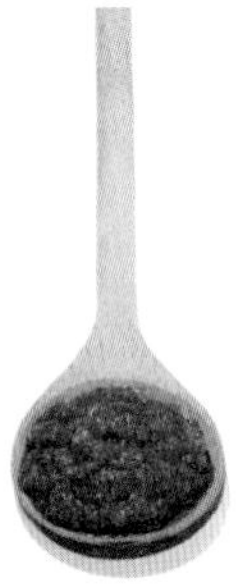

***

CLEANEST

ORGANIC TOMATO SAUCE WITHOUT ADDED SUGARS

Low-sugar organic sauce is delicious and packs a good dose of vitamin C and lycopene, an antioxidant that may help reduce risk of heart disease, cancer, and macular degeneration. Want to make your own (and can't find grandma's recipe)? Try our homemade Tomato-Basil Marinara on the opposite page.

TOMATO-BASIL MARINARA

- **1½ tablespoons olive oil**
- **1½ cups diced onion**
- **3 cloves garlic, chopped**
- **¼ teaspoon dried oregano**
- **½ teaspoon kosher salt**
- **½ teaspoon black pepper**
- **1 can (28 ounces) good-quality whole peeled tomatoes (San Marzano, DOP certified if possible)**
- **¼ teaspoon red-pepper flakes**
- **½ cup fresh basil leaves, roughly torn**

1. HEAT the olive oil in a large deep skillet over medium heat. Add the onion and cook until soft and sweet, 12 to 15 minutes.

2. ADD the garlic, oregano, and ¼ teaspoon each of the salt and pepper. Stir to combine and cook until the garlic is fragrant, about 1 minute.

3. ADD the tomatoes and, using a potato masher or your hands, gently crush the tomatoes. Add the red-pepper flakes and basil leaves and stir to combine. Let simmer, partially covered, until the sauce thickens, about 25 minutes.

4. BLEND the sauce in the skillet with an immersion blender, leaving some texture and some smooth, or to desired consistency.

MAKES 4 SERVINGS ||| Prep time: 10 minutes ||| **Total time: 40 minutes**

HEALTHY HACK

Make a quick and super healthy "cream" sauce by using pureed avocado instead of dairy products. Simply combine 1 large avocado, 4 teaspoons lemon juice, and ¼ cup pasta water in a blender or food processor and puree until smooth. Toss with pasta and enjoy!

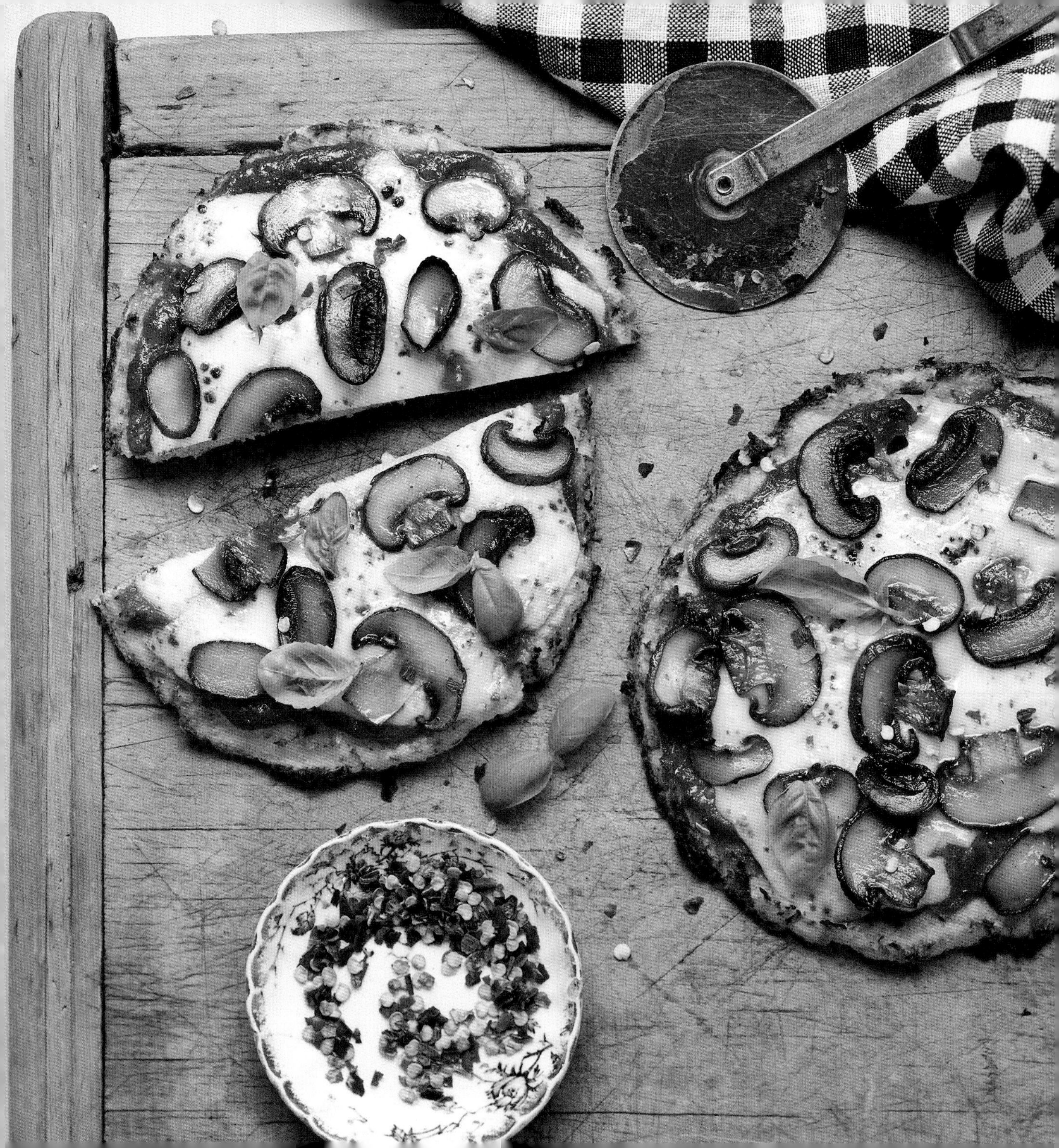

CAULIFLOWER CRUST PIZZA WITH MARINARA, FRESH MOZZARELLA & SAUTÉED MUSHROOMS

CRUST

- 1 teaspoon olive oil
- 3 cups chopped cauliflower (1 medium to large head)
- 1 egg, beaten
- ½ cup fresh grated Parmesan
- 3 tablespoons soft goat cheese
- ½ teaspoon dried oregano

TOPPINGS

- 2 teaspoons olive oil
- 1 cup sliced cremini mushrooms
- ⅓ cup low-sugar organic tomato sauce
- ½ cup fresh mozzarella, cut into thin slices
- ¼ cup fresh basil leaves

1. **HEAT** the oven to 400°F and place a baking sheet in the oven to heat. Cut a piece of parchment paper to fit the baking sheet and grease with 1 teaspoon olive oil. Set the parchment paper aside on a cutting board.

2. **MAKE** the crust: Pulse the cauliflower in a food processor or blender until it has a quinoa-like texture and size.

3. **MICROWAVE** the cauliflower "quinoa" in a loosely covered microwaveable dish until lightly steamed, about 4 minutes. Drain the cauliflower in a fine-mesh sieve. Press on it with the back of a wooden spoon to remove all excess moisture.

4. **TRANSFER** the cauliflower to a large bowl and stir in the egg, Parmesan, goat cheese, and oregano.

5. **DIVIDE** the mixture in half and form into two compact balls. Place on the parchment paper and press into 2 circles, 6 inches in diameter and ¼ inch thick. Bake until the crust begins to turn golden, 10 minutes, then flip and bake another 7 minutes, or until the crust is lightly golden and firm.

6. **HEAT** the olive oil in a medium skillet over medium-high heat. Add the mushrooms and cook until tender, about 5 minutes.

7. **SPREAD** the crusts evenly with the marinara, then top with slices of mozzarella, basil, and cooked mushrooms. Bake until the cheese begins to bubble, 5 to 10 minutes.

MAKES 2 INDIVIDUAL PIZZAS ||| Prep time: 20 minutes ||| **Total time: 45 minutes**

LASAGNA BAKED INTO A SPAGHETTI SQUASH

- **1 spaghetti squash (4 to 5 pounds), halved lengthwise, seeds and membranes removed**
- **1 teaspoon olive oil**
- **1 cup chopped cremini mushrooms**
- **2 cups chopped baby spinach**
- **⅓ cup part-skim ricotta**
- **¼ teaspoon kosher salt**
- **¼ teaspoon black pepper**
- **1 tablespoon chopped fresh parsley**
- **2 tablespoons chopped fresh basil**
- **1 cup Tomato-Basil Marinara (page 159)**
- **½ cup shredded whole-milk mozzarella**

1. HEAT the oven to 400°F. Line a baking sheet with foil.

2. ARRANGE the spaghetti squash halves, cut side down, on the baking sheet. Bake until the flesh is tender to the touch, about 1 hour. Set aside until cool enough to handle.

3. HEAT a medium skillet over medium-high heat. Add the olive oil and the mushrooms and cook until browned, 5 to 7 minutes. Add the spinach and cook until wilted, about 1 minute longer.

4. COMBINE the ricotta, salt, pepper, parsley, and 1 tablespoon of the basil in a small bowl.

5. HOLD the squash halves over a medium bowl and gently remove the strands of flesh by pulling them out with a fork. Add the marinara sauce and stir to combine.

6. FILL each squash shell with the squash and marinara. Top evenly with dollops of ricotta, then with the mozzarella cheese. Bake until the cheese is melted and starting to bubble and brown, 15 to 20 minutes. Garnish with the remaining basil.

MAKES 2 SERVINGS ||| Prep time: 15 minutes ||| **Total time: 1 hour 30 minutes**

Mayo

Mayo gets a bad reputation, but this classic sandwich spread can actually be part of a clean diet if you know what to look for. The secret is finding a product that keeps ingredients simple—eggs, oil, vinegar, and a bit of salt—and uses high-quality oils (like our homemade version on page 166).

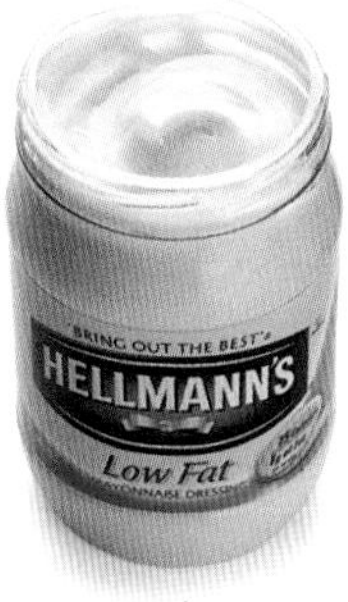

✱

NOT CLEAN

REDUCED-FAT MAYO

While it's tempting, resist the urge to cut calories with low-fat mayos. These generally include dangerous ingredients like high fructose corn syrup and fillers like xanthan gum to add texture in fat's absence, making it an unwelcome addition to a clean diet.

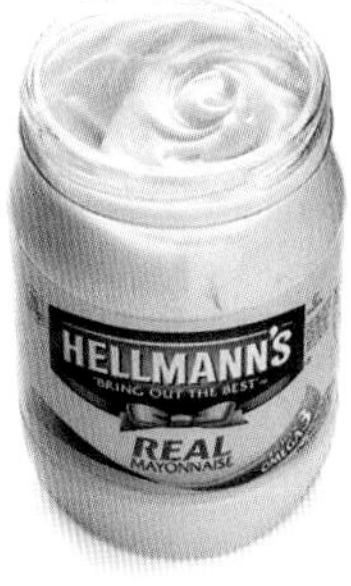

✱✱

CLEAN

REGULAR MAYO

Typical supermarket mayonnaise is often heavily processed and likely to contain genetically modified ingredients (thanks to soybeans), as well as sugar or corn syrup, but it is generally free of funky fillers.

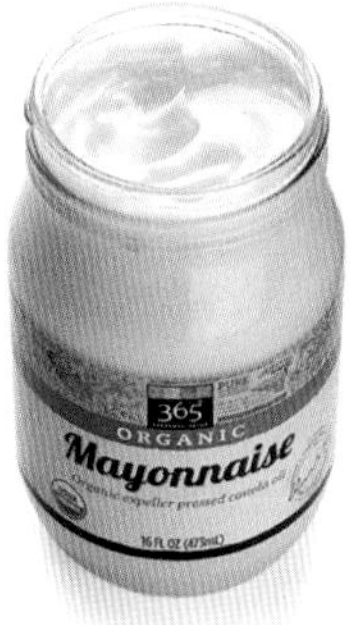

✱✱✱

CLEANEST

ORGANIC MAYO MADE WITH NON-GMO EXPELLER-PRESSED OIL

Unlike conventional and reduced-fat mayonnaise, organic and expeller-pressed mayonnaise is free of GMOs and uses oil that is extracted via pressure as opposed to potentially dangerous chemical solvents. Whole Foods' 365 Organic brand or Spectrum Organic Mayonaise are both good choices.

CREAMY GREEN GOODNESS DRESSING

- **2 tablespoons mayonnaise**
- **¼ cup rice vinegar**
- **1 clove garlic, peeled**
- **½ avocado, pitted and peeled**
- **½ cup fresh dill**
- **½ cup fresh mint**
- **½ cup cilantro**
- **½ cup scallion greens**
- **¼ cup olive oil**
- **½ cup water**
- **½ teaspoon fine sea salt**

BLEND all the ingredients in a blender or food processor until smooth. Store covered in a refrigerator up to 4 days. Serve over salad or use for dipping vegetables.

MAKES 4 SERVINGS ||| Prep time: 5 minutes ||| **Total time: 5 minutes**

SMART SWAP

For an even healthier sandwich, consider slathering your bread with hummus or guacamole. Either spread will increase your protein and fiber intake while adding a bit of Mediterranean or Mexican flair.

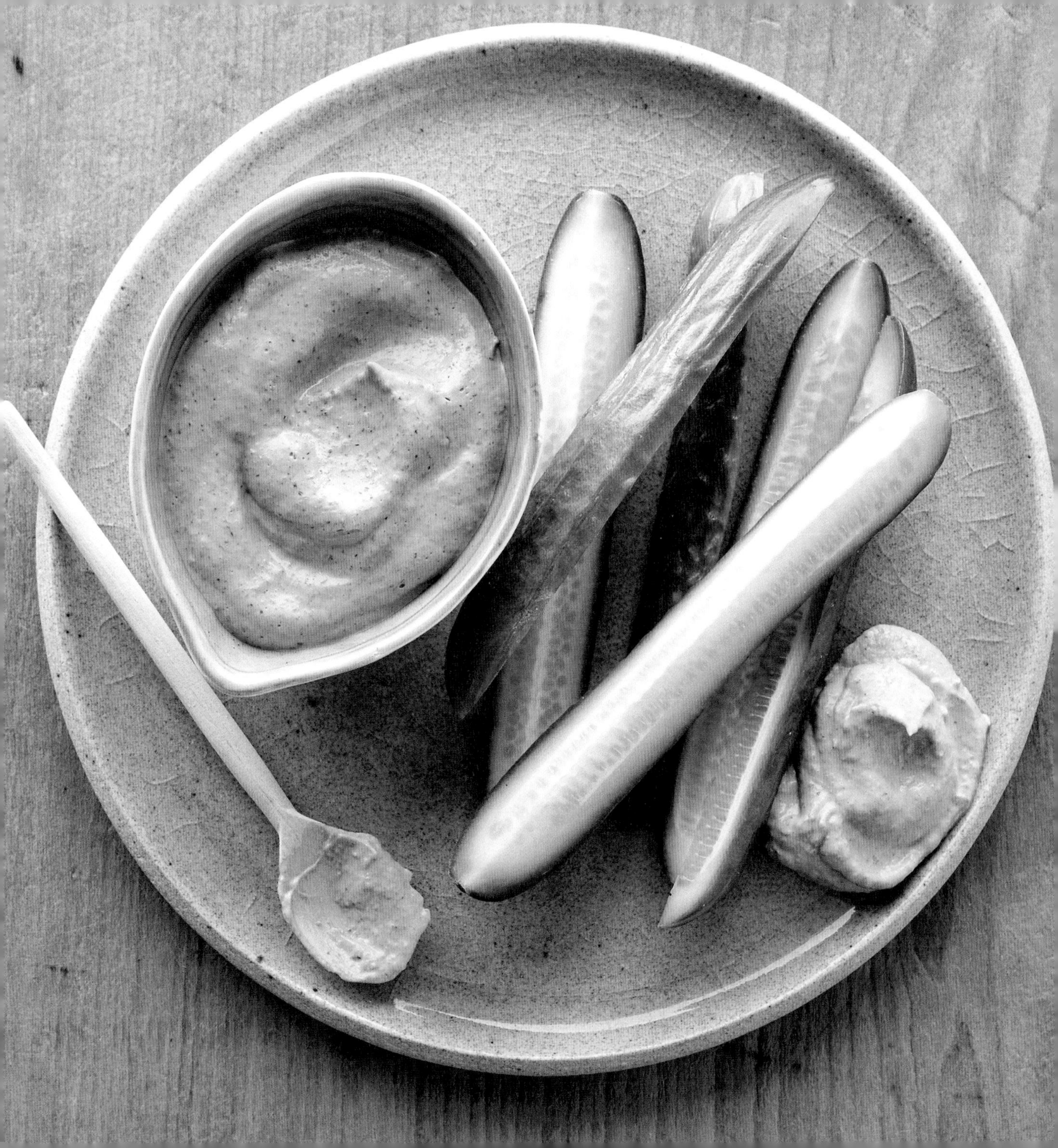

GARLIC & ONION SANDWICH SPREAD

- **2 tablespoons mayonnaise**
- **2 tablespoons 2% plain Greek yogurt**
- **¼ teaspoon garlic powder**
- **¼ teaspoon onion powder**
- **¼ teaspoon dried minced onion**
- **1 teaspoon dried or fresh chives**
- **⅛ teaspoon fine sea salt**

COMBINE all the ingredients in a small bowl, stirring until evenly mixed. Spread on a sandwich or use as a dipping sauce for veggies. Refrigerate leftovers.

MAKES 2 SERVINGS ||| Prep time: 5 minutes ||| **Total time: 5 minutes**

OLIVE OIL MAYO

- **1 large egg, at room temperature**
- **1 tablespoon fresh lemon juice**
- **1 teaspoon Dijon mustard**
- **¼ teaspoon fine sea salt**
- **¼ teaspoon garlic powder**
- **⅓ cup extra virgin olive oil**

PLACE the room-temperature egg, lemon juice, mustard, salt, and garlic powder in a blender and turn on high for 10 seconds. With the machine running, start drizzling in the olive oil and blend for an additional 30 seconds. (Alternatively, place all the ingredients in a cup or narrow bowl and use an immersion blender. Or whisk by hand in a bowl until thick and creamy.) Refrigerate to make firmer.

⅔ CUP YIELD ||| Prep time: 5 minutes ||| **Total time: 5 minutes**

BBQ Sauce

Barbecue sauce can make an amazing marinade and dip,

but—watch out—some actually contain high fructose corn syrup as the first ingredient! The gold standard is an organic low-sugar sauce that's packaged in glass. Or do it yourself and whip up a batch of our Spicy Ginger-Soy BBQ Sauce (page 171).

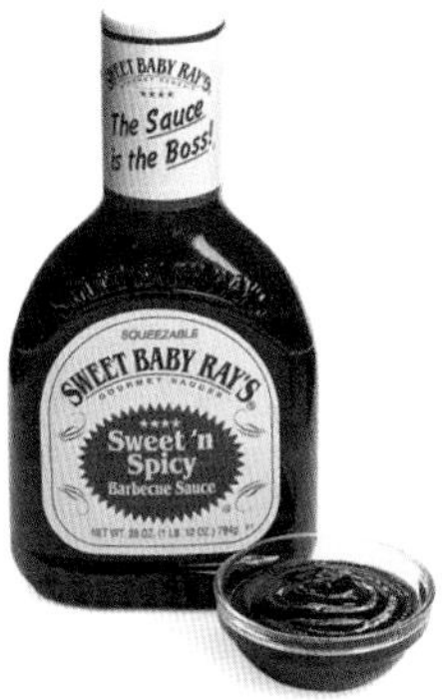

*

NOT CLEAN

CONVENTIONAL HIGH-SUGAR SAUCE IN A PLASTIC JAR

Conventional barbecue sauce is full of added sugars like high fructose corn syrup (often the first ingredient), along with artificial colors and preservatives. They can also pack 70 calories and 16 grams of sugar in just 2 tablespoons.

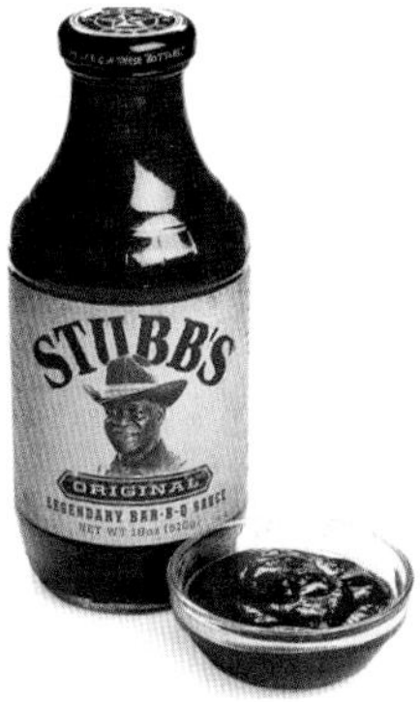

**

CLEAN

CONVENTIONAL SAUCE, WITH NATURAL SWEETENERS, IN A GLASS JAR

If you buy conventional sauce, it's best to choose one that comes in a glass jar and does not contain artificial sweeteners or high fructose corn syrup. Maple syrup, honey, and cane sugar are better sources of sweet.

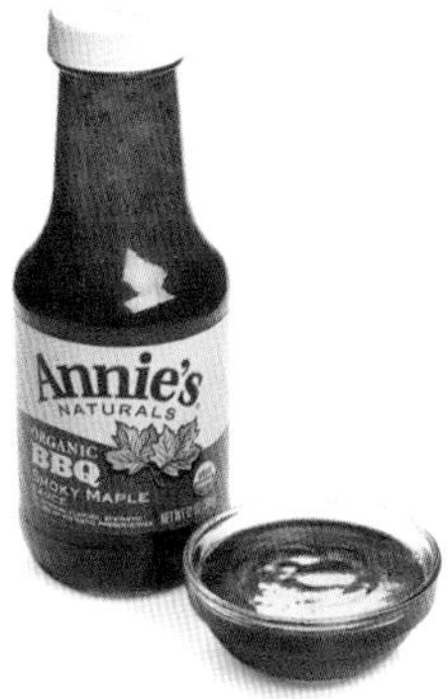

***

CLEANEST

ORGANIC LOW-SUGAR SAUCE IN A GLASS JAR

Look for an organic brand that contains less than 40 calories and 8 grams of sugar per 2 tablespoons. And buy it in a glass jar because the BPA in plastic food packaging can leach into your food—this is especially true of acidic tomato products, which can draw out more chemicals.

BBQ ALMOND CLUSTERS

1 cup skin-on raw almonds
½ cup sliced almonds
½ cup rolled oats
½ cup barbecue sauce

1. HEAT the oven to 350°F.

2. SPREAD the whole almonds on a baking sheet and toast in the oven for 10 minutes. Leave the oven on.

3. TRANSFER the toasted almonds to a bowl and add the sliced almonds, oats, and barbecue sauce. Spread the mixture back on the baking sheet and roast, stirring to redistribute every 10 minutes, for 20 minutes longer.

4. TURN off the oven and allow the nuts to sit in the oven for 30 minutes. Remove from the oven and let cool to room temperature before storing in a closed container.

MAKES 4 SERVINGS ||| Prep time: 10 minutes ||| **Total time: 1 hour 5 minutes**

SPICY GINGER-SOY BBQ SAUCE

½ cup canned tomato sauce
2 tablespoons wheat-free tamari
Juice of ½ lime
1 tablespoon honey
1 inch fresh ginger, grated
½ teaspoon garlic powder
½ teaspoon onion powder
½ teaspoon smoked paprika
¼ teaspoon cayenne

COMBINE all the ingredients in a small bowl, stirring until mixed. Store covered in the refrigerator for up to 1 week.

MAKES 2 SERVINGS ||| Prep time: 5 minutes ||| **Total time: 5 minutes**

Yogurt

Buying yogurt is almost as confusing as buying eggs. There are so many varieties and claims slapped on them that it's hard to know what to focus on—Greek, probiotic, low-fat, plain, or fruit-filled. The solution happens to be refreshingly simple.

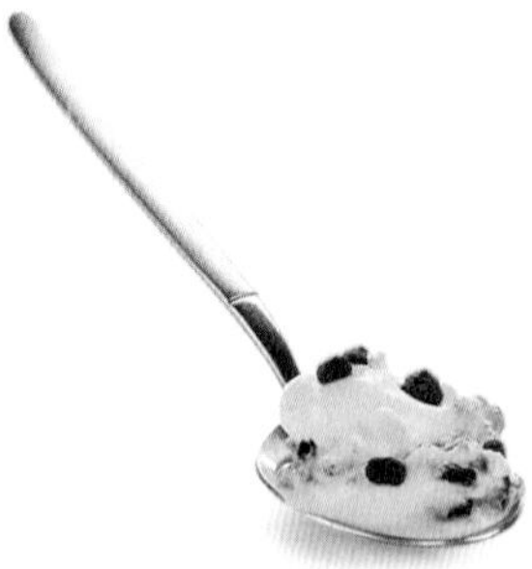

*

NOT CLEAN

SWEETENED YOGURT WITH MIX-INS, OR ARTIFICIALLY SWEETENED YOGURT

Sweetened yogurts with mix-ins like granola or crushed cookies should be avoided at all costs. These yogurts are laden with added sugar and artificial ingredients–many can contain more of the sweet stuff than a candy bar. Also avoid yogurts that include artificial sweeteners like sucralose (Splenda) or aspartame.

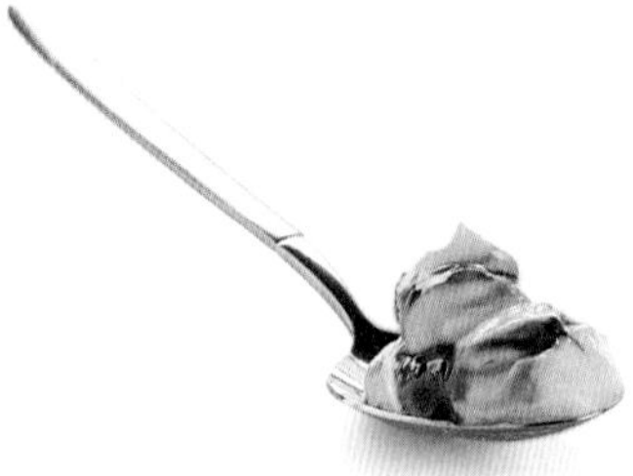

**

CLEAN

NATURALLY SWEETENED YOGURT

If you want a yogurt with some flavor, look for "fruit" listed as an actual ingredient–otherwise you're just getting fruit flavoring. Or try a yogurt sweetened with honey or stevia, a natural no-calorie sweetener. But always avoid yogurts that list sugar as the first or second ingredient.

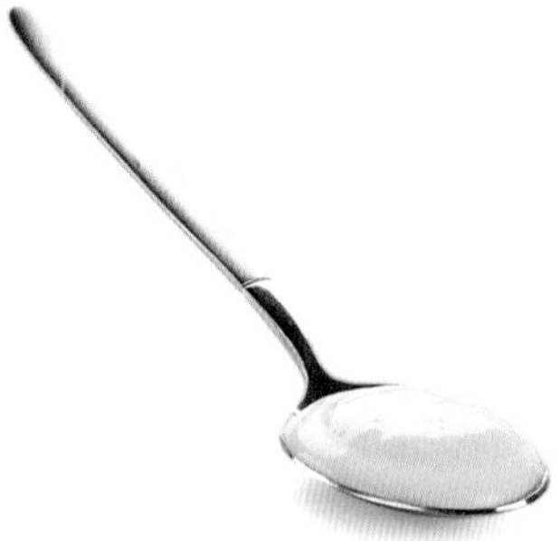

***

CLEANEST

PLAIN YOGURT

When choosing a yogurt, a plain and ideally organic yogurt (of any variety you like–Greek, Icelandic, whatever) is your most nutritious option. Plain will provide a healthy dose of protein and calcium without any added sugar, and organic will ensure that no hormones, antibiotics, or GMO ingredients are present. For some flavor, add your own clean ingredients like walnuts, blueberries, and a drizzle of honey.

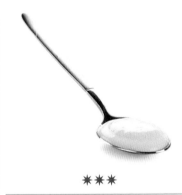

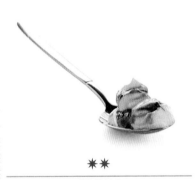

CHICKPEA & EGGPLANT CURRY

- 4 teaspoons grapeseed oil
- 2 cups cubed unpeeled eggplant
- ½ cup chopped yellow onion
- ½ cup chopped tomatoes
- 1 teaspoon cumin seeds
- 1 teaspoon minced garlic
- 1 teaspoon minced fresh ginger
- 2 teaspoons curry powder
- 1½ teaspoons minced fresh jalapeño (or more to taste)
- 1 cup cooked or canned chickpeas
- ¼ cup low-fat plain yogurt
- 2 tablespoons chopped cilantro

1. HEAT 2 teaspoons of the oil in a large skillet over medium heat. Add the eggplant and onion and cook for about 3 minutes. Stir in the tomatoes, cover, and reduce the heat to low for about 5 minutes to let the flavor meld, while you prepare the spice mixture.

2. HEAT the remaining 2 teaspoons oil in a small skillet over medium-low heat. Add the cumin seeds, garlic, ginger, curry powder, and jalapeño. Cook, stirring frequently, until the jalapeño softens and the mixture becomes fragrant, about 2 minutes.

3. ADD the spice mixture and the chickpeas to the eggplant and tomatoes. Cover and let simmer until the eggplant is very soft and the mixture has thickened slightly, about 20 minutes. Stir in the yogurt and cilantro just before serving.

MAKES 2 SERVINGS ||| Prep time: 10 minutes ||| Total time: 30 minutes

Did You Know?

Whole-milk yogurt may be healthier for you than fat-free and low-fat varieties. A recent study links the consumption of whole-fat yogurt (but not low-fat) to a reduced risk of diabetes, while another study finds that low-fat dairy isn't any better at helping people lose weight than whole fat. In fact, people eating the low-fat stuff were more likely to eat more carbs to make up for the difference in calories.

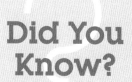

DILL & BASIL YOGURT BREAD

- **1½ cups spelt flour**
- **1½ cups whole wheat flour**
- **1½ teaspoons minced onion (optional)**
- **2 teaspoons dried basil or 2 tablespoons finely chopped fresh**
- **2 teaspoons dried dill weed or 2 tablespoons finely chopped fresh**
- **1 teaspoon fine sea salt**
- **¼ teaspoon baking soda**
- **2 tablespoons evaporated cane juice**
- **1 envelope (2¼ teaspoons) rapid rise yeast**
- **1 cup low-fat plain yogurt**
- **¼ cup water**
- **1 tablespoon grapeseed oil**
- **1 large egg, lightly beaten**

1. COMBINE the spelt flour, wheat flour, onion (if using), basil, dill, salt, baking soda, evaporated cane juice, and yeast in a large bowl. Set aside.

2. STIR together the yogurt, water, and grapeseed oil in a microwaveable medium bowl. Heat in the microwave until warm, about 45 seconds to 1 minute. Stir in the beaten egg.

3. USING an electric mixer with a dough hook on medium speed, slowly mix the yogurt mixture into the flour mixture. Mix until uniform, about 3 minutes. (Or, stir the yogurt mixture and flour mixture by hand until the flour is incorporated and then knead until smooth, about 5 minutes.) The dough will be stiff. Cover and let rise until doubled in bulk, about 45 minutes to 1 hour.

4. HEAT the oven to 375°F. Lightly grease a 9 x 5-inch loaf pan.

5. TRANSFER the dough to the pan. Bake for 25 to 30 minutes, or until golden brown. Let the bread cool for 5 minutes. Remove from pan and let cool another 5 minutes before slicing.

MAKES 12 SLICES ||| Prep time: 15 minutes |||
Total time: 55 minutes + 1 hour rise time

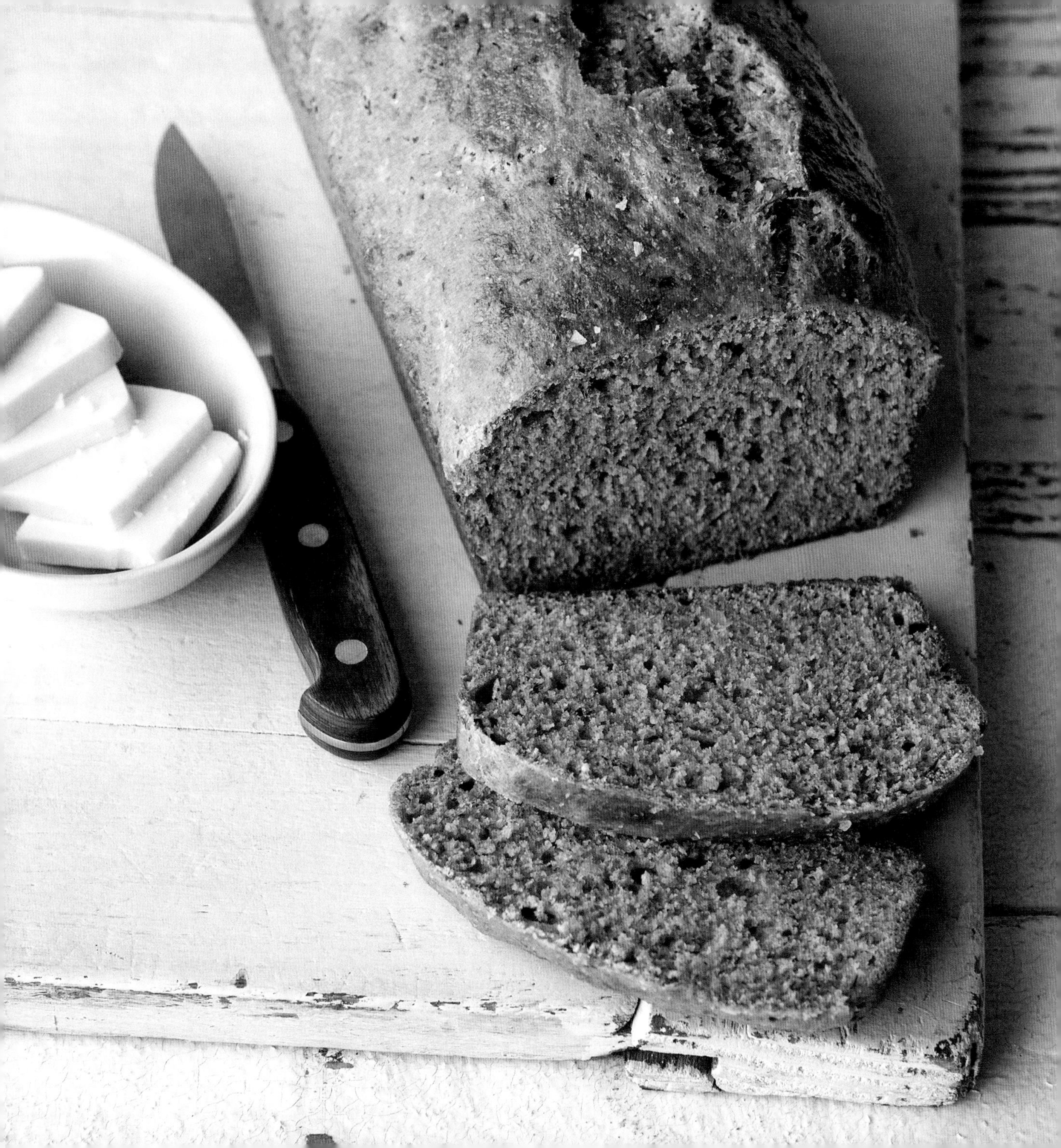

CITRUS GARLIC AIOLI

- ½ cup unsalted dry-roasted cashews
- ½ cup plain low-fat yogurt
- 1 tablespoon minced garlic
- ½ teaspoon grated lemon zest
- 1 teaspoon fresh lemon juice
- 1 teaspoon fresh lime juice
- Fine sea salt and black pepper

1. **PROCESS** the cashews in a food processor until they start to form a paste-like consistency, scraping down the sides every few minutes.

2. **ADD** the yogurt, garlic, lemon zest, lemon juice, and lime juice. Season with salt and pepper to taste. Process until the yogurt and cashew paste are mixed smoothly together. Use as a sandwich spread or dipping sauce. Store in an airtight container in the refrigerator.

MAKES ABOUT ¾ CUP ||| Prep time: 5 minutes ||| **Total time: 5 minutes**

Nuts

Yes, you have permission to go nuts! This perfectly portable snack is loaded with protein, healthy fats, and an array of phytonutrients that may help boost heart and brain health. But how they're processed is definitely important.

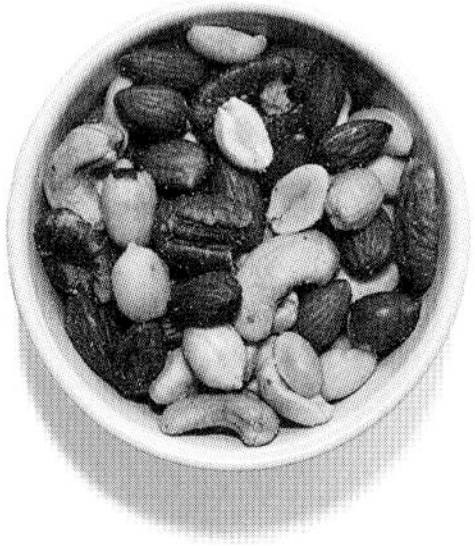

*

NOT CLEAN

OIL-ROASTED OR SUGAR-COATED NUTS

Conventional nuts roasted in oil and coated in sugar or salt aren't clean. In addition to pesticides, you're getting loads of empty calories and excess sodium—nuts are delicious enough already, don't mask their flavor!

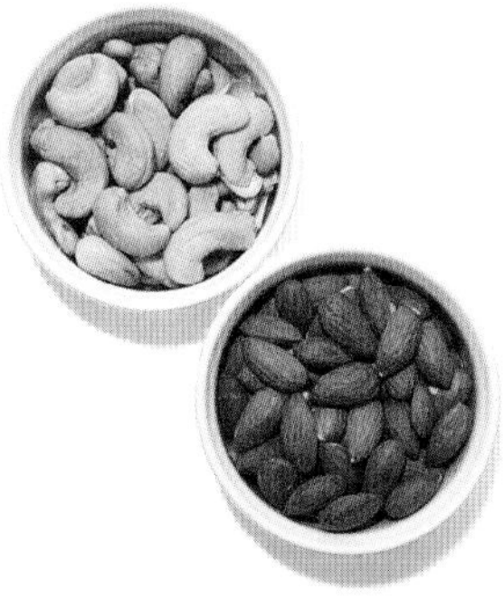

**

CLEAN

CONVENTIONAL RAW OR DRY-ROASTED NUTS

An important difference between organic and nonorganic nuts is that the conventional nuts are treated with pesticides such as endosulfan or phosmet. Both of these pesticides have been shown to have toxic effects. Of course, the experts can't yet say how risky they are when you ingest them via food.

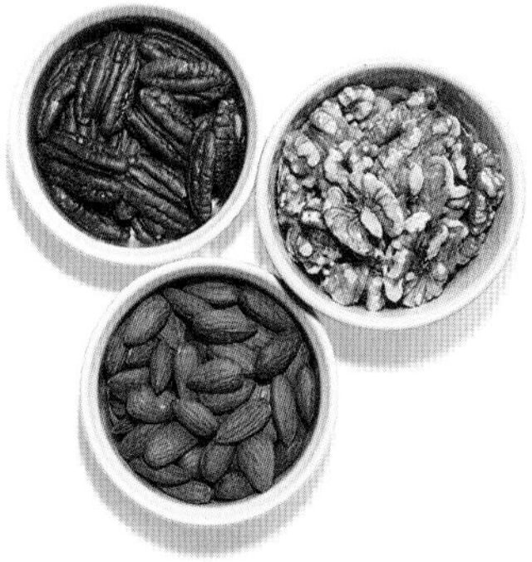

***

CLEANEST

ORGANIC RAW OR DRY-ROASTED NUTS

For maximum nutrition, go for organic nuts (raw or dry-roasted), which aren't treated with pesticides or loaded with added sugars and salt. Most roasted nuts are roasted in low-quality oil, so be sure to read your labels and make sure the only ingredient is nuts.

TWICE-BAKED SWEET POTATOES WITH PECAN-WALNUT CRUMBLE

2 medium sweet potatoes

2 tablespoons pure maple syrup

¼ cup unsweetened plain almond milk

1 large egg

½ teaspoon cinnamon

½ teaspoon ground ginger

¼ teaspoon nutmeg

Fine sea salt and black pepper

¼ cup plus 2 tablespoons chopped pecans

¼ cup plus 2 tablespoons chopped walnuts

1. HEAT the oven to 400°F. Line a baking sheet with foil.

2. POKE 6 holes in each sweet potato with a small knife. Microwave on high until soft, turning once, about 6 minutes total. Let cool.

3. MAKE a slice across the top of each baked sweet potato. Carefully scoop out the flesh and add to a medium bowl.

4. ADD the maple syrup, almond milk, egg, cinnamon, ginger, nutmeg, a dash of salt and pepper, ¼ cup of the pecans, and ¼ cup of the walnuts to the bowl of sweet potato. With a potato masher, mash the ingredients until combined.

5. SCOOP the sweet potato mixture back into the empty sweet potato shells. Place the filled sweet potatoes on the baking sheet and bake for 20 minutes. Remove from the oven and top each sweet potato with the remaining 2 tablespoons pecans and 2 tablespoons walnuts. Return to the oven and bake until the nuts are lightly toasted, about 10 minutes.

MAKES 2 SERVINGS ||| Prep time: 15 minutes ||| **Total time: 55 minutes**

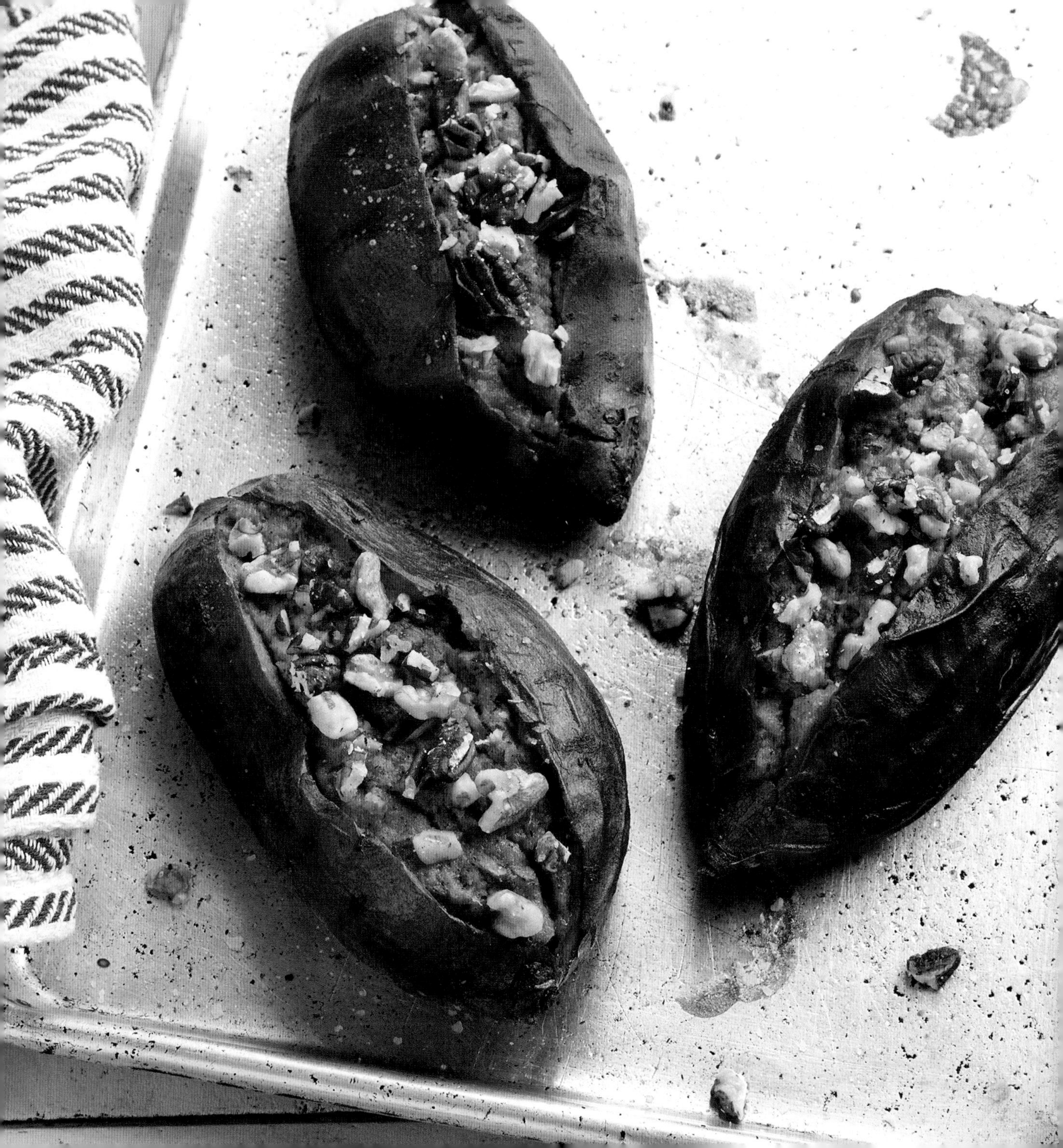

CHERRY, PEAR & PECAN CRISP

- 2 **Medjool dates, pitted and finely chopped**
- ¼ **cup chopped pecans**
- 1 **tablespoon coconut oil, melted, plus more for the ramekins**
- 1 **tablespoon whole wheat flour**
- 1 **tablespoon unsweetened plain almond milk or milk of your choice**
- ½ **cup rolled oats**
- 1 **cup chopped pears**
- 1 **cup pitted dark sweet cherries**
- ¼ **teaspoon ground cardamom**
- 1 **teaspoon vanilla extract**
- 1 **tablespoon pure maple syrup**

1. HEAT the oven to 400°F. Lightly oil two 8-ounce ramekins.

2. COMBINE the dates, pecans, coconut oil, flour, milk, and ¼ cup of the oats in a food processor. Process until crumbly, 1 to 2 minutes. Set the pecan topping aside.

3. TOSS together the the pears, cherries, cardamom, and remaining ¼ cup oats in a medium bowl. Drizzle the vanilla and maple syrup over the mixture and stir to combine. Divide the pear and cherry mixture between the ramekins. Sprinkle the pecan topping evenly over the fruit.

4. COVER each ramekin with foil and bake for 15 minutes. Remove the foil and bake until the topping is lightly browned and the cherry-pear mixture is bubbling, 10 to 15 minutes longer.

Makes 2 servings ||| Prep time: 10 minutes ||| **Total time: 40 minutes**

HEALTHY HACK

Sure, buying nuts in bulk is cost effective, but their high fat content means they'll go rancid if you don't eat them up within a few weeks. Foresee yourself taking longer? Store nuts in an airtight container in the fridge for up to a year, or in the freezer for up to 2 years. To liven up the flavor before you eat them, spread them on a baking sheet and toast for 10 minutes at 350°F.

BARLEY, BRUSSELS SPROUTS & PINE NUT PILAF

- **3 teaspoons grapeseed oil**
- **2 cups brussels sprouts, each sprout sliced into thirds**
- **½ cup chopped red or yellow onion**
- **1 tablespoon minced garlic**
- **½ cup pearl barley**
- **1½ cups low-sodium vegetable broth or water**
- **2 tablespoons dry white wine**
- **2 tablespoons pine nuts**
- **½ teaspoon fresh lemon juice**
- **Fine sea salt and black pepper**
- **¼ cup grated Parmesan (optional)**

1. **HEAT** the oven to 400°F. Grease a baking sheet with 1 teaspoon of the grapeseed oil.

2. **SPREAD** the brussels sprouts evenly on the baking sheet. Roast for 25 minutes. Turn the oven to broil and broil for a few minutes, until crispy. Watch carefully to avoid burning. Set aside.

3. **HEAT** the remaining 2 teaspoons oil in a medium skillet over medium heat. Add the onion and garlic and cook until the onion is translucent and soft, about 5 minutes. Stir in the barley and cook, stirring, until lightly browned, about 2 minutes. Add the broth and bring to a boil. Reduce the heat to low and simmer, uncovered, until the liquid is absorbed and barley is mostly cooked, about 30 minutes. Add the wine and cook until absorbed, about 10 minutes.

4. **TRANSFER** the barley to a medium bowl. Add the brussels sprouts, pine nuts, lemon juice, salt to taste, and a dash of pepper. If desired, top with Parmesan.

MAKES 2 SERVINGS ||| Prep time: 15 minutes ||| **Total time: 1 hour 15 minutes**

Energy Bars

Bars are probably the most convenient way to curb hunger on the go. Keep a few in your car so you don't end up double-fisting 2-for-1 McDonald's apple pies. But because the bar industry is exploding, there are options that are awesome, horrible, and every shade in between. So read your labels, and don't fall victim to good marketing.

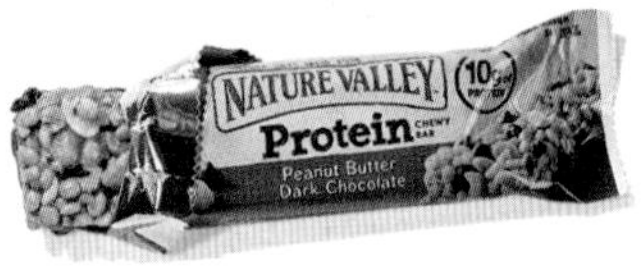

✱

NOT CLEAN

BARS WITH SYNTHETIC INGREDIENTS

Stay away from bars that contain artificial sweeteners, high fructose corn syrup, partially hydrogenated oils, and other synthetic or overly processed ingredients, such as soy protein isolate, and artificial colors and flavors. These are often no better than a candy bar—sometimes worse.

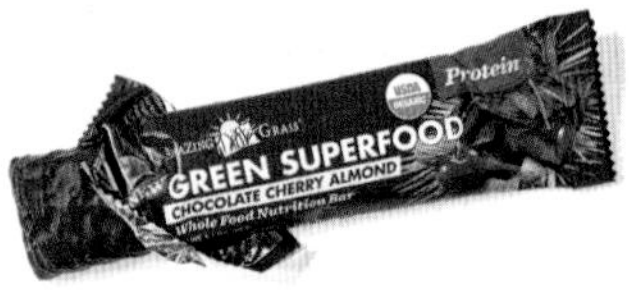

✱✱

CLEAN

BARS MADE FROM ALL WHOLE-FOOD INGREDIENTS

If your bar has more than 10 ingredients, make sure they're all real foods—nothing artificial or overly processed. This includes fruits, nuts, whole grains, protein concentrates (not isolates), and some natural sweeteners like cane sugar, honey, or maple syrup.

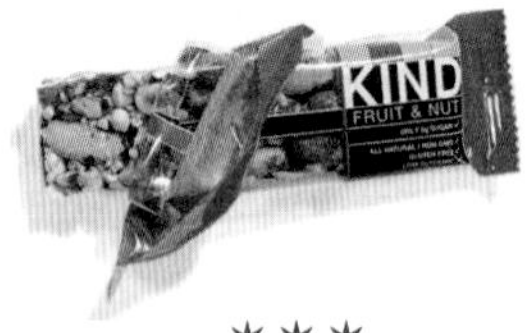

✱✱✱

CLEANEST

BARS WITH FEWER THAN 10 INGREDIENTS AND 10 GRAMS OF SUGAR

The cleanest bars are made from mostly whole-food ingredients, contain no added sugar or artificial ingredients, and boast a balance of fat, protein, and carbs to keep you feeling energized and full. As a general rule, pick bars that have less than 10 ingredients and 10 grams of sugar and at least half as many grams of protein as carbs. Another safe bet? Make your own.

CHOCOLATE CHIP COOKIE DOUGH ENERGY BITES

- **1 cup rolled oats**
- **¼ cup unsweetened shredded coconut**
- **⅓ cup chopped dates**
- **¼ cup pure maple syrup**
- **¼ cup cashew butter**
- **3 tablespoons unsweetened vanilla almond milk**
- **1 teaspoon vanilla extract**
- **½ cup mini chocolate chips**

1. **PULSE** the oats and coconut in a blender or food processor until a flour has formed. Add the dates, maple syrup, cashew butter, almond milk, and vanilla and pulse until combined.

2. **STIR** in the chocolate chips gently.

3. **ROLL** the dough into 10 balls and place on a plate lined with parchment paper. They will be soft at first but will firm up in the refrigerator.

4. **REFRIGERATE** for at least 1 hour before serving. Store refrigerated in an airtight container.

MAKES 10 BITES ||| Prep time: 5 minutes ||| **Total time: 10 minutes**

TREND ALERT!

Meat bars—yes, as in animal meat—are all the rage, thanks to the surge in popularity of Paleo and low-carb diets. Most, like EPIC bars, are made from organic or grass-fed beef, along with spices and dried fruit. The result is clean, unprocessed protein, real meat flavor, and a soft texture, with a hint of natural sweetness.

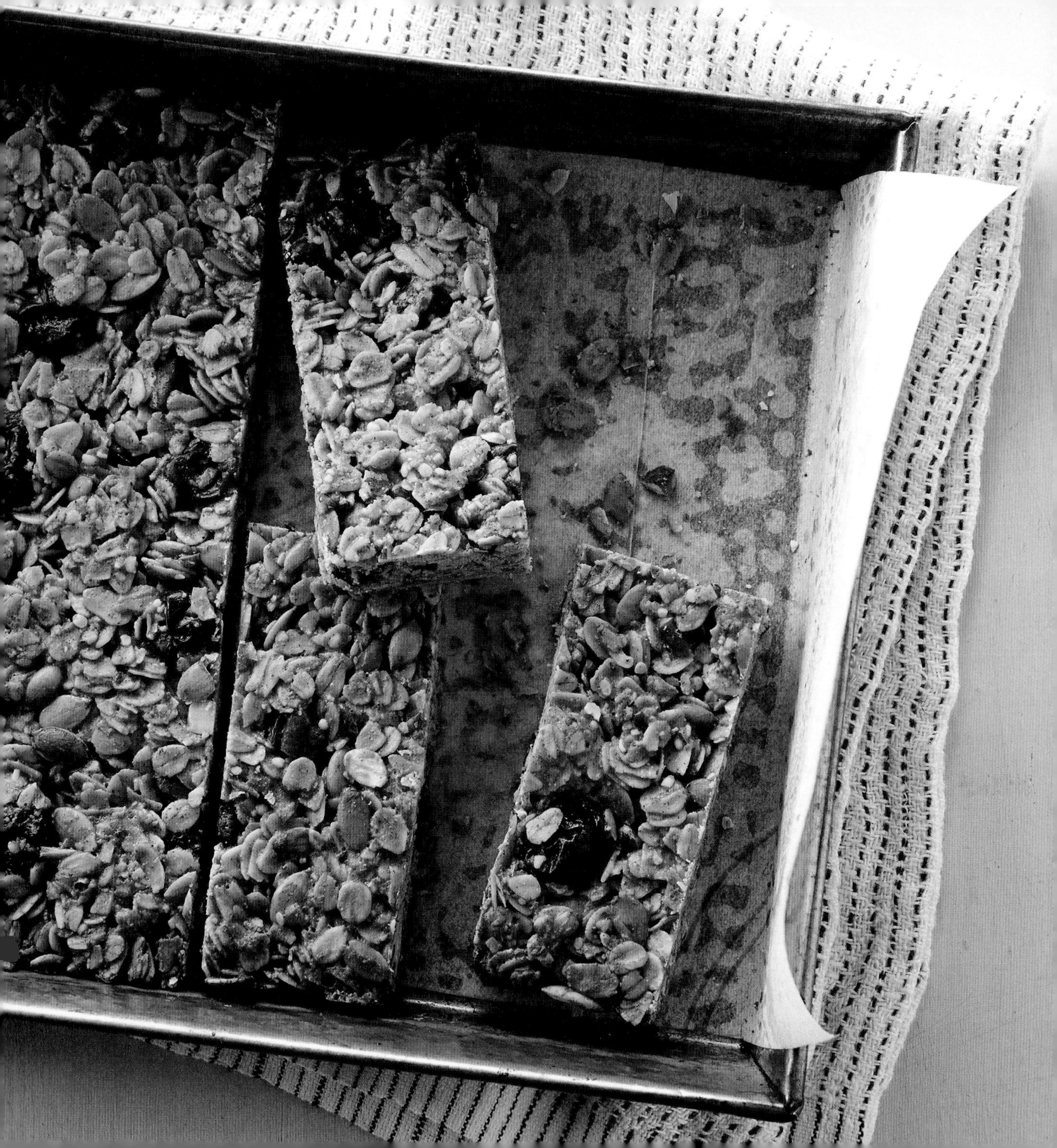

PUMPKIN SEED, CHERRY & PECAN GRANOLA BARS

- 2 cups rolled oats
- ⅓ cup pumpkin seeds
- ⅓ cup chopped pecans
- ¼ cup unsweetened shredded coconut
- ½ cup dried cherries
- 2 tablespoons hemp seeds
- ¾ teaspoon cinnamon
- ¼ teaspoon kosher salt
- ⅓ cup honey
- ¼ cup almond butter
- 3 tablespoons coconut oil, melted
- 1 teaspoon vanilla extract

1. **HEAT** the oven to 350°F. Lightly coat an 8 x 8-inch baking pan with vegetable oil and line the bottom with parchment paper.

2. **PLACE** the oats, pumpkin seeds, pecans, and coconut on a large rimmed baking sheet and toast until fragrant, about 8 minutes, being careful not to let burn. Leave the oven on.

3. **MIX** the cherries, hemp seeds, cinnamon, and salt in a large bowl. Add the toasted oats, nuts, and seeds to the bowl and mix together.

4. **COMBINE** the honey, almond butter, melted coconut oil, and vanilla in a small microwaveable bowl. Microwave for 30 seconds to warm the mixture, then stir together well and pour over the dry ingredients. Stir all the ingredients together until uniformly coated with the wet ingredients.

5. **SPREAD** the mixture in the baking pan and bake for 20 minutes, or until the bars are lightly golden on top.

6. **COOL** completely in the pan, at least 30 minutes, then cut into 10 rectangular bars.

MAKES 10 BARS ||| Prep time: 10 minutes ||| **Total time: 35 minutes + 30 minutes cooling time**

PRESSED FRUIT & NUT COOKIE BARS

- **1 cup chopped cashews**
- **¾ cup pitted dates**
- **½ cup dried cherries**
- **2 tablespoons unsweetened cocoa powder**
- **½ teaspoon cinnamon**
- **½ teaspoon Himalayan pink salt**

1. **COMBINE** all of the ingredients in a food processor or high-powered blender. Pulse until well combined, scraping down the sides as needed, about 5 minutes.

2. **SPREAD** into an 8-inch square, about ½ inch thick, on a piece of parchment paper or a cutting board. Cut into ten 2 x 3-inch rectangular bars.

3. **REFRIGERATE** for 1 hour to set.

4. **STORE** in the refrigerator in a container between layers of parchment paper or in individual bags so that the bars don't stick together.

MAKES 10 BARS ||| Prep time: 10 minutes ||| **Total time: 1 hour 10 minutes**

Veggie Chips

Veggie chips sound healthy, right? While they can be a good alternative to conventional greasy potato chips, it's important to pick varieties that are actually an improvement on the original, and not just dressed-up corn and potato flour.

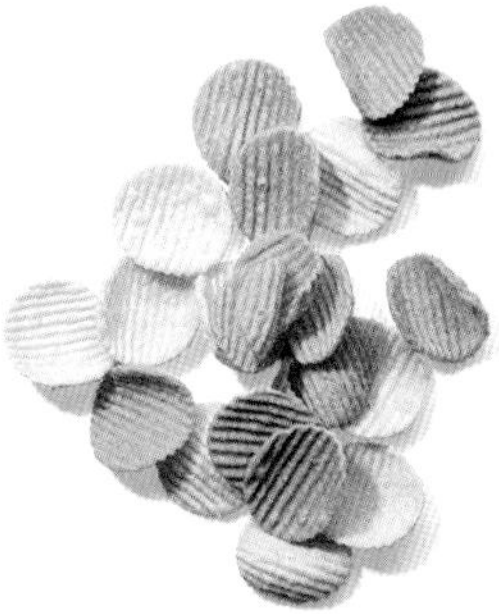

✱

NOT CLEAN

STORE-BOUGHT VEGGIE CHIPS MADE WITH CORN OR POTATO FLOUR

Veggie chips made with corn or potato flour are best left on the shelf—many of these chips are high in fat, calories, and sodium, and they're actually more processed than conventional potato chips. Talk about deceptive.

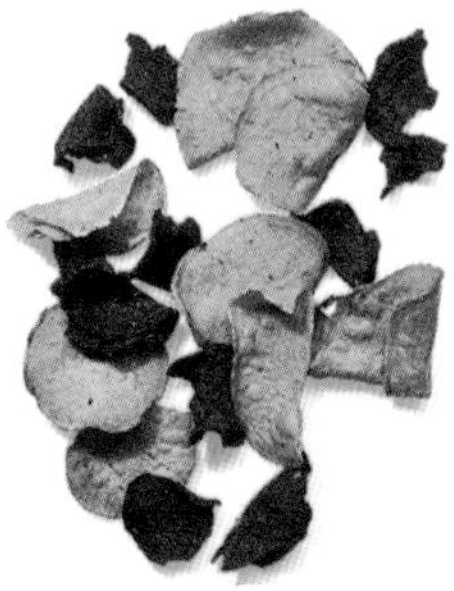

✱✱

CLEAN

STORE-BOUGHT WHOLE-VEGGIE CHIPS

If you buy premade kale or other veggie chips, an actual vegetable should be listed as the first ingredient, followed by ingredients like oil, salt, and spices. The shorter the list, the better the chips.

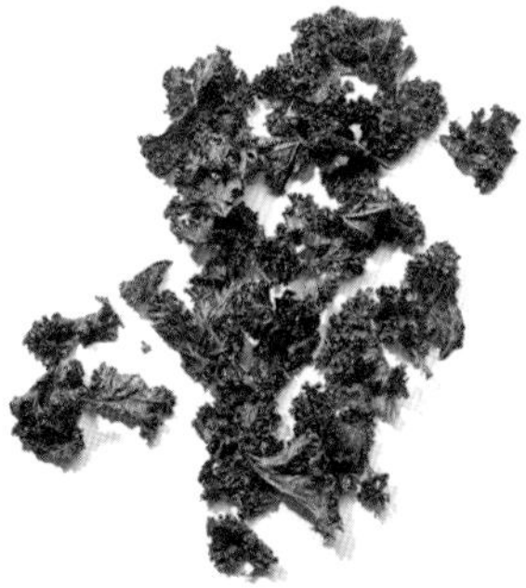

✱✱✱

CLEANEST

HOMEMADE KALE, SWEET POTATO, OR BEET CHIPS

DIY chips offer the most nutrients and fewest funky ingredients per crunch since you get to control how much oil, salt, and other seasonings you use. The easiest: kale chips. Just rinse, pat dry, coat in oil and spices, and bake. Kick 'em up a notch with one of the three crazy-delicious varieties starting on page 188. Bonus: Kale is packed with vitamin K, which helps build strong bones and ensure your blood clots normally.

CHILI-LIME KALE CHIPS

- **6 cups roughly chopped kale (tough ribs removed)**
- **1 tablespoon grapeseed oil**
- **⅛ teaspoon fine sea salt (or more to taste)**
- **⅛ teaspoon chili powder (or more to taste)**
- **1 teaspoon grated lime zest (or more to taste)**

1. HEAT the oven to 350°F. Lightly oil a baking sheet or line with parchment paper.

2. PLACE the kale in a large bowl. Drizzle with the grapeseed oil and sprinkle with ⅛ teaspoon salt. Use your hands to massage the oil and salt into the kale until evenly coated.

3. ARRANGE the kale in a single layer on the baking sheet. Bake for 10 minutes. Remove the baking sheet from the oven and carefully flip the kale chips over. Return the baking sheet to the oven and bake until crispy, about 5 minutes longer.

4. SPRINKLE with ⅛ teaspoon chili powder and the lime zest. If desired, season with more salt and chili powder to taste. Serve immediately.

MAKES 2 SERVINGS ||| Prep time: 10 minutes ||| **Total time: 25 minutes**

COOL TOOL!

With a dehydrator, you can morph any veggie into a "chip," without the need for loads of added oil. A temperature-control dehydrator (which is what you want) will run you around $80, but with quality veggie chips going for around $8 per pound at Whole Foods and similar stores, that will pay for itself quickly.

SALT & PEPPER KALE CHIPS

- **6 cups roughly chopped kale (tough ribs removed)**
- **1 tablespoon grapeseed oil**
- **⅛ teaspoon fine sea salt (or more to taste)**
- **⅛ teaspoon black pepper (or more to taste)**

1. **HEAT** the oven to 350°F. Lightly oil a baking sheet or line with parchment paper.

2. **PLACE** the kale in a large bowl. Drizzle with the grapeseed oil and sprinkle with the salt. Use your hands to massage the oil and salt into the kale until evenly coated.

3. **ARRANGE** the kale in a single layer on the baking sheet. Bake for 10 minutes. Remove the baking sheet from the oven and carefully flip the kale chips over. Return the baking sheet to the oven and bake until crispy, about 5 minutes longer.

4. **SPRINKLE** with the pepper. If desired, season with more salt and pepper to taste. Serve immediately.

MAKES 2 SERVINGS ||| Prep time: 10 minutes ||| **Total time: 25 minutes**

PIZZA KALE CHIPS

- ¼ **cup dry-packed sun-dried tomatoes**
- ⅓ **cup unsalted dry-roasted cashews**
- 1 **tablespoon tahini**
- 2 **cloves garlic, minced**
- 2 **tablespoons finely chopped fresh basil**
- 1½ **teaspoons finely chopped fresh oregano**
- 1 **tablespoon fresh lemon juice**
- ¼ **cup grated Parmesan or nutritional yeast**
- ⅛ **teaspoon red-pepper flakes**
- **Fine sea salt**
- 6 **cups roughly chopped kale (tough ribs removed)**

1. SOAK the sun-dried tomatoes in ½ cup hot water for 30 minutes. Drain, reserving the soaking liquid.

2. HEAT the oven to 300°F. Lightly oil a baking sheet.

3. PLACE the cashews in a food processor and grind to a fine powder, about 3 minutes. Add the tahini, garlic, basil, oregano, lemon juice, cheese, sun-dried tomatoes, pepper flakes, and a dash of salt and blend until smooth, up to 5 minutes, depending on your processor. If necessary to help it blend, add the reserved tomato soaking water to the mixture, 1 tablespoon at a time, and no more than ¼ cup.

4. TRANSFER the sauce to a large bowl and add the chopped kale. Use your hands to massage the sauce into the kale until well coated.

5. ARRANGE the kale in a single layer on the oiled baking sheet. Bake for 20 minutes. Remove the baking sheet from the oven and carefully flip the kale chips over. Return the baking sheet to the oven and bake until crispy, about 20 minutes longer.

MAKES 2 SERVINGS ||| Prep time: 15 minutes ||| **Total time: 55 minutes**

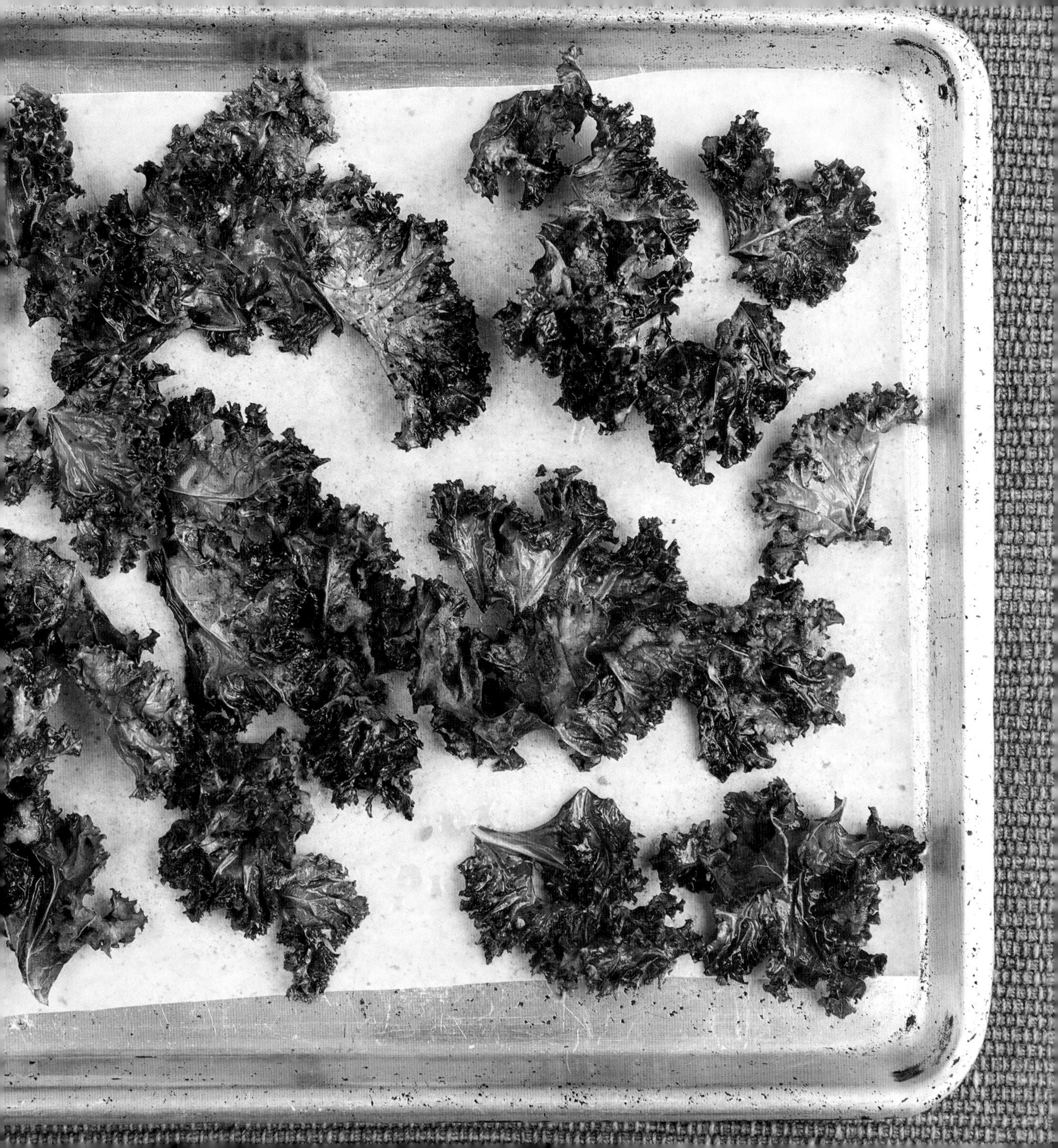

Pita Chips

Pita chips are the perfect accompaniment to clean spreads and dips. And if you have some semistale pita bread lying around, you've got almost everything you need to make your own. Store-bought brands can be tricky, with some seemingly wholesome options being more processed than potato chips.

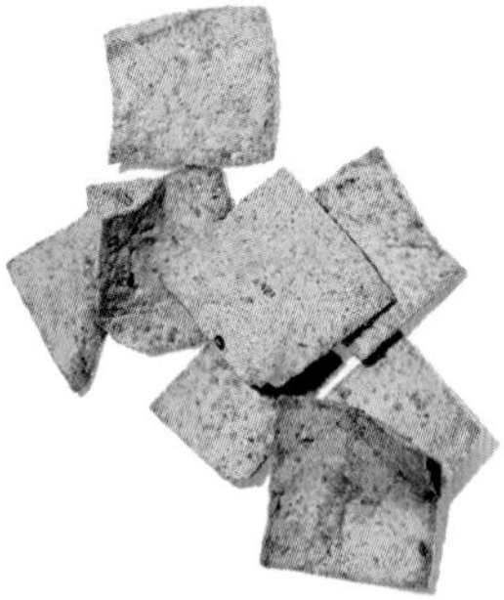

*

NOT CLEAN

PITA CHIPS MADE FROM ENRICHED WHEAT FLOUR

Most "natural" pita chips are made with enriched wheat flour and can have just as many calories and as much unhealthy fat as other chips do. This kind of flour is going to cause a quick blood sugar spike and leave you dragging shortly after.

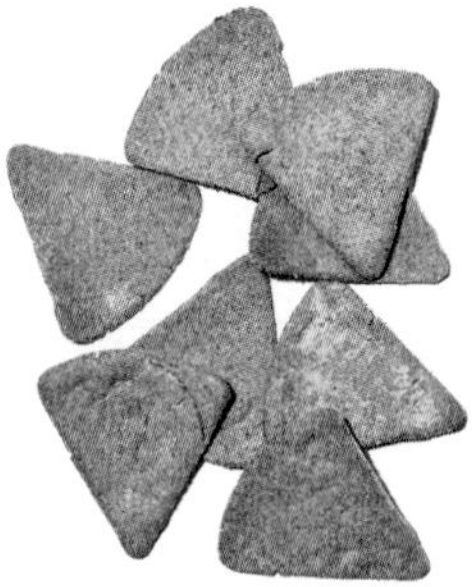

**

CLEAN

WHOLE-GRAIN STORE-BOUGHT PITA CHIPS

If you go the store-bought route, look for chips that list a whole grain as the first ingredient. These will ensure you're not losing out on all that beneficial fiber and protein.

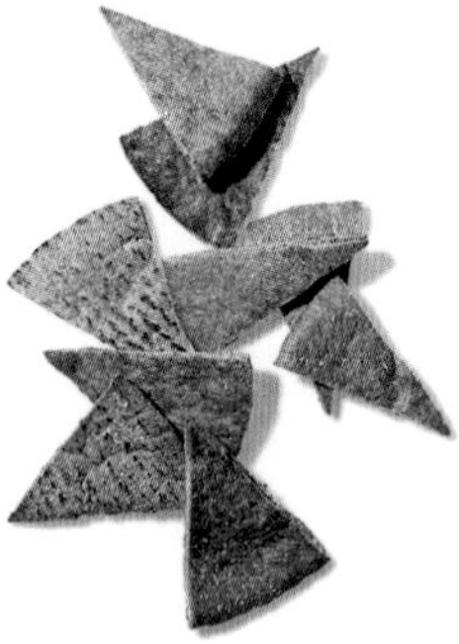

***

CLEANEST

HOMEMADE AND BAKED WITH OLIVE OIL AND SALT

The best no-junk chips are the ones you make at home. Simply slice up your favorite whole-grain pita, brush with organic expeller-pressed olive oil, top with a dash of sea salt, and bake until crisp. You'll avoid excess salt and get the benefit of cholesterol-lowering whole grains and heart-healthy monounsaturated fats from olive oil. Spice things up with the easy and sure-to-impress recipes that follow.

CINNAMON-SUGAR PITA CHIPS

- **2 teaspoons grapeseed oil**
- **1 teaspoon unsalted butter, melted**
- **1 teaspoon light brown sugar**
- **¼ teaspoon cinnamon**
- **⅛ teaspoon coarse sea salt**
- **1 large whole wheat pita (6- to 7-inch)**

1. **HEAT** the oven to 350°F.

2. **COMBINE** the oil, melted butter, brown sugar, cinnamon, and salt in a large bowl.

3. **CUT** the pita into 8 wedges and gently split the pocket edges of each triangle into 2 triangles.

4. **BRUSH** each side of the triangles with the oil mixture. Spread in a single layer on a baking sheet.

5. **BAKE,** turning once, until the chips are lightly browned and crisp, 15 to 20 minutes.

MAKES 2 SERVINGS ||| Prep time: 5 minutes ||| **Total time: 20 minutes**

PITA CHIPS WITH OLIVE OIL & SEA SALT

- **1 tablespoon olive oil**
- **⅛ teaspoon garlic powder**
- **1 large whole wheat pita (6- to 7-inch)**
- **¼ teaspoon coarse sea salt**

1. **HEAT** the oven to 350°F.

2. **COMBINE** the olive oil and garlic powder in a small bowl.

3. **CUT** the pita into 8 wedges and gently split the pocket edges of each triangle into 2 triangles.

4. **BRUSH** each side of the triangles with the oil mixture. Spread in a single layer on a baking sheet and sprinkle a small pinch of the sea salt on each triangle.

5. **BAKE,** turning once, until the chips are lightly browned and crisp, 15 to 20 minutes.

MAKES 2 SERVINGS ||| Prep time: 5 minutes ||| **Total time: 20 minutes**

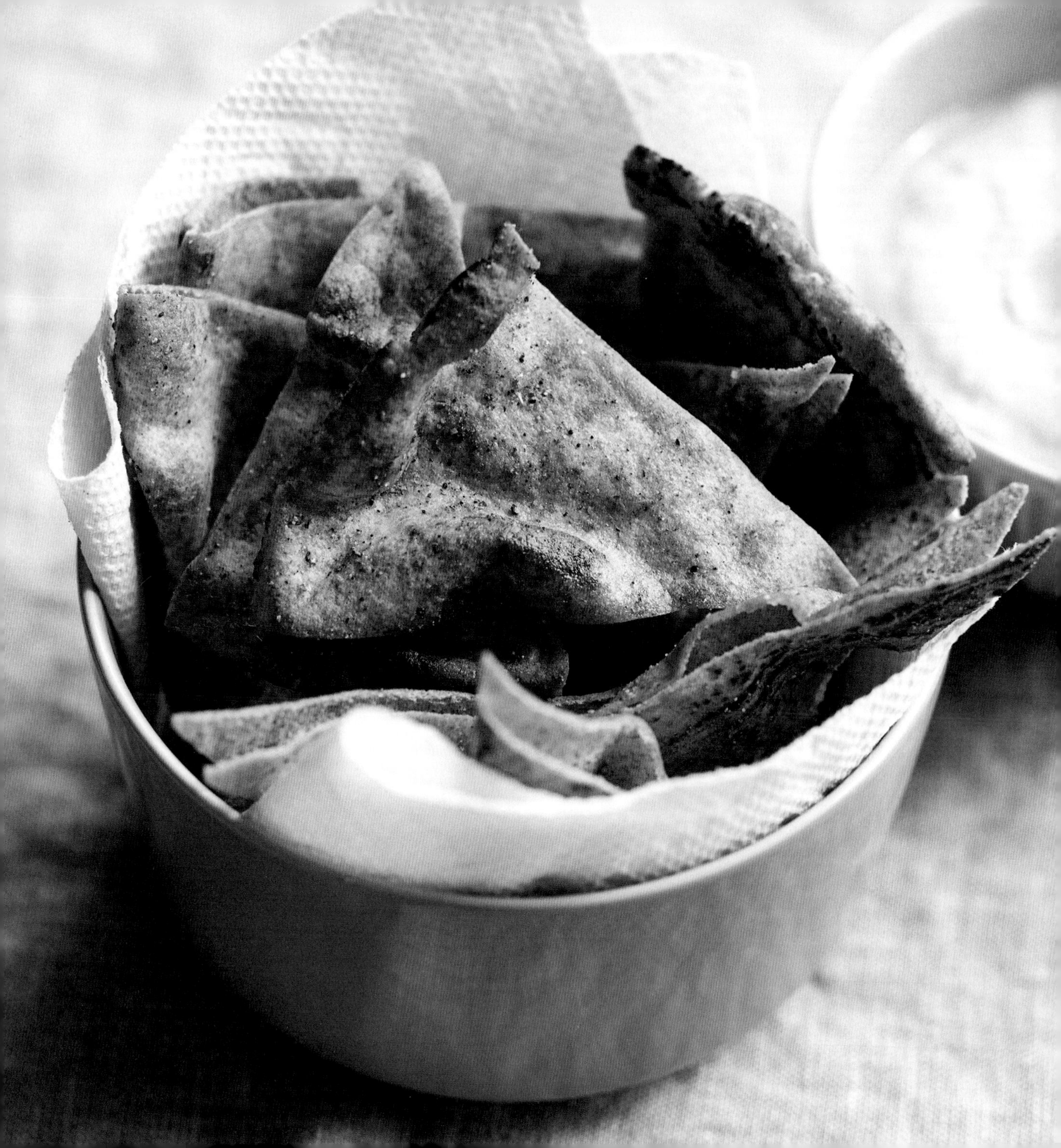

SWEET CHILI PITA CHIPS

- 2 **teaspoons olive oil**
- ¼ **teaspoon ground cumin**
- ¼ **teaspoon ground coriander**
- ¼ **teaspoon chili powder**
- ¼ **teaspoon light brown sugar**
- ¼ **teaspoon garlic powder**
- ⅛ **teaspoon black pepper**
- ⅛ **teaspoon kosher salt**
- 1 **large whole wheat pita (6- to 7-inch)**

1. HEAT the oven to 350°F.

2. COMBINE the olive oil, all the spices, and the salt in a bowl.

3. CUT the pita into 8 wedges and gently split the pocket edges of each triangle into 2 triangles.

4. BRUSH each side with the oil mixture. Spread in a single layer on a baking sheet.

5. BAKE, turning once, until the chips are lightly browned and crisp, 25 to 30 minutes.

MAKES 2 SERVINGS ||| Prep time: 5 minutes ||| Total time: 35 minutes

HEALTHY HACK

Try to always pair pita chips with a healthy dip like guacamole or hummus. Both have protein or fat and fiber that help stabilize the blood sugar spike you can get by eating the carbs in chips, and thus help minimize subsequent cravings.

Popcorn

Eating clean doesn't mean forgoing your "movie and popcorn" habit. Plain popcorn is actually a great whole-grain snack that's loaded with fiber. Bonus: A cup of air-popped popcorn only has 30 calories. But most movie theater and microwavable stuff is another story. We've got three exciting flavor combos for you to try starting on the opposite page.

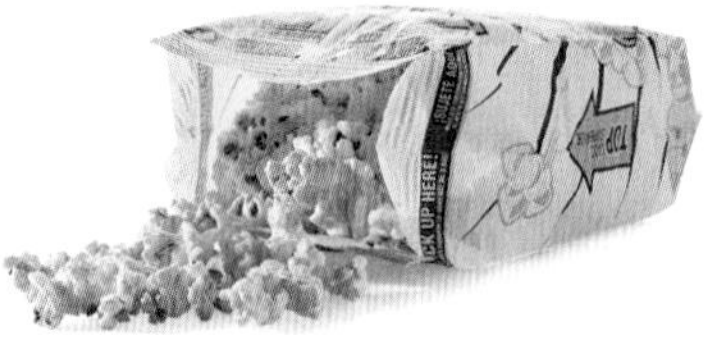

✱

NOT CLEAN

MICROWAVE POPCORN

Conventional microwaved popcorn is actually pretty sketchy. That smell that hits you after you open the bag comes from a chemical called diacetyl, or synthetic butter flavoring. Even worse, the bag is typically lined with a chemical called perfluorooctanoic acid (PFOA)—the same chemical used on nonstick pots and pans. Research shows PFOA in the blood is linked to health problems like high cholesterol and various cancers. Steer clear.

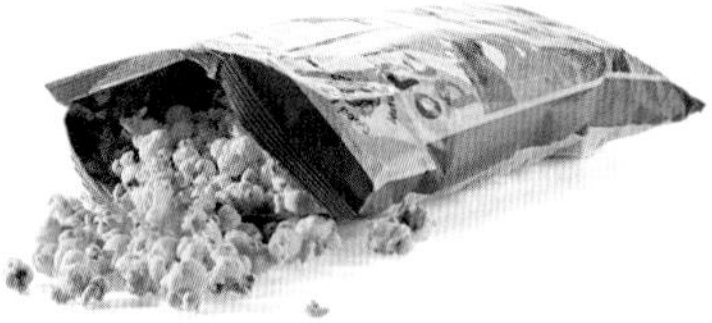

✱✱

CLEAN

ORGANIC BAGGED POPCORN

For convenience, organic bagged popcorn is a great alternative. It will be free of pesticides, genetically modified corn, and synthetic ingredients, but it may still contain salt and oils—not necessarily "unclean" ingredients, but you won't be able to control how much you're getting.

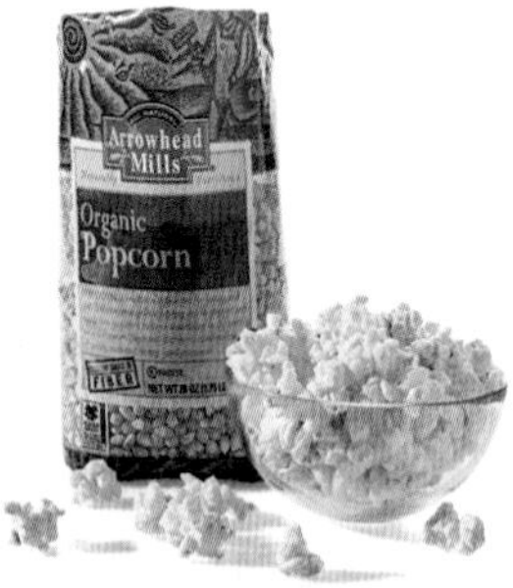

✱✱✱

CLEANEST

STOVE-TOP NON-GMO POPPED CORN WITH OLIVE OIL AND SEA SALT

Simply buy organic kernels and pop them in a saucepan with olive oil, then top with sea salt. You'll avoid pesticides, genetically modified corn, and funky chemicals used to make popcorn's smell more appealing.

OLIVE OIL & SEA SALT POPCORN

- ¼ **cup popcorn kernels**
- 2 **tablespoons plus 2 teaspoons olive oil**
- ⅛ **teaspoon coarse sea salt**

1. MEASURE the popcorn kernels and 2 tablespoons of the oil into a large Dutch oven. Set over medium-high heat, cover, and wait until the kernels begin to pop, about 2 minutes. Leave the pot over the heat, gently shaking the pot, until the popping sounds slow to every 2 to 3 seconds.

2. REMOVE from the heat, uncover, and pour the contents into a large bowl. Drizzle with the remaining 2 teaspoons olive oil, sprinkle with the salt, and toss gently to disperse.

MAKES 2 SERVINGS ||| Prep time: 5 minutes ||| Total time: 5 minutes

SMOKED PAPRIKA & PARMESAN POPCORN CROUTONS

- 1 **cup stove-top popped popcorn**
- ⅛ **teaspoon smoked paprika**
- 2 **tablespoons shredded Parmesan**

1. HEAT the oven to 350°F.

2. COAT a baking sheet with olive oil spray and spread the popcorn out in a single layer. Spray the popcorn with oil. Sprinkle the paprika and Parmesan over the popcorn evenly.

3. BAKE, stirring once, until the Parmesan has melted and the popcorn is lightly golden, about 15 minutes.

MAKES 1 CUP ||| Prep time: 5 minutes ||| Total time: 20 minutes

MEXICAN CHOCOLATE POPCORN BALLS

- ⅓ **cup honey**
- 2 **tablespoons light brown sugar**
- 2½ **tablespoons unsweetened cocoa powder**
- ½ **teaspoon cinnamon**
- ¼ **teaspoon cayenne**
- **Pinch of fine sea salt**
- 5 **cups stove-top popped popcorn**
- **Olive oil**

1. COMBINE the honey, brown sugar, cocoa, cinnamon, cayenne, and salt in a small saucepan and bring to a simmer over medium heat. Simmer until the mixture darkens and thickens, about 2 minutes.

2. POUR the mixture over the popcorn in a large bowl and use a rubber spatula to gently stir the popcorn to evenly coat.

3. COAT your hands with olive oil and form the mixture into 4 balls, pressing gently to ensure that each ball is well stuck together. Let set for at least 20 minutes before eating.

MAKES 4 BALLS ||| Prep time: 5 minutes ||| **Total time: 10 minutes**

HEALTHY HACK

Next time you want to add some cheesy flavor to popcorn, skip the Parmesan and try sprinkling your snack with nutritional yeast. This gluten- and dairy-free powder, which is simply vitamin-fortified inactive yeast made from cane or beet molasses, is packed with B vitamins and 6 grams of a protein in every 45-calorie ¼ cup (compare that to the 110 calories in the same amount of Parmesan).

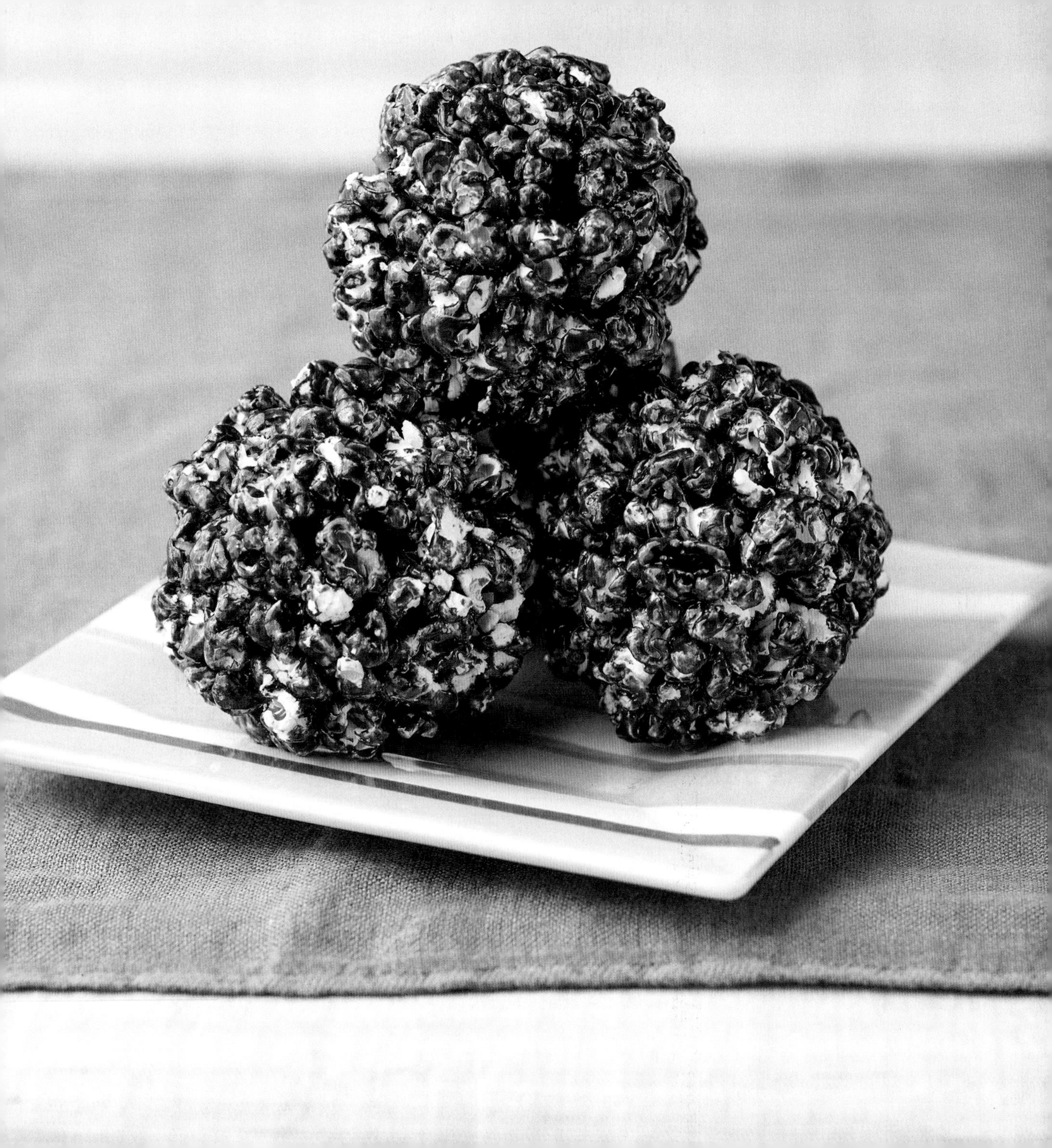

Baked Goods

Everybody needs dessert now and then . . . and no, we're not talking some lame sliced fruit with a drizzle of honey. We mean the good stuff like freshly baked apple pie. Luckily, that can be part of a clean diet if you're using high-quality ingredients.

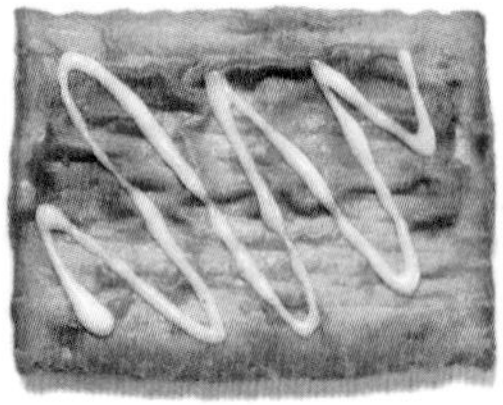

*

NOT CLEAN

APPLE-FLAVORED TOASTER PASTRY

Like we even have to explain this one. Apple-flavored pastries are likely made with artificial sweeteners, trans fats, and preservatives—and contain none of the nutritional benefits of apples.

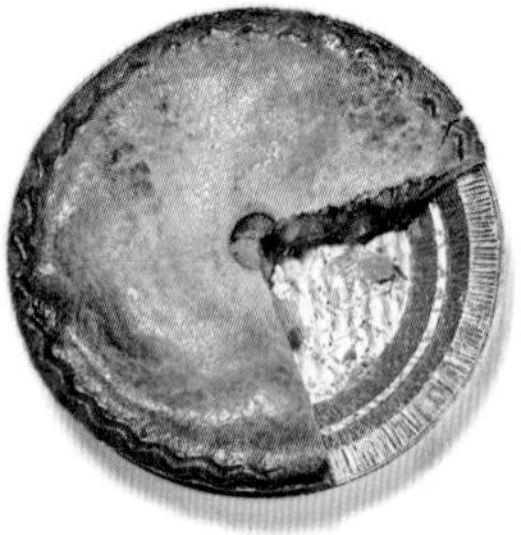

**

CLEAN

FARMERS' MARKET APPLE PIE

Resist temptation to buy grocery store pie. It's likely to be laden with excess sugar and unhealthy trans fats—the fat most closely linked to an increased risk of heart disease. If you have to buy premade, hit up your local farmers' market, where you can chat with the bakers to see what kinds of ingredients their products contain.

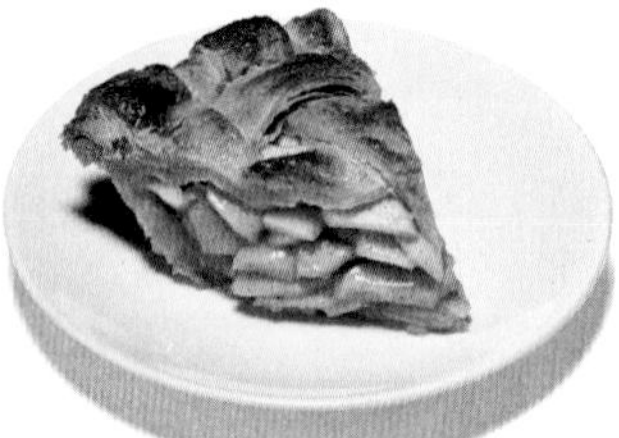

***

CLEANEST

HOMEMADE APPLE PIE

A homemade apple pie with a crust made with organic grass-fed butter and your favorite variety of local in-season apples is nothing to feel guilty about. Apples are full of heart-healthy fiber, and by using the freshest, most flavorful varieties you can find, you'll be able to use less sugar.

CINNAMON APPLE PIE WITH OAT CRUMBLE CRUST

CRUST

- ¾ **cup rolled oats**
- ½ **cup chopped walnuts**
- **2 tablespoons pure maple syrup**
- ¼ **cup coconut oil**
- **Pinch of sea salt**

FILLING

- **2 tablespoons coconut oil**
- **6 Pink Lady apples, sliced**
- **8 pitted Medjool dates, soaked in warm water for 30 minutes**
- **2 tablespoons cinnamon**
- **Pinch of nutmeg**
- **Pinch of ground cloves**
- **1 teaspoon fresh lemon juice**
- **2 tablespoons orange juice**

1. **HEAT** the oven to 350°F.

2. **MAKE** the crust: Place the oats, walnuts, maple syrup, coconut oil, and salt in a blender or food processor and pulse until the oats are broken up but not powdery. Add 1 tablespoon water and pulse a few times until the dough sticks together. Scrape into an 8- or 9-inch pie plate and press into the bottom and up the sides.

3. **BAKE** the crust until light brown, about 25 minutes. Leave the oven on and increase the temperature to 375°F.

4. **MAKE** the filling: Heat 1 tablespoon of the coconut oil in a large skillet over medium heat. Add the apples and cook until golden and just soft, about 15 minutes.

5. **DRAIN** the dates. Add them to a blender along with the cinnamon, nutmeg, cloves, lemon juice, orange juice, 3 to 4 tablespoons fresh water, and the remaining 1 tablespoon coconut oil in a blender and process until smooth. Pour over the apples and gently toss to coat.

6. **POUR** the apple mixture into the pie shell and bake until the pie is golden, about 40 minutes. Let cool completely before serving.

MAKES 8 SERVINGS ||| Prep time: 25 minutes ||| **Total time: 1 hour 25 minutes**

APPLE PIE PARFAIT

- **1 teaspoon vanilla extract**
- **1 tablespoon pure maple syrup**
- **1⅓ cups low-fat plain yogurt**
- **⅓ cup rolled oats**
- **2 tablespoons almond butter**
- **¼ teaspoon nutmeg**
- **¼ teaspoon ground ginger**
- **1 teaspoon cinnamon**
- **2 teaspoons coconut oil**
- **1 Pink Lady apple, diced**

1. HEAT the oven to 350°F.

2. STIR the vanilla and maple syrup into the yogurt. Cover and refrigerate until serving.

3. MIX together the oats, almond butter, nutmeg, ginger, and ½ teaspoon of the cinnamon until evenly dispersed. Spread the mixture out onto a baking sheet and bake until golden brown and fragrant, about 15 minutes. Remove from the oven and set the oat crumble aside.

4. HEAT the coconut oil in a medium skillet over medium heat. Add the diced apple and remaining ½ teaspoon cinnamon and cook until the apple is tender and golden, about 10 minutes.

5. SPOON ⅓ cup of the yogurt mixture into the bottom of each of 2 parfait glasses. Top each with ¼ of the apple mixture and a heaping tablespoon of the oat crumble. Repeat the layering.

MAKES 2 SERVINGS ||| Prep time: 25 minutes ||| Total time: 30 minutes

HEALTHY HACK

Calorie-packed pies, crisps, cobblers, and crumbles aren't the only option when you want an apple dessert. To get the taste of these treats without all the calories, sauté organic apples in a skillet with a bit of coconut oil and finish with a sprinkle of cinnamon. The result is a delicious, healthy dessert that will help control blood sugar and satisfy cravings.

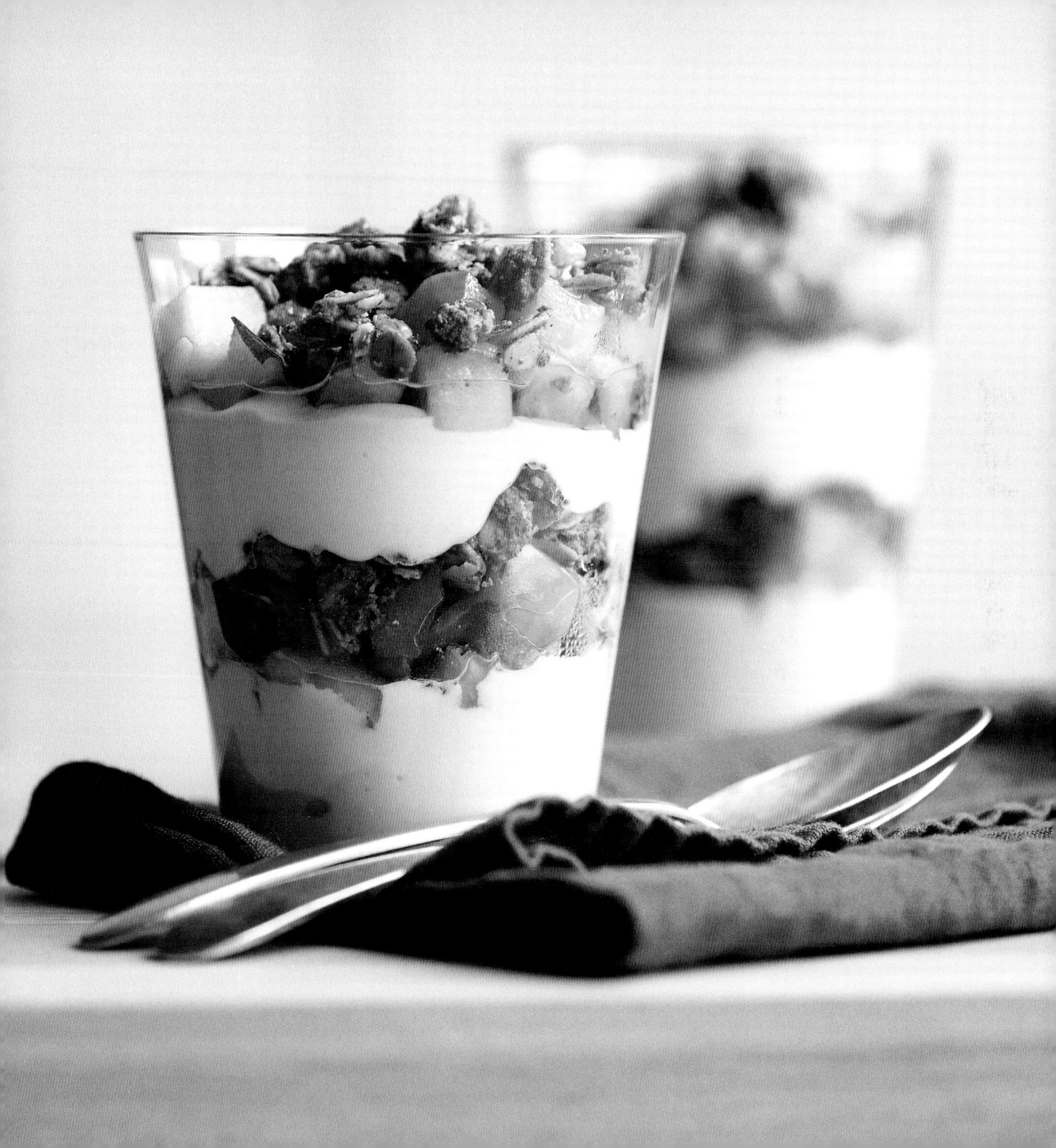

APPLE PIE SMOOTHIE

- **1½ Cortland or Honeycrisp apples, chopped**
- **2 teaspoons cinnamon**
- **10 ounces unsweetened plain almond milk**
- **½ very ripe banana**
- **¼ cup almond butter**
- **½ cup rolled oats**
- **1 cup ice**

1. COMBINE the apple pieces, ¼ cup water, and ½ teaspoon of the cinnamon in a microwaveable bowl. Microwave until the apples are soft, about 5 minutes, stirring halfway through. Let cool completely.

2. BLEND the almond milk, cooled apples, banana, almond butter, oats, and remaining 1½ teaspoons cinnamon on high speed in a blender until smooth, about 1½ minutes.

3. ADD the ice and blend until thick and smooth, another minute.

MAKES 2 SERVINGS ||| Prep time: 5 minutes ||| **Total time: 10 minutes**

Chocolate

Nutella may never make it onto our "clean" list (yeah, we're bummed, too), but there's definitely a whole bunch of chocolate out there that you can feel good about eating. Cocoa beans contain the antioxidants known as flavonols, which have been found to protect skin from sun damage, reduce blood pressure, and improve cardiovascular function.

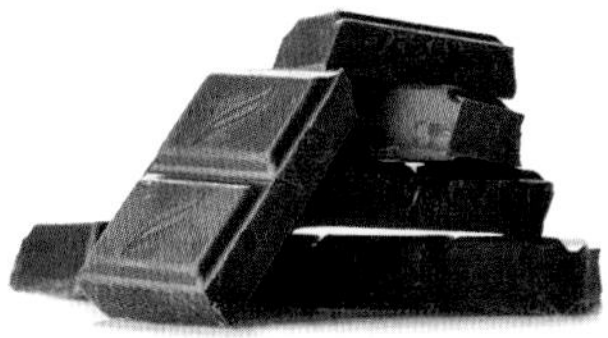

*

NOT CLEAN

MILK CHOCOLATE

Since milk chocolate doesn't have the same cocoa content, it doesn't offer the cardiovascular benefits you'd get from dark chocolate. Milk chocolate is also full of added sugars, putting you at risk for weight gain and obesity.

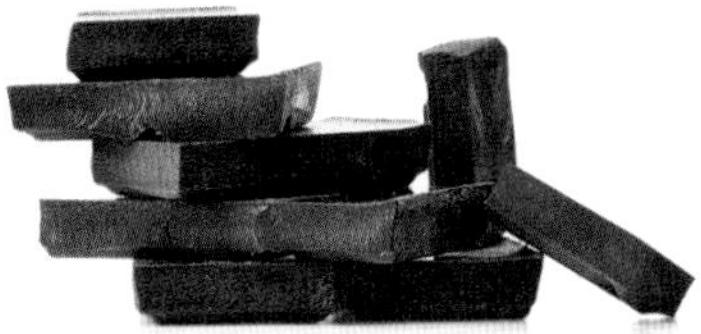

**

CLEAN

REGULAR DARK CHOCOLATE

Regular dark chocolate is certainly better than milk chocolate, but it may still contain pesticide residue, and you'll have to watch out for added sugars.

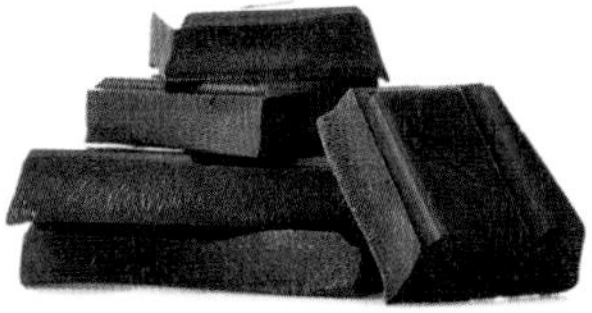

***

CLEANEST

ORGANIC 80% CACAO DARK CHOCOLATE

The next time you treat yourself with chocolate, make it organic dark chocolate with at least 80% cacao. You'll be avoiding lindane, a pesticide used in cocoa production that's been shown to cause reproductive and neurotoxic issues in animals. Plus, the darker the chocolate, the more health benefits.

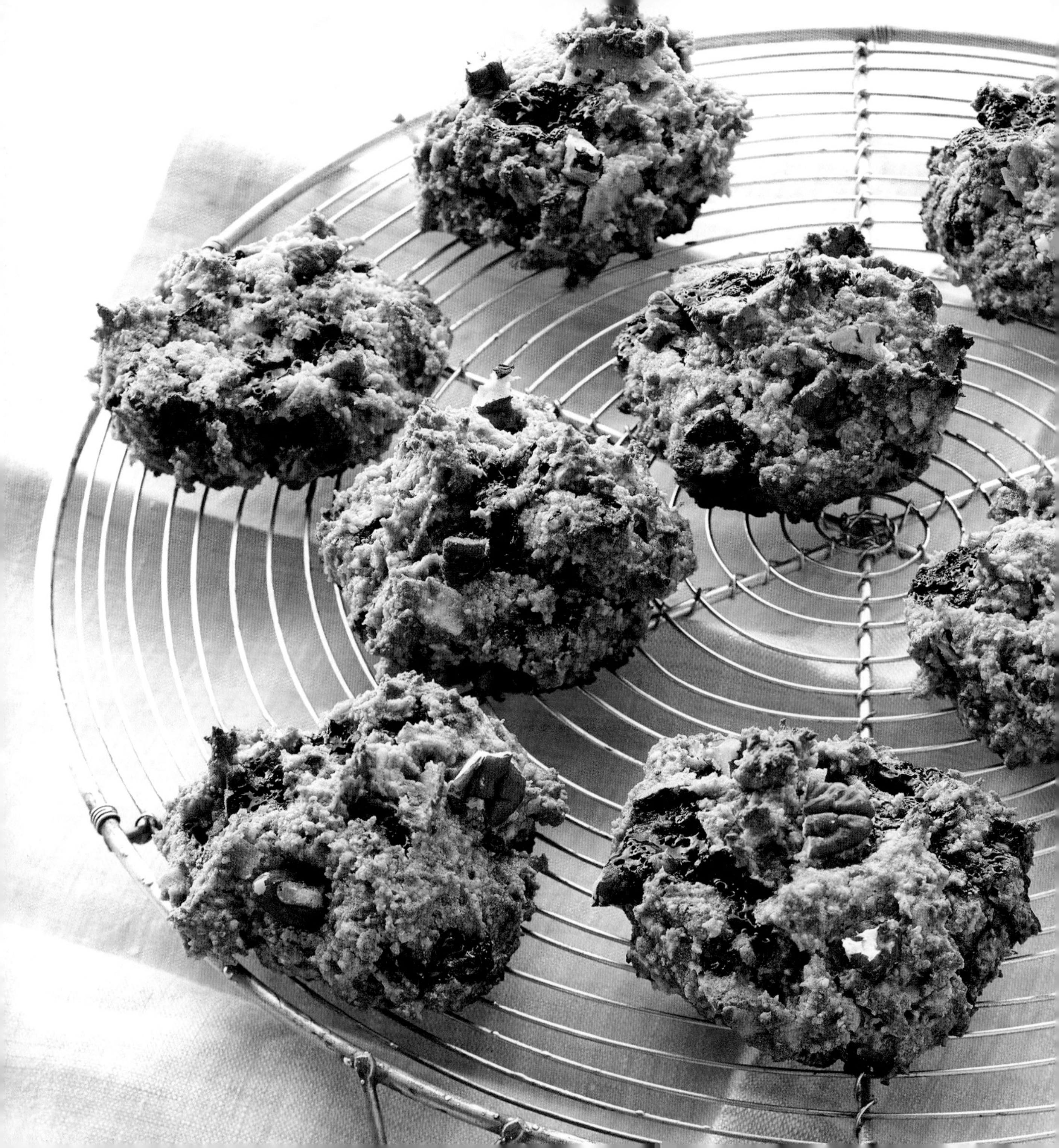

ORANGE–DARK CHOCOLATE CHUNK COOKIES

- 1 **cup almond meal/flour**
- 2 **tablespoons raw sugar**
- 1½ **teaspoons baking powder**
- ¼ **teaspoon fine sea salt**
- ½ **pound Medjool dates, pitted**
- 1 **large egg**
- 2 **tablespoons coconut oil, melted**
- 1 **tablespoon vanilla extract**
- 1½ **teaspoons grated orange zest**
- ¼ **cup chopped pecans**
- ¼ **cup unsweetened coconut flakes**
- ¼ **cup plus 2 tablespoons chopped dark chocolate (at least 80% cacao)**

1. HEAT the oven to 375°F. Line a baking sheet with parchment paper.

2. STIR together the almond meal, sugar, baking powder, and salt in a medium bowl.

3. PROCESS the dates in a food processor for 2 minutes, scraping down the sides frequently. Add the egg, coconut oil, vanilla, and orange zest and process until a smooth puree is formed.

4. STIR the puree into the dry ingredients slowly. Once the dough is evenly mixed, stir in the pecans, coconut flakes, and chocolate.

5. USE a 1½-tablespoon cookie scoop to measure cookie dough onto the prepared baking sheet, spacing them 2 inches apart.

6. BAKE until the edges begin to brown, 15 to 17 minutes. Let cool on a rack before serving. Once cooled, store leftovers in an airtight container.

MAKES 15 COOKIES ||| Prep time: 15 minutes ||| Total time: 30 minutes + cooling time

VANILLA MAPLE–CASHEW CREAM DARK CHOCOLATE PUDDING

- **½ cup Vanilla Maple–Cashew Cream (page 249)**
- **¾ cup canned lite coconut milk**
- **1½ teaspoons unsweetened cocoa powder**
- **1 tablespoon evaporated cane juice or date sugar**
- **1½ ounces chopped dark chocolate (at least 80% cacao)**
- **2 teaspoons vanilla extract**
- **Fine sea salt**

1. **HEAT** the cashew cream and coconut milk in a small saucepan over low heat just until warmed. Stir in the cocoa powder and evaporated cane juice. Continue to heat until the sugar is dissolved, stirring constantly.

2. **ADD** the chopped chocolate and stir over low heat until the chocolate is melted and the pudding is smooth. Stir in the vanilla and a dash of salt.

3. **SERVE** immediately or cover and refrigerate until chilled.

MAKES 2 SERVINGS ||| Prep time: 15 minutes ||| **Total time: 15 minutes**

HEALTHY HACK

A no-cal way to get the skin-care benefits of cocoa's flavonols: Use it as a bath soak. To do so, add 2 tablespoons unsweetened cocoa powder, which also nourishes dry skin, and ⅓ cup instant fat-free dry milk to your tub.

DARK CHOCOLATE–SEA SALT TRUFFLES

- **4 ounces chopped dark chocolate (at least 80% cacao)**
- **¼ cup plus 2 tablespoons canned lite coconut milk**
- **1 tablespoon coconut oil**
- **2 teaspoons vanilla extract**
- **⅛ teaspoon fine sea salt**
- **⅓ cup unsweetened shredded coconut**

1. COMBINE the chocolate, coconut milk, and coconut oil in a medium microwaveable bowl. Microwave in 15-second intervals, stirring in between, until melted and smooth. Stir in the vanilla and salt. Cover the bowl and refrigerate for about 1 hour, or until firm.

2. PLACE the shredded coconut in a shallow bowl. Roll 1 teaspoon of the chilled chocolate mixture between your palms to form a ball. Drop the ball in the bowl of coconut and roll around until entirely coated. Set aside on a cutting board or parchment paper and repeat with the rest of the mixture. Store in an airtight container in the refrigerator.

MAKES 15 TRUFFLES ||| Prep time: 10 minutes ||| Total time: 10 minutes + 1 hour chilling time

Milk

Milk is a convenient source of protein and essential nutrients. One cup contains 8 grams of protein, 30% of your Daily Value of bone-building calcium, and 40% of your vitamin B_{12}. But milk from conventionally raised cows may not be worth the perks.

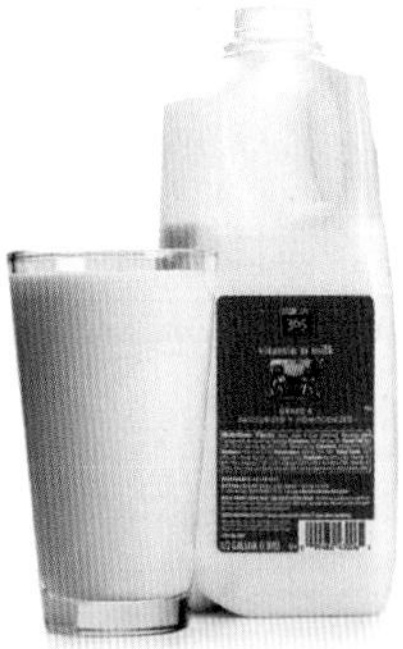

✷

NOT CLEAN

CONVENTIONAL MILK

Conventional milk comes from cows fed a processed diet containing GMO grain, and will lack the omega-3 fatty acids you'll get from higher-quality milk. If you have buy it, try to at least choose a brand that's rBGH and rBST free—cows given these growth hormones are more likely to require antibiotics.

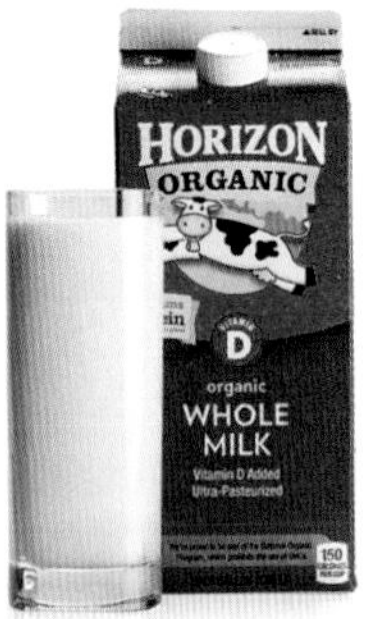

✷✷

CLEAN

ORGANIC 1% OR 2% MILK

Non-grass-fed organic milk will still provide protein and be free of dangerous growth hormones such as rBGH or rBST, but you're not going to get the amazing benefits of fat- and inflammation-fighting fatty acids. Opt for 1% or 2%, which has some fat to boost satiety and keep you fuller longer than skim.

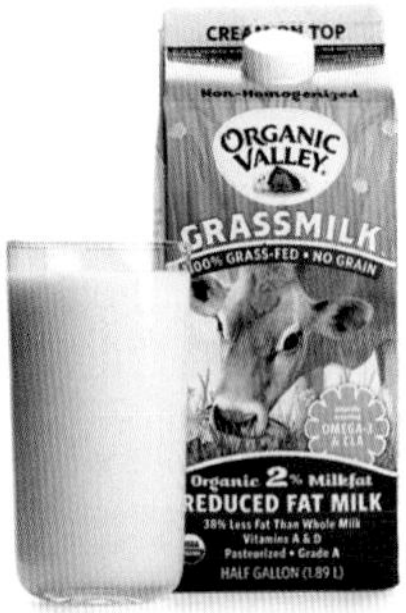

✷✷✷

CLEANEST

ORGANIC GRASS-FED 2% MILK

Grass-fed cows graze in pastures and are not pumped with growth hormones or fed a processed diet—this results in milk with more omega-3 fatty acids, vitamin E, beta-carotene, and conjugated linoleic acid (CLA), a fatty acid associated with reduced body fat and inflammation. To reap the benefits, pick a milk with adequate fat—we like 2%.

CREAMY PARMESAN, CAULIFLOWER & LEEK SOUP

- 2 teaspoons grapeseed oil
- ¼ cup chopped carrots
- 1 leek, chopped
- 1 cup chopped cauliflower
- 1 teaspoon minced garlic
- 1 tablespoon finely chopped fresh dill
- 1 tablespoon finely chopped fresh parsley
- 1½ teaspoons unsalted butter
- 1½ teaspoons whole wheat flour
- 1 cup 2% milk, slightly warmed
- ¼ cup plus 2 tablespoons grated Parmesan
- Fine sea salt and black pepper

1. **HEAT** the oil in a medium saucepan over medium-high heat. Add the carrots, leek, and cauliflower. Cook, stirring frequently, until lightly browned, 5 to 10 minutes. Stir in the garlic and cook until the garlic becomes fragrant, about 1 minute. Add 1 cup water and bring to a boil. Reduce the heat, cover, and simmer until thickened, about 20 minutes.

2. **USE** an immersion blender to puree the soup in the pot (or transfer to a stand blender and puree). Stir in the dill and parsley. Keep warm over low heat while you make the white sauce.

3. **HEAT** the butter in a small saucepan over low heat. Stir in the flour and cook, whisking constantly for 2 minutes to remove the raw flour taste. Slowly whisk in the warm milk, whisking thoroughly to prevent lumps from forming.

4. **ADD** the white sauce and Parmesan to the vegetable puree. Gently stir to combine. Season with salt and pepper to taste. Serve hot.

MAKES 2 SERVINGS ||| Prep time: 25 minutes ||| **Total time: 45 minutes**

HEALTHY HACK

Go ahead, give goat milk a whirl. It doesn't have a huge presence in the United States, but it does worldwide—and it holds its own against the cow. With less lactose and a chemical structure similar to that of breast milk, it's usually easier to digest for sensitive stomachs. Plus, it has more calcium, potassium, and vitamin A. Cow milk, on the other hand, delivers more B vitamins and selenium.

HOMEMADE RICOTTA CHEESE

- ½ **gallon (8 cups) 2% milk**
- 1 **teaspoon fine sea salt**
- 2 **tablespoons distilled white vinegar or lemon juice**

1. **LINE** a fine-mesh sieve with two layers of ultrafine cheesecloth. Place the sieve over a large bowl and set aside.

2. **COMBINE** the milk and salt in a large saucepan and heat over medium heat to 165° to 175°F. Use an instant-read thermometer to frequently check the temperature.

3. **REMOVE** from the heat and slowly stir in the vinegar. Once it is all stirred in, let the mixture sit for about 20 minutes. The mixture should separate into solid white curds and translucent liquid whey.

4. **SCOOP** up the curds with a slotted spoon or skimmer into the lined sieve, leaving as much of the liquid whey behind as possible. Cover the sieve with plastic wrap and let drain until it reaches the desired consistency. Use the ricotta immediately or transfer the contents of the sieve to a bowl (discard the whey liquid) and refrigerator. It will keep for up to a week.

MAKES ABOUT 2 CUPS ||| Prep time: 10 minutes |||
Total time: 40 minutes + draining time

Did You Know?

Raw milk is either a superfood or a super good way to get sick, depending on whom you ask. Often derived from organic, grass-fed dairy but never pasteurized, raw milk can contain pathogens like E. coli. Recently, the CDC announced that the number of raw milk-related outbreaks is rising: About 1,000 people fell ill between 2007 and 2012. While the CDC is antiraw, some experts are torn. Some experts say that the good bacteria in raw milk can be healthy for the gut and help immune function. Others say drinking it is "like playing Russian roulette." But most agree: Children, pregnant women, and the immunocompromised should avoid it.

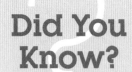

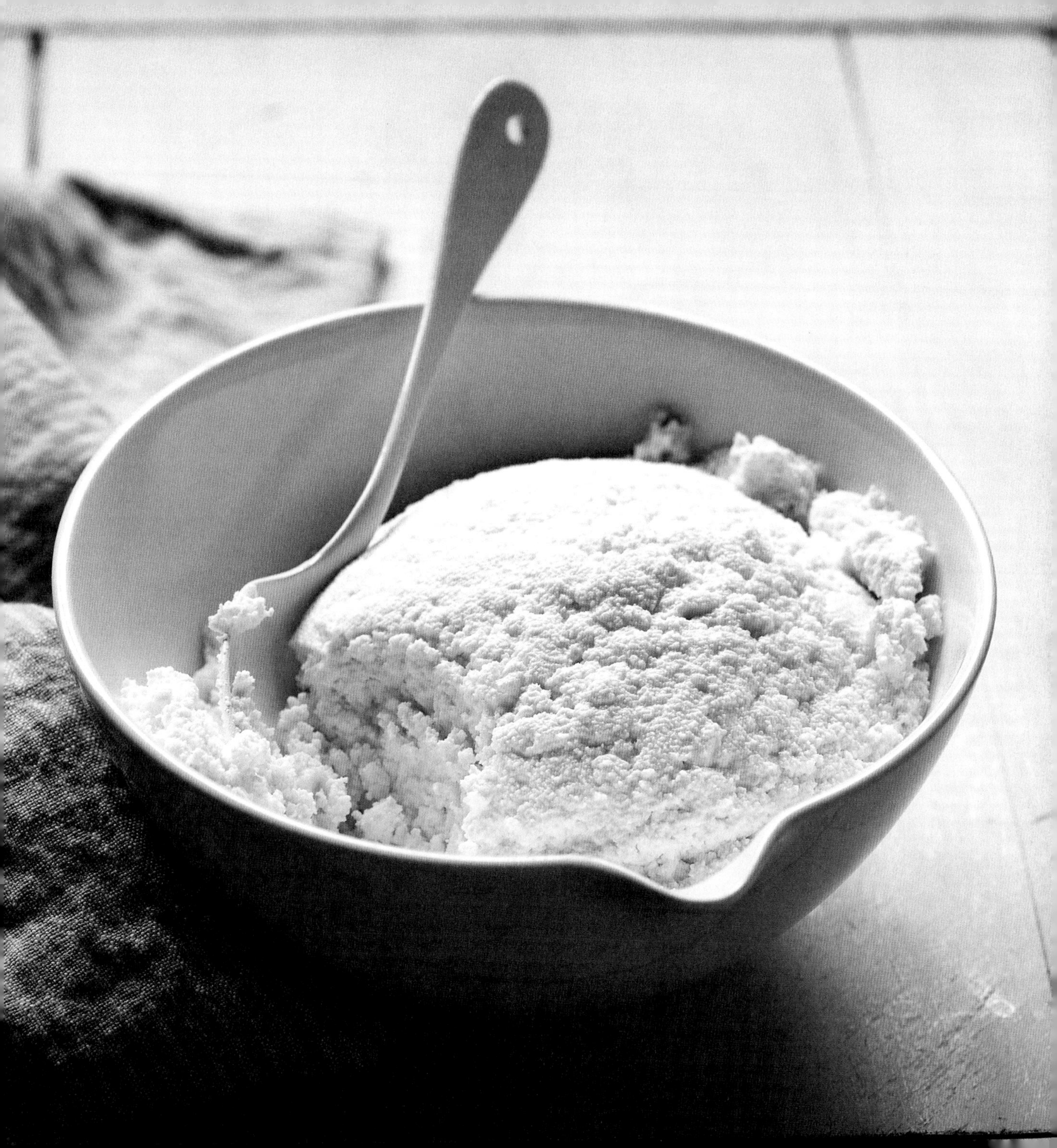

CREPES WITH COCOA-HAZELNUT BUTTER & BANANAS

- **1 large egg, lightly beaten**
- **¼ cup plus 2 tablespoons 1% milk**
- **1½ tablespoons plus 1 teaspoon unsalted butter, melted**
- **1 teaspoon vanilla extract**
- **½ cup whole wheat flour**
- **1 tablespoon confectioners' sugar**
- **¼ teaspoon cinnamon**
- **Nutmeg**
- **Fine sea salt**
- **¼ cup Homemade Cocoa-Hazelnut Butter (page 146)**
- **2 bananas, sliced**

1. COMBINE ¼ cup water, the egg, milk, 1½ tablespoons of the melted butter, the vanilla, flour, sugar, cinnamon, and a dash each of nutmeg and salt in a blender and pulse for about 30 seconds, or until blended and smooth. Refrigerate the batter for at least 1 hour, but no more than 2 days.

2. PLACE a nonstick medium skillet over medium-high heat and add ¼ teaspoon of the melted butter to the pan. Pour ⅓ cup batter into the pan and swirl to spread evenly. Cook for 30 seconds on one side, and 10 seconds on the other side. Set aside on a plate or cutting board. Repeat until all of the batter has been used, adding more butter for each crepe. You should have 4 crepes total.

3. SPREAD 1 tablespoon of the hazelnut butter in a line across the diameter of the crepe, then spread the hazelnut butter as far toward the edges as possible. Spread the slices from ½ banana evenly across the center. Fold the crepe in half and roll up, starting with the folded side. Repeat with remaining crepes and fillings.

MAKES 2 SERVINGS (2 CREPES EACH) ||| Prep time: 20 minutes ||| **Total time: 1 hour 20 minutes**

Milk Alternatives

If you don't drink cow's milk, the bevy of nondairy options

can be totally overwhelming. Most are at least fortified, so they've got you covered in terms of calcium and vitamin D, but you need to be careful about added sugars, flavorings, and other additives.

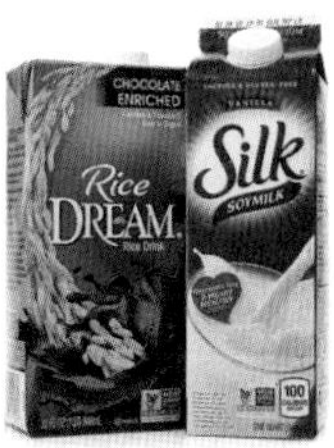

✱

NOT CLEAN

FLAVORED AND SWEETENED ALTERNATIVE MILKS

Flavored nondairy milks tend to have even higher sugar content than "original" varieties—one brand of chocolate almond milk has a whopping 17 grams! That's more sugar than a chocolate frosted donut from Dunkin' Donuts (13 grams).

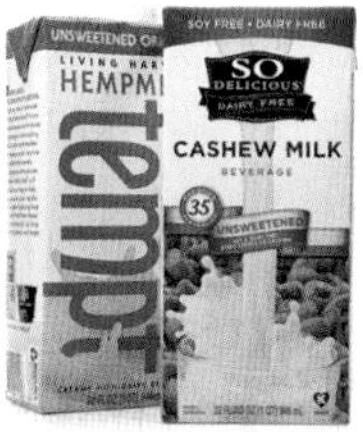

✱✱

CLEAN

"ORIGINAL" ALTERNATIVE MILKS, PREFERABLY WITHOUT CARRAGEENAN

So-called "original" nondairy milks usually have around 7 grams of added sugar in the form of cane sugar. Not totally outrageous, but if you're using it frequently, those calories and sugar grams will add up fast. Carrageenan-free options exist even among nonorganic varieties, so opt for those.

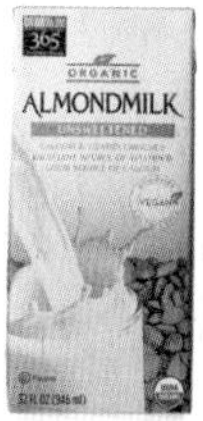

✱✱✱

CLEANEST

ORGANIC UNSWEETENED ALTERNATIVE MILKS WITHOUT CARRAGEENAN

Nearly all "original" varieties of these nondairy milks contain added sugars, so ideally you should opt for "unsweetened." Choose organic varieties to avoid pesticide residue and, if possible, steer clear of brands with carrageenan—a controversial thickening agent that has been linked to GI inflammation in animals.

ALMOND CHAI SCONES

- 1 cup sliced almonds, ground (or almond meal/flour)
- 2 cups whole wheat or white whole wheat flour
- 2 teaspoons baking powder
- ¼ cup granulated sugar
- 2 tablespoons Chai Seasoning
- Fine sea salt
- 4 tablespoons coconut oil, solid
- ⅔ cup unsweetened vanilla almond milk
- 1 egg
- 1 teaspoon almond extract
- 2 tablespoons raw sugar

CHAI SEASONING

- 1 tablespoon ground cloves
- 1 tablespoon ground cardamom
- 1 tablespoon cinnamon
- 1 tablespoon ground ginger
- 1 tablespoon ground anise
- 1 teaspoon black pepper

1. **HEAT** the oven to 350°F. Line a baking sheet with parchment paper.

2. **COMBINE** all the ingredients for the chai seasoning in a bowl. Store any leftovers in an airtight container.

3. **PROCESS** the almonds, 1½ cups of the whole wheat flour, the baking powder, sugar, chai seasoning, and a dash of salt in a food processor until thoroughly mixed and even in texture.

4. **ADD** the solid coconut oil and pulse again until evenly distributed into fine crumbs. Pour in the almond milk, egg, and almond extract and pulse 8 to 10 times until the dough is uniform and sticky.

5. **DUST** a clean, flat surface with the remaining ½ cup flour and scrape the dough on top. Gently knead the dough to incorporate enough flour so the dough is not sticky. Pat into a round that is roughly 2 inches tall and 8 inches in diameter. Slice into 6 wedges and place each on the lined baking sheet.

6. **SPRINKLE** the wedges with the raw sugar and pat gently into the dough. Bake until golden with a light crust, about 20 minutes. Remove from the pan and cool on a wire rack.

MAKES 6 SCONES ||| Prep time: 20 minutes ||| **Total time: 40 minutes + cooling time**

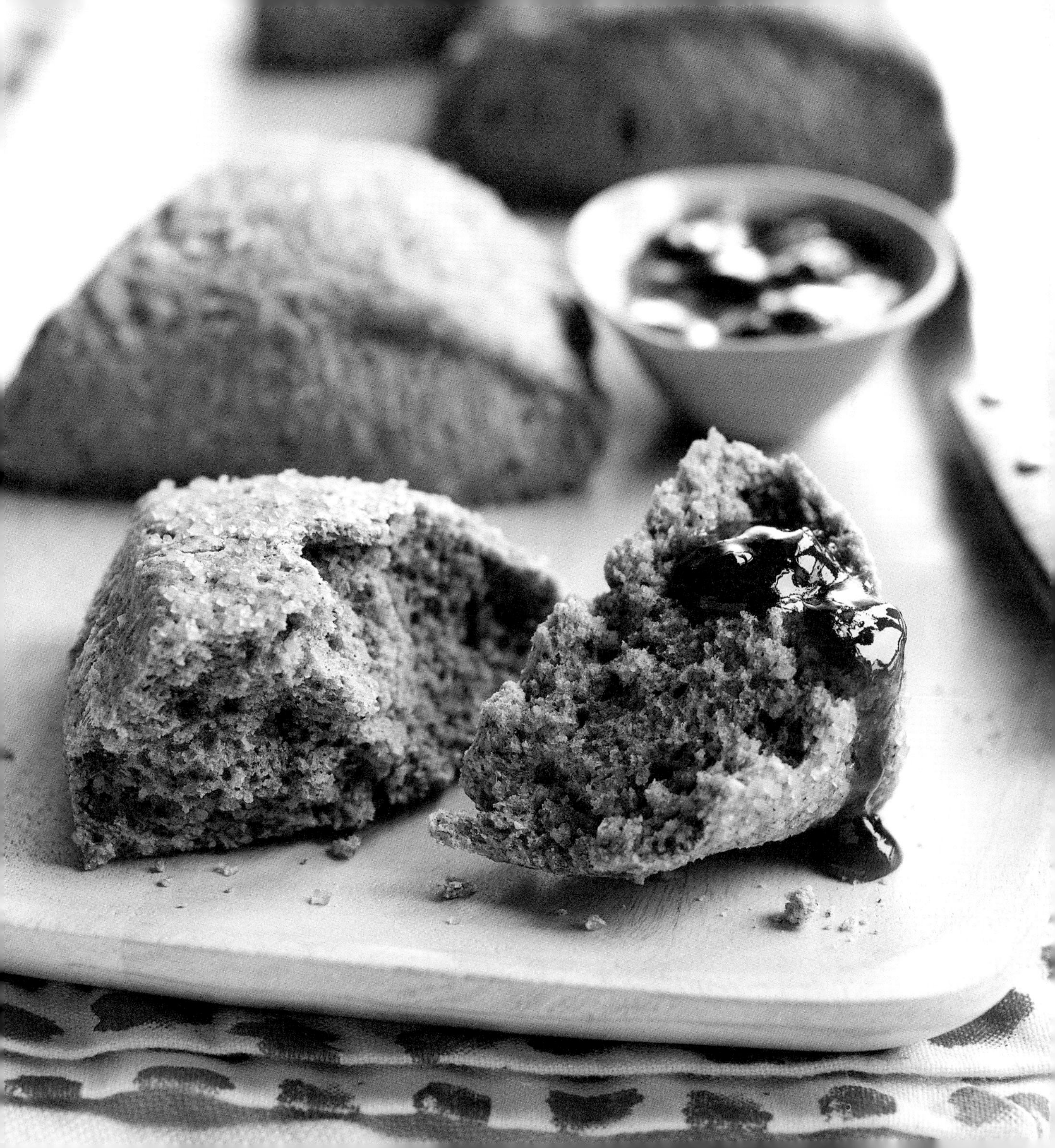

COCONUT RICE PUDDING WITH CHIA

- **½ cup brown basmati rice**
- **¾ cup coconut milk**
- **¼ cup sugar**
- **2 teaspoons vanilla extract**
- **3 tablespoons chia seeds**
- **Sliced mango or other fruit (optional)**

1. COMBINE the brown rice, ¾ cup water, the coconut milk, sugar, and vanilla in a medium pot and bring to a boil. Reduce to a simmer, cover, and cook, stirring occasionally, for 20 minutes.

2. FOLD in the chia seeds, remove from the heat, and let sit covered for 10 minutes longer, until all the liquid is absorbed. If desired, serve with sliced mango.

MAKES 2 SERVINGS ||| Prep time: 10 minutes ||| **Total time: 40 minutes**

HEALTHY HACK

It's actually supereasy to make your own nondairy nut milk. Soak 1 cup of raw almonds in enough water to cover for 4 hours, or up to overnight. Drain the almonds and blend in a blender with 4 cups of water until smooth, about 1 minute. Strain through cheesecloth. Refrigerate in a covered container and enjoy for up to 3 days.

PUMPKIN SPICE CASHEW CREAM

1½ cups cashews
½ teaspoon ground ginger
½ teaspoon cinnamon
¼ teaspoon ground cloves
¼ teaspoon nutmeg
1 tablespoon honey

1. SOAK the cashews overnight in 3 cups water.

2. DRAIN the cashews and transfer to a blender or food processor. Add 2½ cups fresh water, the spices, and honey and puree until smooth and the consistency of heavy cream. Add more water to thin to desired consistency. Store covered in the refrigerator for up to 4 days.

MAKES 4 SERVINGS (8 OUNCES EACH) ||| Prep time: 5 minutes ||| **Total time: 5 minutes + overnight soaking**

Juice

Fruit juice can be a great way to start your morning. Orange juice, for example, is naturally high in the B vitamins thiamin and folate, potassium, and vitamin C, which plays an essential role in immune system function. But if you're getting it from a carton or bottle, you could be missing out.

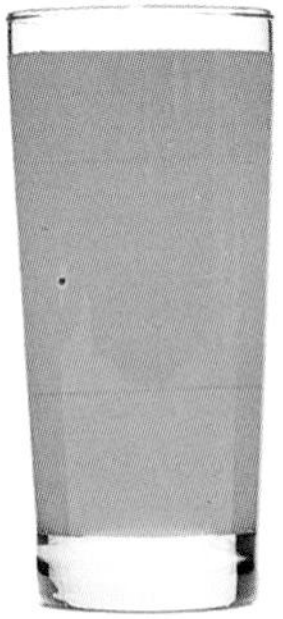

✷

NOT CLEAN

ORANGE-FLAVORED DRINKS

Don't be fooled by orange-flavored beverages or sports drinks. They contain high fructose corn syrup and little or no actual fruit juice. This means you'll miss out on all the benefits of natural vitamin C, and you'll be slurping empty calories and excess sugar.

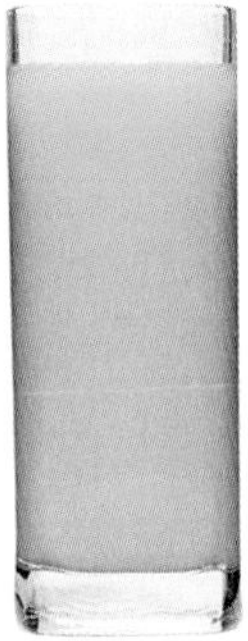

✷✷

CLEAN

100% ORANGE JUICE, PREFERABLY ORGANIC

You never know how long packaged orange juice has been sitting in that refrigerated case, meaning all those awesome nutrients have likely degraded and are far less potent than they once were. If you go this route, at least make it organic OJ, made from oranges that haven't been doused in pesticides.

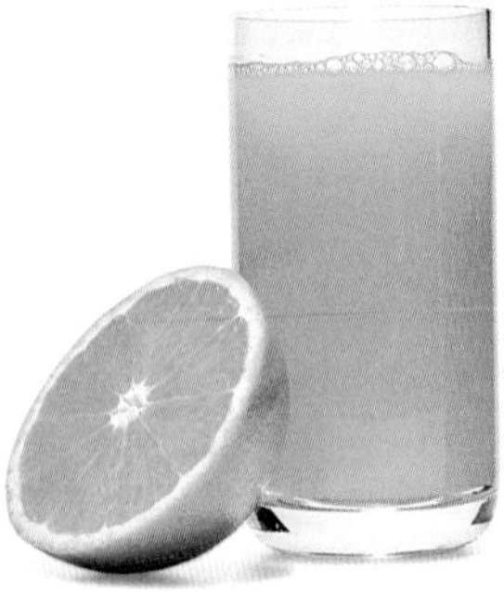

✷✷✷

CLEANEST

FRESHLY SQUEEZED OJ

Simply squeezing an orange at breakfast guarantees you'll be drinking the freshest most nutrient-packed juice possible, sans any added sugars or preservatives. It's been shown that the level of vitamin C present in juice is higher the fresher it is.

PULPY GINGER-ORANGE "WHOLE JUICE"

- 2 **large oranges, peeled and segmented**
- ½ **teaspoon grated fresh ginger**

COMBINE 1 cup filtered water, the orange segments, and ginger in a blender and blend on high until fully pureed, about 2 minutes.

MAKES 2 SERVINGS ||| Prep time: 5 minutes ||| **Total time: 5 minutes**

ORANGE-MISO SALAD DRESSING

- 2 **tablespoons fresh orange juice**
- 1 **tablespoon reduced-sodium wheat-free tamari**
- 1 **tablespoon rice vinegar**
- 1 **tablespoon sunflower seed oil**
- 1 **teaspoon sesame oil**
- 2 **teaspoons white miso paste**
- ½ **teaspoon minced garlic**
- **Pinch of black pepper**

WHISK all the ingredients together. Store in a sealed jar in the refrigerator.

MAKES $^1/_3$ CUP ||| Prep time: 5 minutes ||| **Total time: 5 minutes**

LABEL, DECODED!

Ever wonder what that "No HPP" label on your juice bottle means? It refers to a drink that hasn't been subjected to high pressure processing (HPP), a cold pasteurization technique that prevents bacterial growth and extends shelf life. Some juice brands claim that HPP makes a product less fresh and causes beneficial enzymes and nutrients to degrade. Right now, you'll only see this label on superfresh juices sold in juice bars or the stores where they're made.

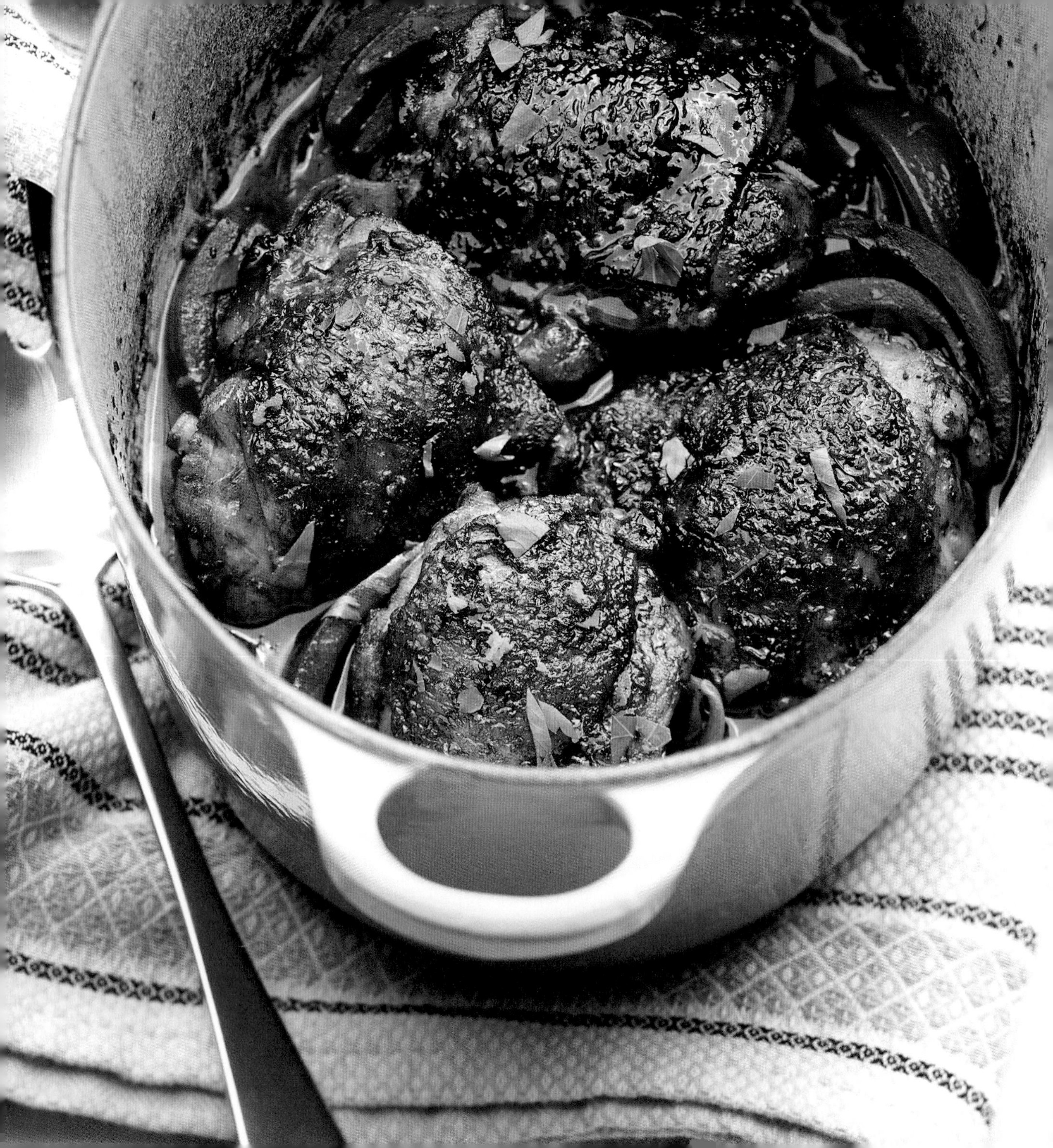

ORANGE-SAGE BRAISED CHICKEN THIGHS

2 tablespoons sunflower oil
4 bone-in chicken thighs
4 teaspoons grated orange zest
1 cup fresh orange juice
2 tablespoons balsamic vinegar
1 medium onion, sliced
1 teaspoon ground dried sage
1 teaspoon fine sea salt

1. HEAT the oven to 375°F.

2. HEAT the oil in a small Dutch oven or ovenproof lidded saucepan over medium-high heat. Add the chicken thighs and cook until browned on each side, about 8 minutes total.

3. WHISK in the orange zest, orange juice, vinegar, onion, sage, and salt and bring to a simmer. Cover and transfer to the oven. Bake for 45 minutes.

4. BASTE the chicken with the cooking juices and bake uncovered until the internal temperature reaches 160°F, 20 minutes longer.

5. SERVE the chicken with cooking juices spooned over the top.

MAKES 2 SERVINGS ||| Prep time: 10 minutes ||| **Total time: 1 hour 15 minutes**

Carbonated Drinks

We don't need to tell you that you should forgo soda

on a clean diet, and diet soda isn't any better. Sometimes, though, you just need a drink with a nice carbonated bite and a bit of flavor. Luckily, healthy options are popping up left and right.

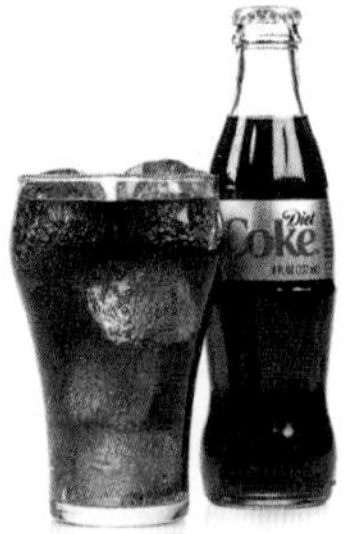

✷

NOT CLEAN

DIET SODA OR SPARKLING WATERS WITH ARTIFICIAL SWEETENERS

There's increasing evidence that artificial sweeteners like aspartame are bad for your health. In fact, a recent study showed that drinking just one diet soda a day is associated with metabolic syndrome and an increased waist circumference—likely because artificial sweeteners disrupt your body's ability to regulate calorie consumption.

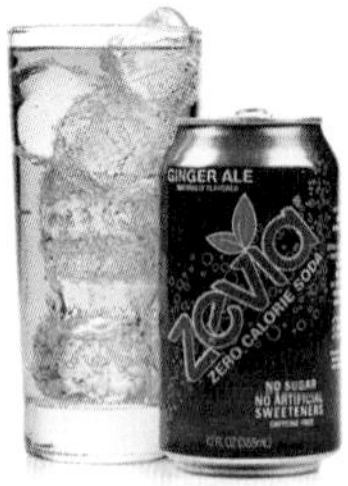

✷✷

CLEAN

STEVIA-FLAVORED SODA OR SELTZER

If you are looking for a diet cola or a sweetened beverage, choose one that contains stevia—likely the safest of all zero-calorie sweeteners, as it's derived from a plant that's been consumed for over a thousand years in South America and not totally concocted in a lab.

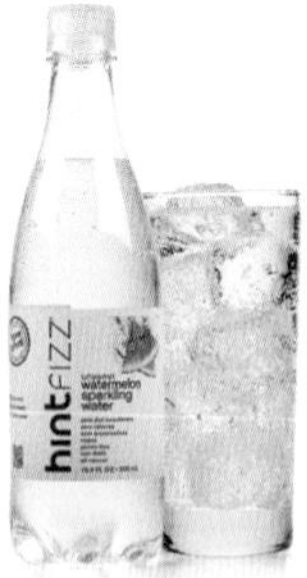

✷✷✷

CLEANEST

NATURALLY FLAVORED SELTZER

There are loads of clean naturally flavored seltzer waters in fun flavors like grapefruit, blackberry, and cherry. These will keep you hydrated, and they're free of potentially dangerous artificial sweeteners. And if you crave a little caffeine to go along with your carbonation, try a caffeinated seltzer.

NEW YORK EGG CREAM

1 cup sweetened vanilla almond milk
1 tablespoon cocoa powder
1 cup seltzer
Optional adult add-ins:
1 ounce Baileys Irish Cream or Kahlúa

WHISK together the almond milk and cocoa (or process in a blender) until smooth. Divide between 2 glasses. Add ½ cup seltzer to each, stirring briskly while pouring. If desired, stir in an adult add-in. Drink immediately.

MAKES 2 SERVINGS ||| Prep time: 5 minutes ||| **Total time: 5 minutes**

GINGER-SPIKED PEACH FIZZ

½ inch fresh ginger, peeled
2 bottles (12 ounces each) peach-flavored seltzer water

GRATE the ginger into 2 tall glasses and pour the seltzer over. Serve immediately.

MAKES 2 SERVINGS ||| Prep time: 5 minutes ||| **Total time: 5 minutes**

BASIL-WATERMELON SELTZER

- **3 large fresh basil leaves, plus sprigs for garnish**
- **1 bottle watermelon-flavored seltzer water**

CHOP the basil leaves, pressing with the side of the knife to mash (or use a bar muddler). Add to watermelon-flavored seltzer water and swirl to mix. Garnish with a sprig of basil leaves.

MAKES 2 SERVINGS ||| Prep time: 5 minutes ||| **Total time: 5 minutes**

SMART SWAP

If you don't mind a few calories (and a unique, tangy taste), consider drinking kombucha to get some added perks along with your carbonation. This fizzy fermented tea is made by adding a SCOBY (symbiotic colony of bacteria and yeast) to brewed tea with a bit of sugar. The SCOBY ferments the sugar and results in a probiotic-packed drink with around 4 grams of sugar and 70 calories per 16 ounces.

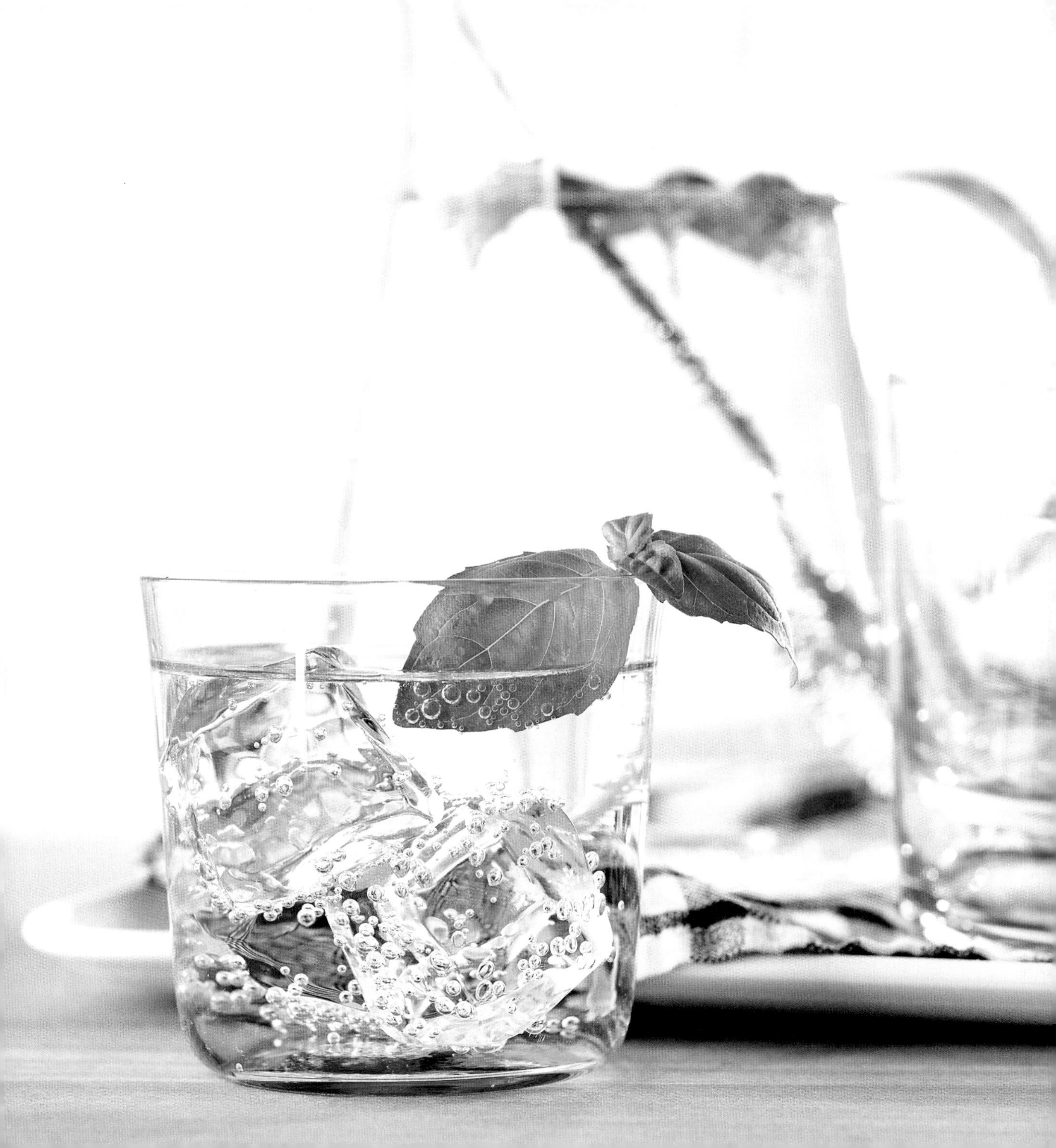

Iced Tea

This summer classic is a perfectly healthy option when you make it yourself. And no, we don't mean from a sugar-loaded powdered mix. Tea can actually have more flavonoids than a piece of fruit, and these powerful antioxidants have been linked to a reduced risk of diabetes, certain cancers, heart disease, and even Alzheimer's.

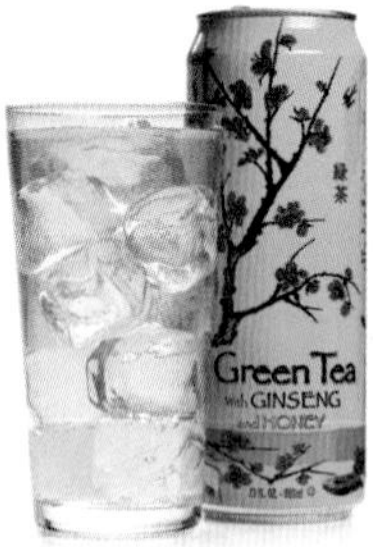

*

NOT CLEAN

SWEETENED WITH SUGAR OR HIGH FRUCTOSE CORN SYRUP

You'll want to avoid premade teas sweetened with sugar or high fructose corn syrup. Some sweetened teas can contain as many as 6 tablespoons of sugar per 16-ounce bottle, which can spike your blood sugar and leave you feeling wiped out rather than energized.

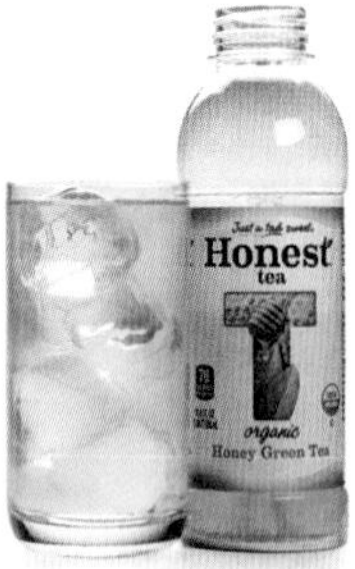

**

CLEAN

SWEETENED WITH HONEY

If you absolutely must have yourself some sweet tea, use a natural sweetener like honey. If you opt for raw unfiltered honey, you'll get some trace nutrients and live enzymes that may promote health.

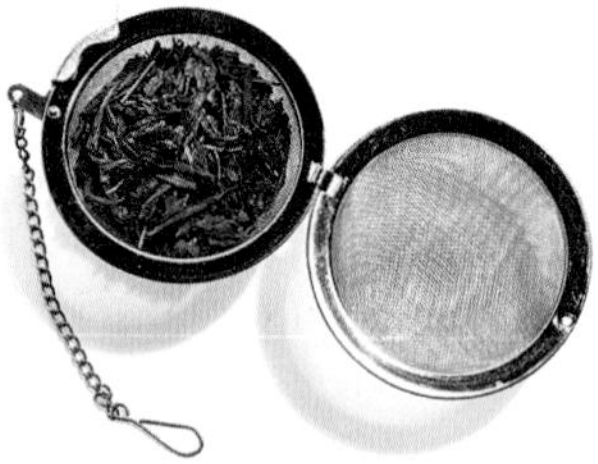

***

CLEANEST

UNSWEETENED

While any tea is going to give you a nice dose of cancer-fighting antioxidants, tea brewed at home has been shown to contain significantly more than bottled. Make it from organic tea leaves and skip the added sugar to keep it even cleaner.

JASMINE MINT ICED TEA

- **3 teaspoons loose jasmine green tea**
- **6 fresh mint leaves**
- **4 teaspoons honey**
- **1 cup ice cubes**

POUR 1 cup steaming hot (but not boiling) water over the loose tea and mint leaves and soak for 3 minutes. Stir in the honey until totally dissolved. Strain and mix with 1 cup cold water and pour into two ice-filled glasses.

MAKES 2 SERVINGS ||| Prep time: 5 minutes ||| **Total time: 5 minutes**

HIBISCUS LEMON-GINGER ICED TEA

- **¼ cup dried hibiscus flowers**
- **1 teaspoon chopped fresh ginger**
- **2 teaspoons honey**
- **1 teaspoon fresh lemon juice**

POUR 2 cups room-temperature or cold water over the hibiscus flowers and ginger. Refrigerate for 3 hours. Strain. Mix the honey with 1 tablespoon warm water and the lemon juice. Stir the mixture into the tea and divide between two glasses.

MAKES 2 SERVINGS ||| Prep time: 5 minutes ||| **Total time: 5 minutes + chilling time**

HEALTHY HACK

If the idea of homemade iced tea isn't thrilling, try getting creative. Any kind of tea can be made into iced tea–mint, green, chamomile, you name it–and fresh herbal additions like mint, rosehips, hibiscus, and lemongrass add instant flavor. You can also toss fresh strawberry or peach slices into the pitcher to give tea a fruity taste and extra antioxidants.

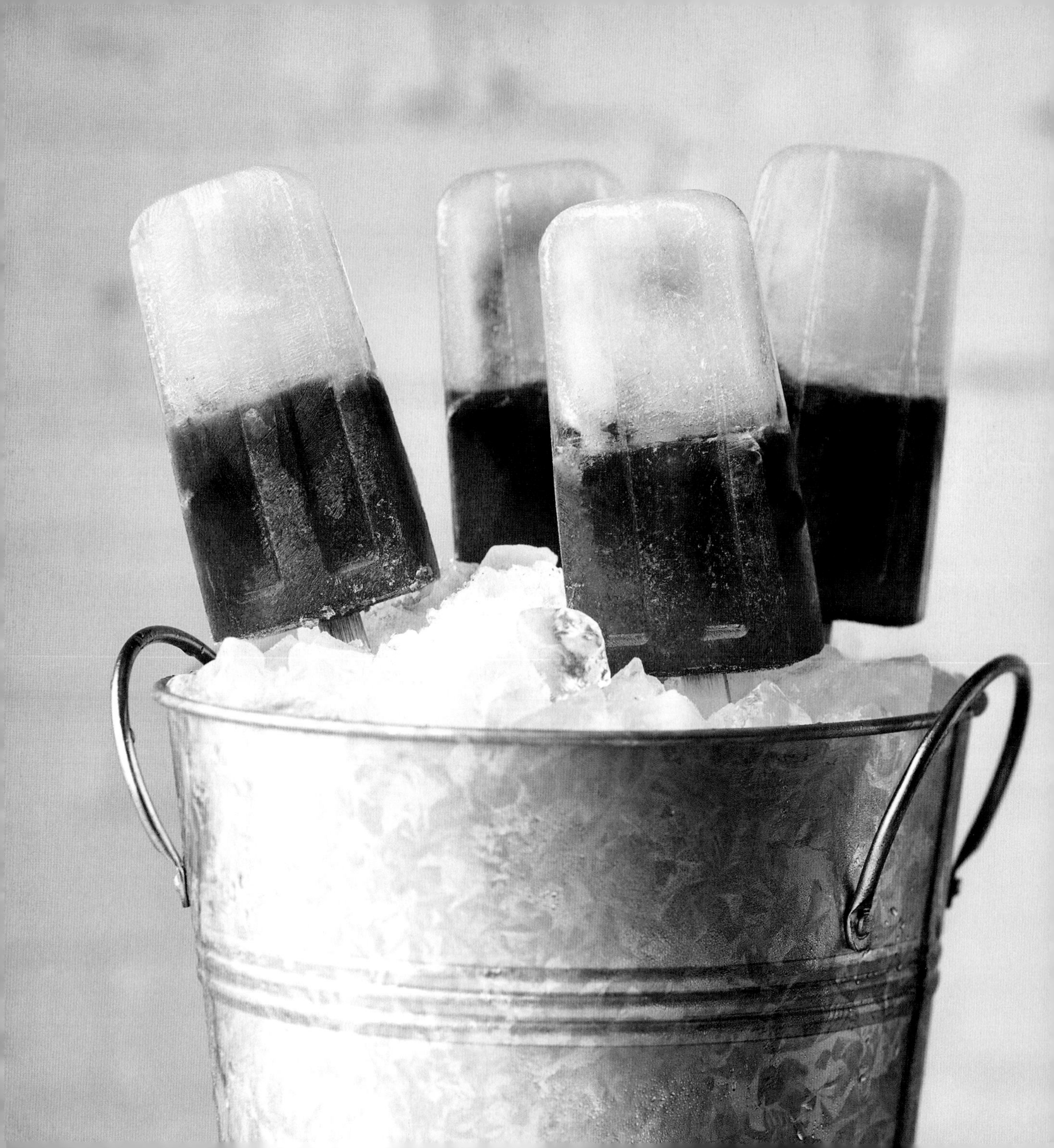

POMEGRANATE GREEN TEA ICE POPS

1½ cups unsweetened iced green tea (see Note)

1½ cups pomegranate juice

½ cup pomegranate seeds

STIR all the ingredients together. Pour into six 4-ounce ice pop molds. Freeze for 4 hours or overnight.

Notes: Brew regular strength green tea or use a prebrewed brand that is unsweetened.

To achieve a two-toned look, pour the iced green tea halfway into the ice pop molds. Freeze until slushy, about 1 hour, then add the stick and the pomegranate juice and seeds. Freeze.

MAKES 6 POPS ||| Prep time: 5 minutes ||| **Total time: 5 minutes + freezing time**

Tea

Sipping on tea throughout your day is a great way to curb hunger and up your intake of disease-fighting antioxidants—not to mention, it's downright delicious. Drinking about 3 cups of green tea per day has been shown to help lower cholesterol and blood pressure. But like everything else, not all tea is created equal.

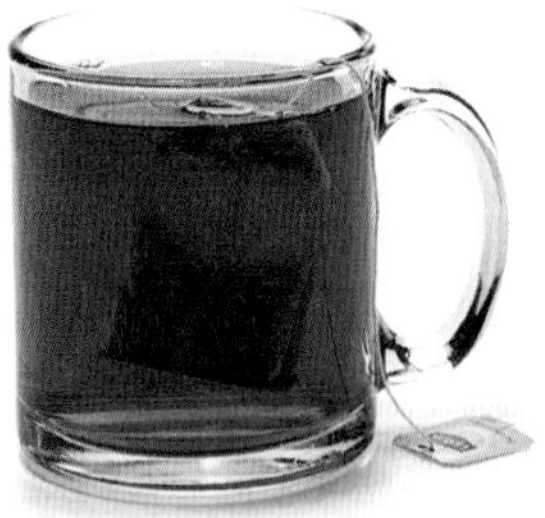

*

NOT CLEAN

CONVENTIONAL PACKAGED TEA

Conventional teas are best avoided since they may have been exposed to pesticides and even hidden soy or GMO ingredients disguised as "natural flavors."

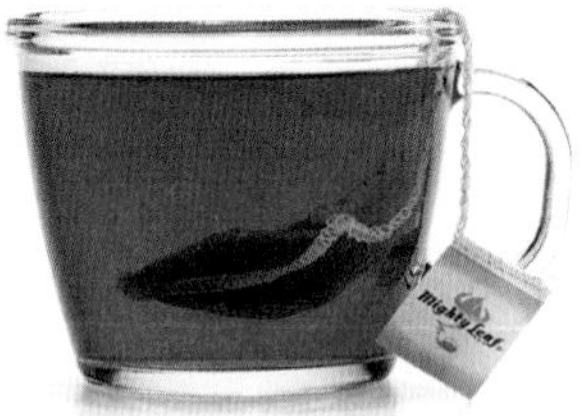

**

CLEAN

ORGANIC TEA BAGS

Organic bagged tea is another option, but there have been some concerns about the tea bags themselves–some actually contain plastic. Given that you're dousing them in boiling water, it's safe to assume some of that plastic is leaching into your brew.

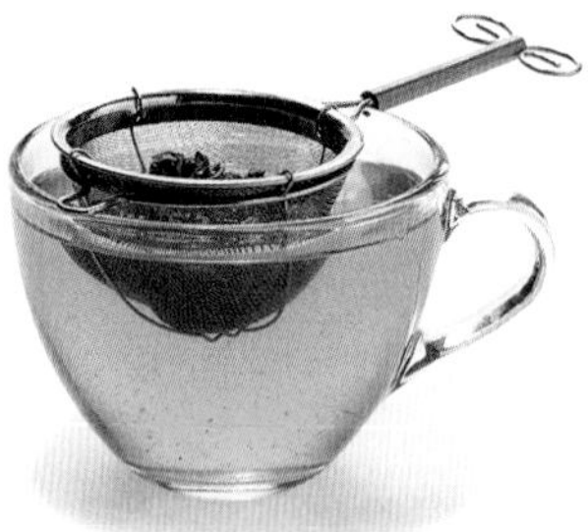

***

CLEANEST

ORGANIC LOOSE-LEAF TEA

Buy organic loose-leaf tea to avoid pesticide residues and funky chemicals that may be in a tea bag. If you don't think pesticide residue is a problem in tea, think again. A recent report found that 91% of the tea tested from one very popular brand had pesticide residues exceeding US limits.

LAVENDER EARL GREY LATTE

- **1½ teaspoons loose-leaf Earl Grey tea**
- **½ teaspoon dried lavender**
- **½ cup 1% milk or unsweetened milk alternative**
- **1 teaspoon honey**
- **¼ teaspoon vanilla extract**

1. BREW the tea leaves and lavender together in 8 ounces of just-boiled water, steeping for about 5 minutes to create a strong brew.

2. HEAT the milk, honey, and vanilla in a small saucepan until just simmering, being careful not to let the milk boil, about 3 minutes.

3. STRAIN the brewed tea into a large mug and add the honey-vanilla milk.

MAKES 1 SERVING ||| Prep time: 5 minutes ||| **Total time: 10 minutes**

Did You Know?

If you're drinking tea for the health benefits and not just the flavor, you may want to skip the added milk. It's a debated issue among scientists, but there is some consensus that milk can bind with the beneficial antioxidants in tea, making it tough for the body to absorb them and get the health benefits. If you do need milk, try to use just a splash—tea's flavorful enough already.

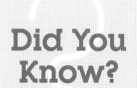

CARDAMOM-GINGER CHAI TEA

- **4 whole green cardamom pods, smashed**
- **2 thin slices (1-inch-diameter) fresh ginger**
- **1 inch cinnamon stick**
- **1 whole clove**
- **1½ cups 1% milk or unsweetened milk alternative**
- **1½ teaspoons loose-leaf black tea**
- **1 teaspoon vanilla extract**
- **1 teaspoon pure maple syrup or honey (optional)**

1. COMBINE 1½ cups water, the cardamom, ginger, cinnamon stick, and clove in a small saucepan. Bring the mixture to a boil. Reduce the heat to low and simmer until the mixture is fragrant, about 3 minutes.

2. ADD the milk, tea leaves, and vanilla and simmer for 1 minute longer. Turn off the heat and let steep for 2 minutes.

3. STRAIN into 2 cups through a fine-mesh sieve (discard the leaves and spices). If desired, sweeten with the maple syrup.

MAKES 2 SERVINGS ||| Prep time: 5 minutes ||| **Total time: 10 minutes**

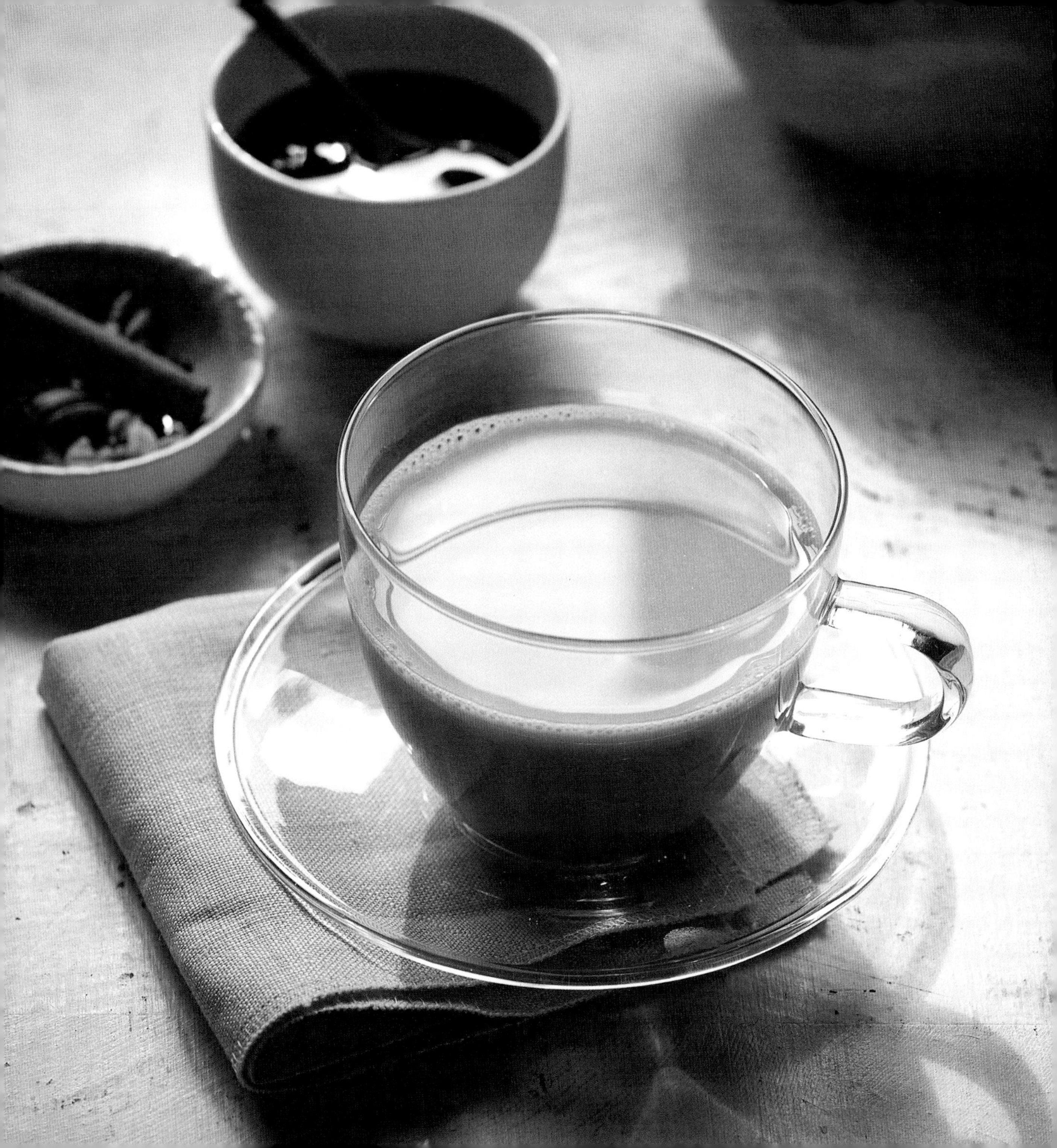

BLACK SESAME BUBBLE TEA

- **1 tablespoon loose-leaf black tea**
- **2 teaspoons honey**
- **½ cup 1% milk or unsweetened milk alternative, such as almond milk**
- **2 tablespoons black sesame paste**
- **2 tablespoons prepared tapioca balls (available online or at Asian markets)**

1. BREW the black tea in 1½ cups just-boiled water. Strain and refrigerate to chill.

2. WHISK the honey into the milk until dissolved.

3. COMBINE the chilled tea, honey-milk, and sesame paste in a container with a lid. Shake together until well combined.

4. DIVIDE between 2 glasses and stir in the tapioca. Sip with a large-diameter bubble tea straw.

MAKES 2 SERVINGS ||| Prep time: 5 minutes ||| **Total time: 5 minutes + chilling time**

Coffee

Coffee is pretty great. The smell, the taste, the fact that it's pretty much undisputedly awesome for you: In fact, coffee has been linked to improved memory and a reduced risk of type 2 diabetes, heart disease, depression, and skin cancer. So keep tipping back that mug, just make sure it contains a quality brew.

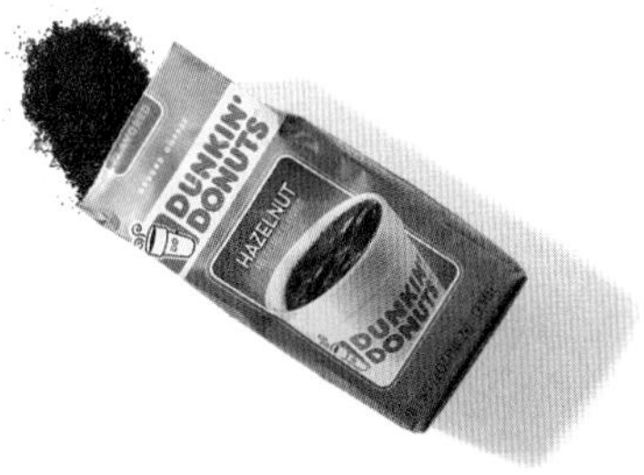

✷

NOT CLEAN

GROUND FLAVORED COFFEE

Flavored coffees—think hazelnut, French vanilla, chocolate frosted donut (yeah, that actually exists)—usually aren't flavored naturally with real hazelnut extract, vanilla beans, or chocolate, but are likely the result of a chemical solvent such as propylene glycol mixed with a flavor compound.

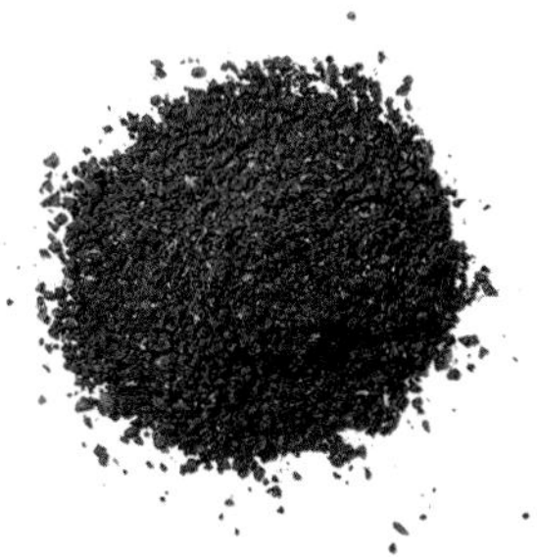

✷✷

CLEAN

WHOLE BEAN OR GROUND COFFEE

When you buy conventional whole bean or ground coffee, you don't really know how it's been processed, or if farmers are getting paid a livable wage. It's still better, however, than flavored varieties.

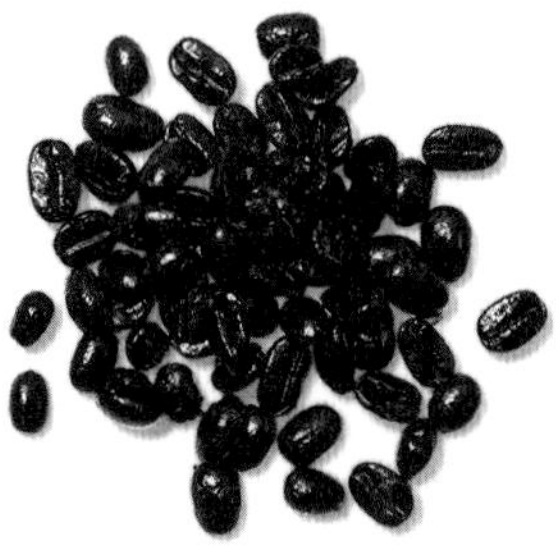

✷✷✷

CLEANEST

ORGANIC FAIR-TRADE WHOLE BEANS THAT YOU GRIND AT HOME

Organic, fair-trade coffee is good for you and the well-being of those who grow it. The Fair Trade certification ensures that coffee farmers are paid a fair price, and organic will ensure that you're limiting your exposure to pesticides and chemicals. Other than that, pick whatever roast you prefer.

TIRAMISU CRÈME

- 1 **cup Homemade Ricotta Cheese (page 212)**
- 1 **tablespoon freshly ground coffee beans**
- 2 **tablespoons sugar**
- ½ **teaspoon cinnamon**
- **Dash of nutmeg**
- 2 **teaspoons vanilla extract**
- 2 **teaspoons unsweetened cocoa powder**

COMBINE all the ingredients in a bowl and mix with a fork or whisk until evenly combined (or puree in a blender or food processor for smoother texture). Chill covered in the refrigerator for at least 1 hour to allow the coffee grounds to soften and the flavors to meld. Serve as a garnish for desserts, or enjoy with a spoon!

MAKES 2 SERVINGS ||| Prep time: 5 minutes ||| **Total time: 5 minutes + chilling time**

Did You Know?

It's actually a myth that dark roast coffees have more caffeine than light. In fact, if you measure your coffee by scoops—like most people do—light roasted coffee will have more caffeine since the beans are denser than a darker roast.

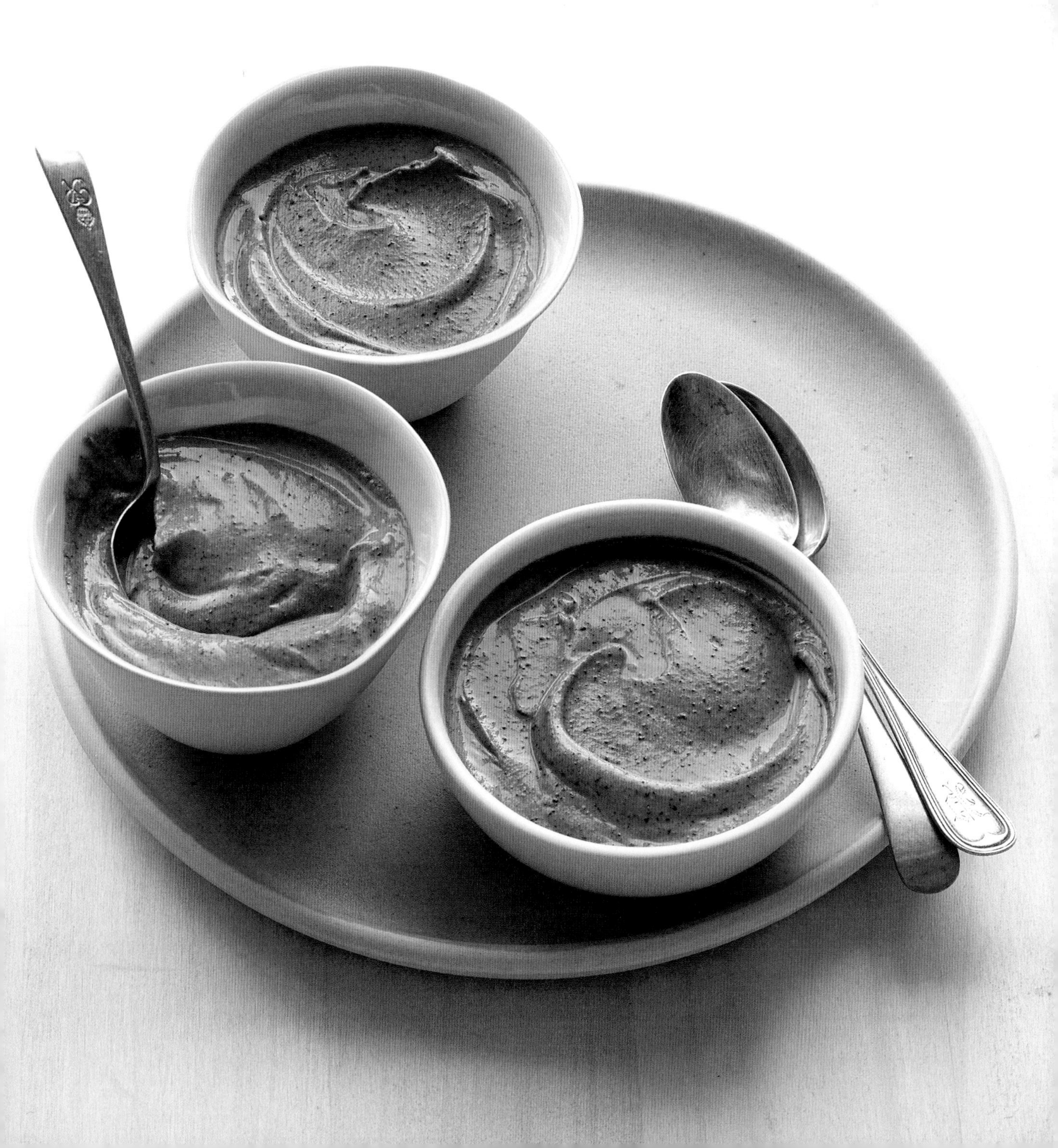

MOCHA PEANUT BUTTER SMOOTHIE

- **3 tablespoons freshly ground coffee beans**
- **½ cup boiling water**
- **¼ cup milk of choice**
- **½ banana (about 4 inches), frozen**
- **1 tablespoon creamy peanut butter**
- **1 tablespoon plus 1 teaspoon unsweetened cocoa powder**
- **1 teaspoon vanilla extract**
- **2 teaspoons sugar**
- **4 ice cubes**

BREW the coffee grounds in a French press with the boiling water for 4 minutes (or brew ½ cup of coffee). Transfer the brewed coffee to a blender and add the milk, banana, peanut butter, cocoa powder, vanilla, sugar, and ice cubes and puree until smooth. Serve immediately.

MAKES 1 OR 2 SERVINGS ||| Prep time: 5 minutes ||| **Total time: 10 minutes**

COFFEE-RUBBED PORK TENDERLOIN & ROASTED BRUSSELS SPROUTS

2 tablespoons freshly ground coffee beans
1 tablespoon ground cumin
½ tablespoon garlic powder
½ tablespoon onion powder
1 tablespoon light brown sugar
½ teaspoon fine sea salt
1 pound pork tenderloin (about 2 inches in diameter and 8 inches long)
2 tablespoons olive oil
2 cups halved brussels sprouts

1. HEAT the oven to 350°F.

2. STIR together the coffee grounds, cumin, garlic powder, onion powder, brown sugar, and ¼ teaspoon of the salt in a bowl.

3. PAT the pork dry and spread the seasonings all over the surface, rubbing in to cover completely.

4. HEAT 1 tablespoon of the olive oil in a skillet over high heat. When hot, add the pork and sear for 1 minute on each of 4 sides, turning until the entire surface is browned.

5. PLACE the brussels sprouts on a nonstick rimmed baking sheet. Sprinkle with the remaining 1 tablespoon oil and remaining ¼ teaspoon salt and toss to coat. Move the sprouts to the sides and place the pork in the center. Roast until the internal temperature of the pork reaches 140°F and the brussels sprouts are dark green and crispy, about 40 minutes. Let the pork stand for 10 minutes before slicing crosswise into ½-inch-thick slices.

MAKES 4 SERVINGS ||| Prep time: 15 minutes ||| **Total time: 1 hour 5 minutes**

Fancy Coffee Drinks

Don't fool yourself: That triple mocha frappuccino is not coffee; it's basically a caffeinated milkshake. But we get it, sometimes you want more than your typical medium roast with a splash of 2%. Luckily, there are ways to feel fancy without all the fat and sugar.

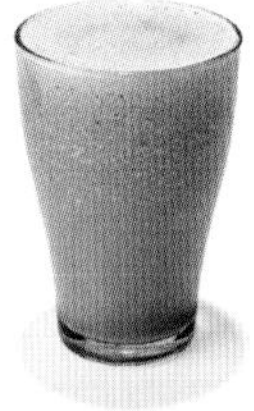

*

NOT CLEAN

FLAVORED AND BLENDED FROZEN COFFEE DRINK

These drinks are absolute no-nos. Some contain more fat and sugar—often in the form of high fructose corn syrup—than the American Heart Association recommends a person consume in an entire day, and as many calories as a meal. Artificial flavors and colors are also common.

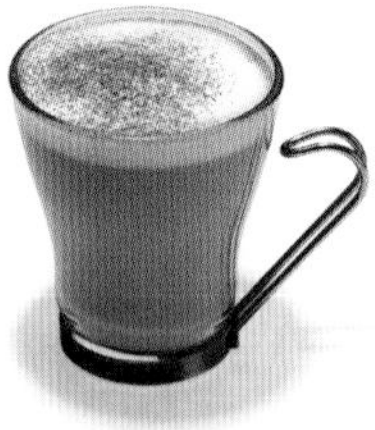

**

CLEAN

REGULAR LATTE

If you can tolerate dairy, a latte is another solid choice, but milk will add fat and calories that you might forget to factor in, and chances are that the milk used won't be organic or grass-fed—of course, you can always ask.

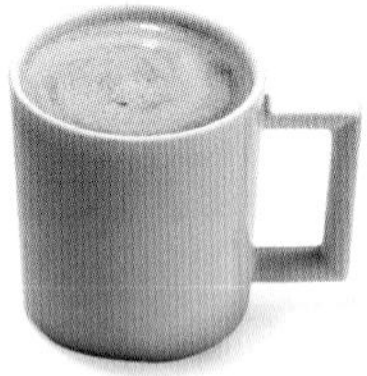

***

CLEANEST

AMERICANO, ESPRESSO, OR COLD BREW

Enjoy a post-dinner espresso instead of that Irish coffee, or have an Americano (simply espresso with hot water) instead of your typical medium roast. Or try a cold-brew iced coffee (coffee grounds slow-steeped in cold water) for a smoother, almost chocolatey tasting version of iced coffee with no extra calories. These are options that maximize flavor without the need for add-ins.

DARK CHOCOLATE ESPRESSO AVOCADO MOUSSE

- ¼ **cup (about 1 ounce) dark chocolate pieces (at least 80% cacao)**
- 1 **avocado, halved and pitted**
- 1 **tablespoon unsweetened vanilla almond milk**
- 1 **tablespoon unsweetened dark cocoa powder**
- 1 **tablespoon honey**
- ¼ **teaspoon vanilla extract**
- 3 **teaspoons espresso**
- **Dash of Himalayan pink salt**

1. MICROWAVE the dark chocolate in a microwaveable bowl in 15-second intervals, stirring in between, until melted and smooth. Set aside to cool slightly.

2. SCRAPE the melted chocolate into a food processor. Scoop the avocado flesh into the processor. Add the almond milk, cocoa powder, honey, vanilla, espresso, and salt. Process until creamy, about 2 minutes.

3. REFRIGERATE for at least 1 hour before serving.

MAKES 2 SERVINGS ||| Prep time: 5 minutes ||| **Total time: 10 minutes**

Did You Know?

Cold-brew coffee has become immensely popular over the last few years, and if you haven't tried it yet, it may be worth the venture. Cold brew tends to be less acidic than regular coffee, so it's gentler on your stomach. Less bite also means it generally needs less milk and sweetener, if you use either, helping to cut down on calories.

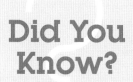

VANILLA ALMOND MOCHA FROZEN FRAPPE

- **4 ounces (2 shots) brewed espresso**
- **2 cups unsweetened vanilla almond milk**
- **1 cup 0% plain Greek yogurt**
- **4 teaspoons honey**
- **4 teaspoons unsweetened cocoa powder**
- **1 teaspoon vanilla extract**

1. POUR the espresso into an ice cube tray and freeze overnight.

2. BLEND the frozen espresso cubes with the almond milk, yogurt, honey, cocoa powder, and vanilla until smooth.

MAKES 2 SERVINGS ||| Prep time: 5 minutes ||| **Total time: 10 minutes + freezing time**

MOCHA BANANA SMOOTHIE

- **2 very ripe bananas, cut into chunks and frozen**
- **¼ cup brewed espresso (or ¼ cup very strong coffee), cooled**
- **½ cup plain 0% Greek yogurt**
- **⅔ cup 1% milk**
- **1 tablespoon unsweetened cocoa powder**
- **Ice cubes (optional)**
- **1 tablespoon cacao nibs**

PROCESS the bananas, espresso, yogurt, milk, and cocoa powder in a blender until smooth. For a frothier smoothie, add ice until you reach your desired consistency. Garnish the smoothie with cacao nibs.

MAKES 2 SERVINGS ||| Prep time: 5 minutes ||| **Total time: 5 minutes**

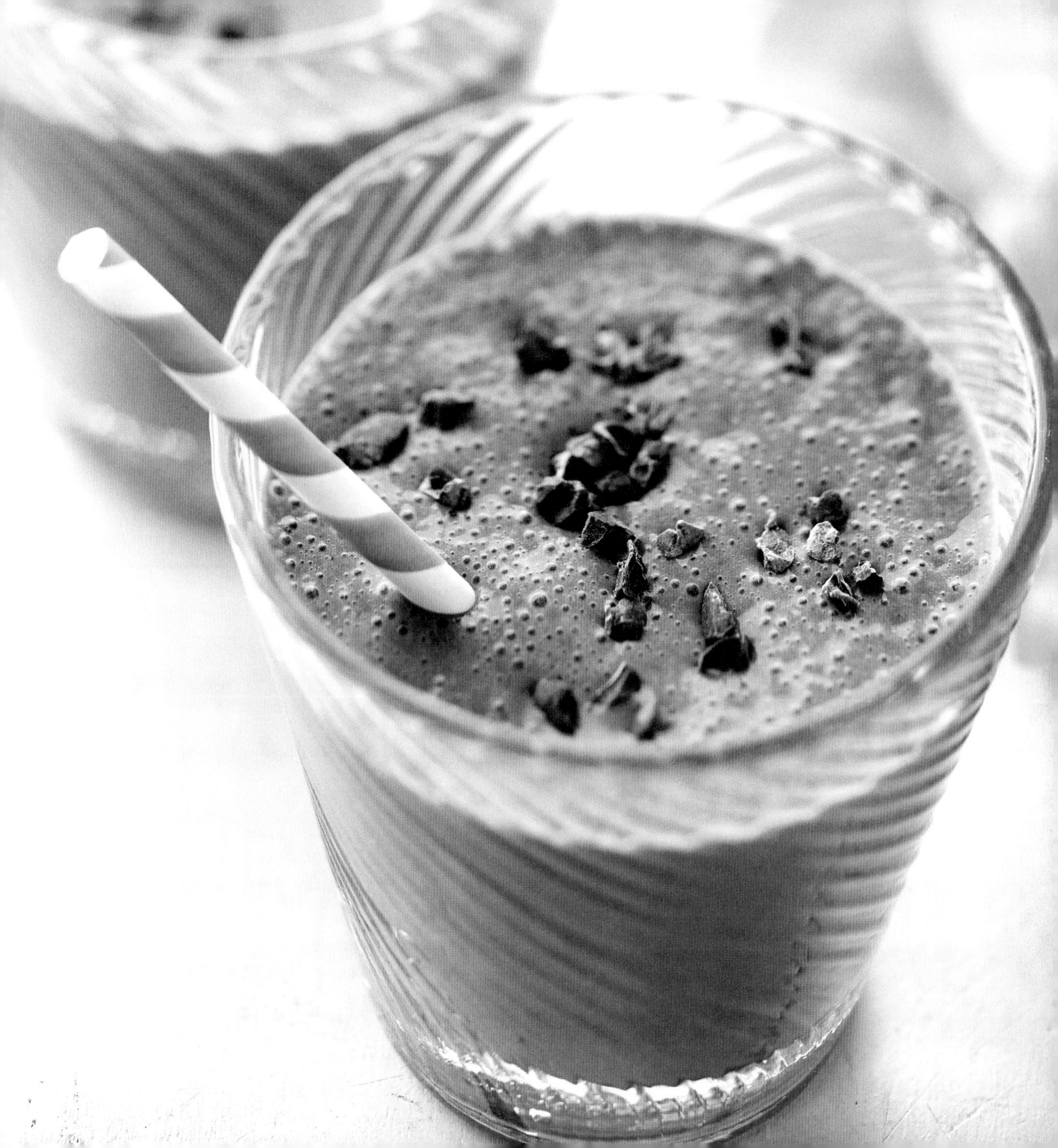

Sugar

We'll be honest, there's no magic sweetener that you can eat with abandon. All should be consumed in moderation and in the context of a healthy diet that emphasizes whole foods. But certain options are certainly less evil and even offer trace nutrients that plain old table sugar doesn't.

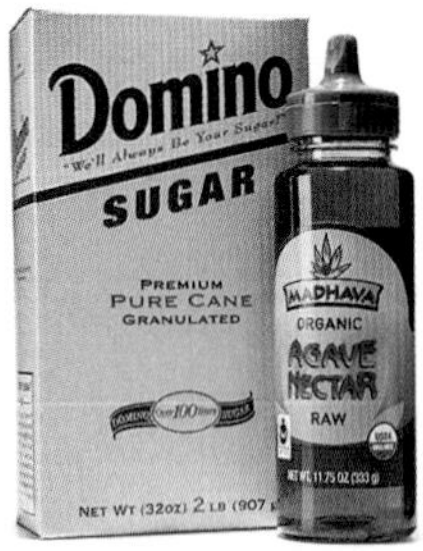

✱

NOT CLEAN

TABLE SUGAR, AGAVE NECTAR

White table sugar consumption has been linked to obesity, type 2 diabetes, dementia, high blood pressure, and heart disease. And agave, once the go-to natural sweetener of the über health conscious, is likely even worse due to it's extremely high fructose content. Too much fructose may contribute to unhealthy changes in liver function, triglyceride levels, and insulin sensitivity.

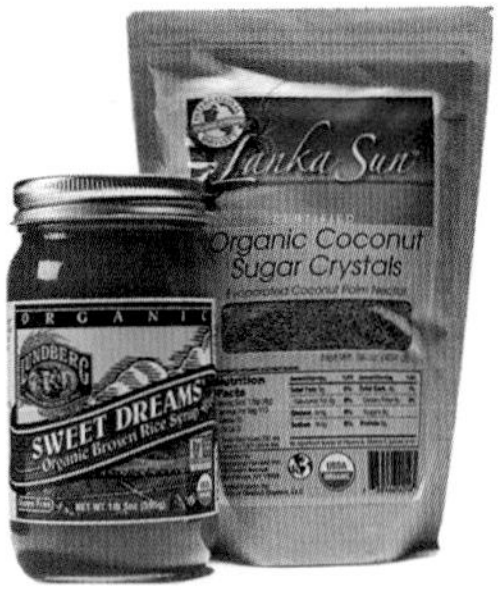

✱✱

CLEAN

COCONUT SUGAR, DATE SUGAR, BROWN RICE SYRUP

Brown rice syrup, date sugar, and coconut sugar are other natural options that are less processed than table sugar, but in terms of added health benefits, they don't offer much, and there's some concern about high levels of arsenic in certain products that contain brown rice syrup.

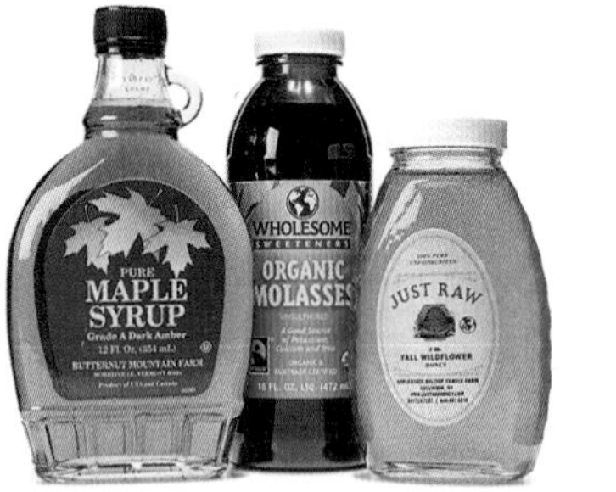

✱✱✱

CLEANEST

RAW LOCAL HONEY, PURE MAPLE SYRUP, OR MOLASSES

Pure maple syrup, raw local honey, and molasses are all clean options that offer trace minerals. Raw honey retains its natural enzymes, and research shows it has antimicrobial properties and may be effective for fighting cold symptoms. Maple syrup and molasses contain antioxidants and an array of minerals such as iron, potassium, magnesium, and calcium.

SPICY MOLASSES BAKED BEANS

- **1 teaspoon grapeseed oil**
- **1 teaspoon minced garlic**
- **¼ cup finely chopped onion**
- **¼ cup low-sodium vegetable broth**
- **2½ tablespoons tomato paste**
- **1 tablespoon plus 1 teaspoon molasses**
- **1 teaspoon honey**
- **1 tablespoon reduced-sodium wheat-free tamari**
- **1½ teaspoons apple cider vinegar**
- **¼ teaspoon yellow mustard**
- **½ teaspoon dried oregano**
- **¼ teaspoon paprika**
- **½ teaspoon chili powder**
- **1 cup cooked navy beans**

1. **HEAT** the oven to 350°F.

2. **HEAT** the oil in a small skillet over medium-low heat. Add the garlic and onion and cook until the onions turn translucent, about 5 minutes.

3. **WHISK** together the broth, tomato paste, molasses, honey, tamari, vinegar, mustard, oregano, paprika, and chili powder in a medium bowl. Stir in the beans and sautéed onion. Pour into a 1-quart baking dish.

4. **BAKE** until the edges start to bubble, 20 to 25 minutes. Serve hot.

MAKES 2 SERVINGS ||| Prep time: 10 minutes ||| **Total time: 40 minutes**

HEALTHY HACK

It may seem a bit counterintuitive, but a tiny pinch of salt can enhance the natural sweetness in many ingredients and dishes, allowing you to use less sweetener. The trick works especially well with fresh fruit, so before you add something to sweeten that next smoothie, try a little salt and taste it again. The natural sweetness will be more pronounced.

HONEY-SOY GLAZED BAKED TOFU WITH VEGGIES

- Half of a 14-ounce block extra-firm tofu, cubed
- 1 teaspoon sesame oil
- 2 teaspoons minced garlic
- ½ teaspoon ground ginger
- ¼ cup low-sodium vegetable broth
- 2 tablespoons reduced-sodium wheat-free tamari
- 2 tablespoons honey
- ⅛ teaspoon red-pepper flakes
- 1 teaspoon grapeseed oil
- 1½ cups chopped broccoli florets
- ½ cup finely chopped onion
- ½ cup chopped red bell pepper
- 2 cups cooked brown rice (optional)

1. **HEAT** the oven to 400°F.

2. **TOSS** the tofu with the sesame oil. Arrange on a baking sheet and bake until the tofu is golden, about 20 minutes, turning over halfway.

3. **COMBINE** the garlic, ginger, broth, tamari, honey, and pepper flakes. Set the glaze aside.

4. **HEAT** the grapeseed oil in a wok or medium skillet over high heat. Add the broccoli, onion, and bell pepper. Cook until the pepper is softened and the onion is translucent, about 5 minutes. Reduce the heat to medium, cover, and let steam until the broccoli and pepper are crisp-tender, about 3 minutes.

5. **POUR** the glaze over the vegetables. Add the tofu and stir. Cook until just a small amount of liquid is left in the pan, about 3 minutes. Serve alone or with brown rice.

MAKES 2 SERVINGS ||| Prep time: 15 minutes ||| **Total time: 25 minutes**

Flour

Chances are you've been getting the same type of flour on autopilot since you started buying your own groceries. But switching from an ultraprocessed and bleached version of this staple to one that incorporates the whole grain can be a huge first step in cleaning up your diet.

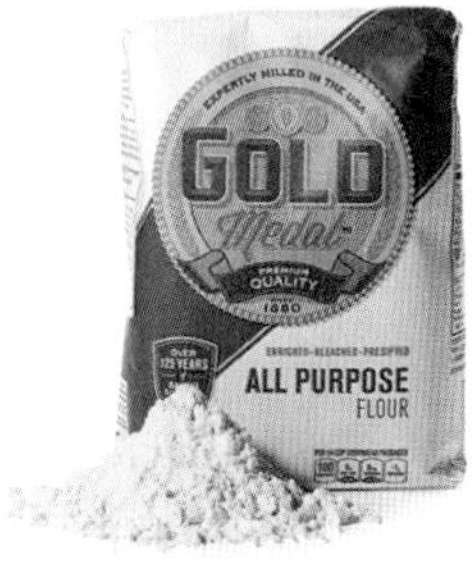

*

NOT CLEAN

REGULAR ALL-PURPOSE FLOUR

Regular all-purpose flour is best avoided as it quickly spikes blood sugar and may contain alloxan, a chemical left over from the bleaching process. Alloxan has been shown to produce diabetes in animals, likely because it can destroy cells in the pancreas, but the effect of small quantities like this on humans is unknown.

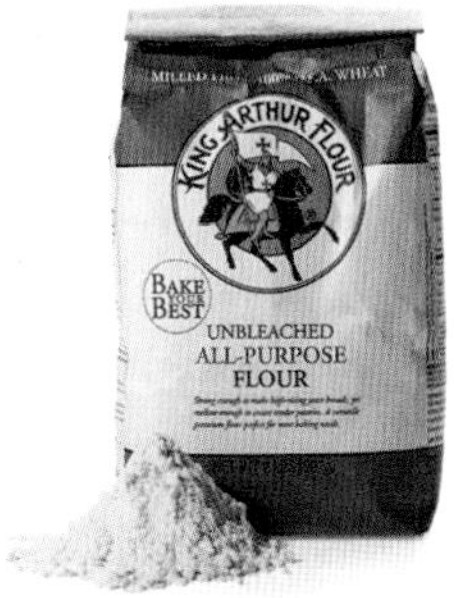

**

CLEAN

UNBLEACHED ALL-PURPOSE FLOUR

These flours are missing the healthiest parts of the plant—the wheat bran and germ—and have little protein and fiber as a result. A diet full of refined flours puts you at greater risk for cardiovascular disease, type 2 diabetes, and obesity. But they are free of the chemical used in the bleaching process, which makes them your second best choice.

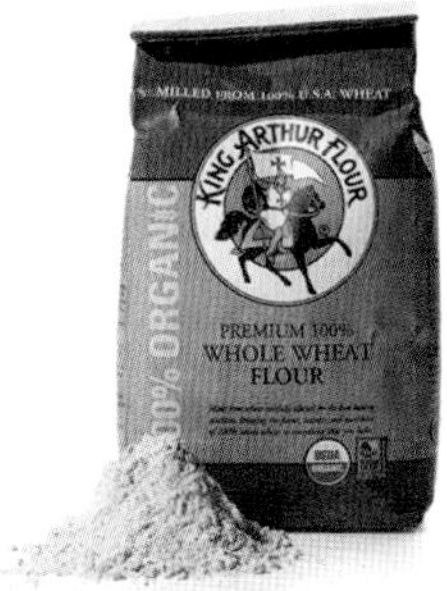

***

CLEANEST

WHOLE-GRAIN FLOUR

Swap out white flour for whole wheat flour. Not only will it add a more complex, nutty flavor to baked goods, but whole grains are nutrient-rich, featuring protein, fiber, B vitamins, antioxidants, and minerals. Bonus: A recent study showed that people who eat whole grains have less abdominal fat.

COCONUT-BANANA PANCAKES

- 1 egg
- ½ cup coconut milk
- 1 teaspoon vanilla extract
- ½ large or 1 small ripe banana
- ¼ cup whole wheat flour
- ¼ cup oat flour (or grind rolled oats in a food processor)
- ¼ cup unsweetened coconut flakes, finely ground
- 2 teaspoons baking powder
- Fine sea salt
- 1 tablespoon coconut oil
- Pure maple syrup, berries, confectioners' sugar, or nut butter, for topping

1. COMBINE the egg, coconut milk, vanilla, and banana in a blender or food processor and puree until smooth. Add the whole wheat flour, oat flour, ground coconut, baking powder, and a dash of salt and pulse 5 to 7 times until evenly combined (but not overmixed).

2. HEAT the oil in a large skillet or griddle over medium-high heat. When hot, pour small dollops of batter (about 4 inches in diameter) onto the oil. When bubbles form on the batter surface, flip and brown the second side.

3. SERVE with toppings of choice.

MAKES 2 SERVINGS (8 TO 10 SMALL PANCAKES TOTAL) ||| Prep time: 5 minutes ||| **Total time: 15 minutes**

Keep it Fresh!

Consider storing your whole-grain flour in the fridge. Unlike all-purpose flour, whole-grain still contains the bran and germ, which are high in nutrients and oils that make them more prone to spoilage. Refrigeration will extend your flour's shelf life and ensure your baked goods have no off flavors.

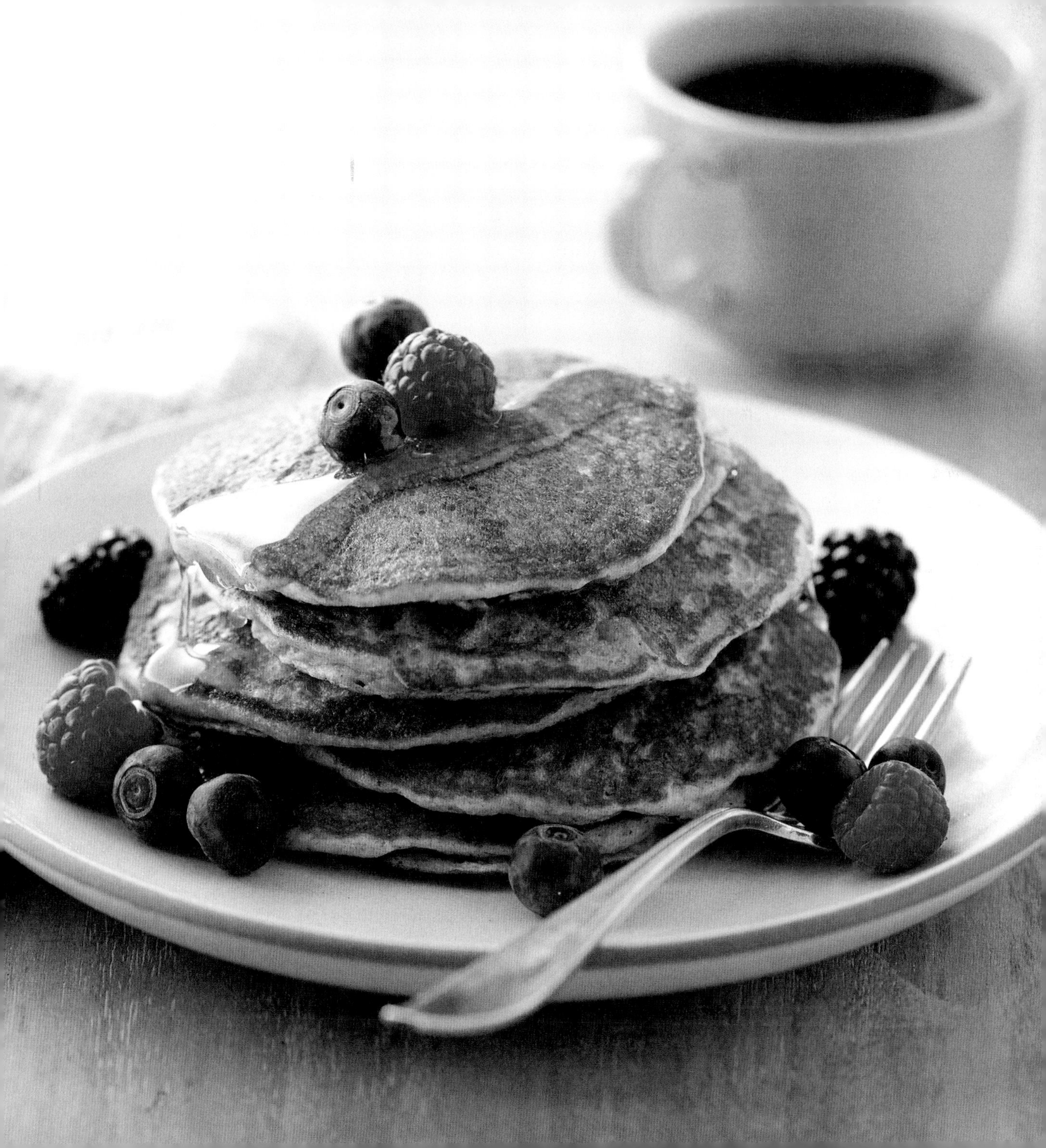

WHOLE WHEAT LUNCH CREPES

- ½ cup 1% milk
- 1 large egg, lightly beaten
- 1 cup whole wheat flour
- ½ teaspoon garlic powder
- 2 tablespoons extra virgin olive oil
- Fillings: Cheese, greens, lunchmeat, or other savory items

1. WHISK together ¼ cup water, the milk, and egg. Gently stir in the flour, garlic powder, and 1 tablespoon of the olive oil.

2. HEAT 1 teaspoon of the remaining oil in a 9-inch skillet over medium-high heat until hot (but not smoking). Pour about ½ cup batter into the pan and tilt to swirl until it evenly reaches the edges of the pan. Cook until small bubbles rise. Flip over once and cook until lightly golden brown. Transfer to a plate. Repeat with the remaining oil and batter.

3. SERVE with fillings of choice.

MAKES 2 SERVINGS (2 CREPES EACH) ||| Prep time: 15 minutes ||| Total time: 15 minutes

WARM BERRY BREAKFAST BARS

- ¼ **cup chia seeds**
- ½ **cup unsweetened coconut flakes**
- ½ **cup whole wheat flour**
- 1 **cup pitted dates**
- 1 **cup rolled oats**
- ¼ **cup light brown sugar**
- 2 **tablespoons coconut oil**
- 1 **cup sliced almonds**
- 3 **tablespoons peanut butter**
- 1 **teaspoon vanilla extract**
- ½ **cup plain 2% Greek yogurt**
- 1 **tablespoon granulated sugar**
- ½ **cup blueberries**

1. **HEAT** the oven to 350°F. Grease a small baking pan (8 x 6 inches works well) or a 9 x 5-inch loaf pan.

2. **STIR** together the chia seeds and 1 cup water in a small bowl. Let sit for 5 minutes until the mixture forms a loose gel.

3. **COMBINE** the coconut flakes, flour, dates, and ½ cup of the oats in a food processor. Pulse until the dates are broken into small crumb-size pieces and distributed evenly. Pulse in the brown sugar and coconut oil to combine. Transfer the flour mixture to a large bowl. Stir in the almonds, peanut butter, vanilla, soaked chia seeds, and the remaining ½ cup oats until thoroughly blended.

4. **PUREE** the yogurt, granulated sugar, and blueberries in a food processor until smooth.

5. **PRESS** the oat mixture evenly into the baking pan. Pour the blueberry yogurt mixture on top. Bake for 55 minutes. Cut into 8 bars.

MAKES 8 BARS ||| Prep time: 15 minutes ||| **Total time: 1 hour 10 minutes**

Cooking Oil

From olive to coconut to flax, it's no secret that oils are having a major culinary moment. Good thing, too, since most of them are rich in healthy fats that'll help keep your heart in tip-top shape. But what's the smartest way to fit all of these different lipids into your kitchen repertoire?

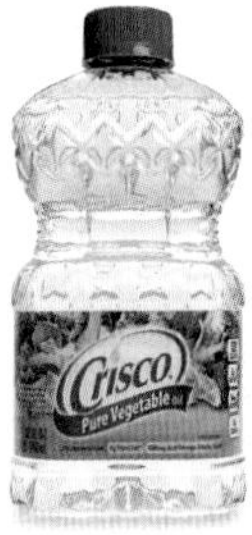

*

NOT CLEAN

CONVENTIONAL (USES HEXANE OR CHEMICAL EXTRACTION)

The chemicals used during this process are toxic—hexane is classified as a neurotoxin by the CDC, as it's destructive to nerve tissue when inhaled (little is known about the effects of consumption). These toxins then need to be removed from the oil in a deordorization, a process that involves steaming oils with extremely high temperatures (often over 500°F), which can damage fatty acids and speed up oxidation, causing oils to go rancid. No thanks.

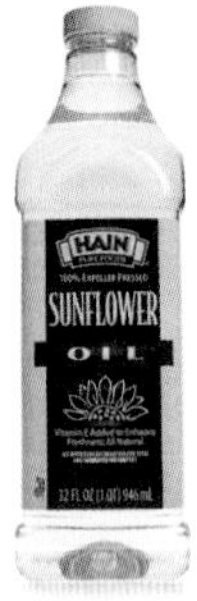

**

CLEAN

EXPELLER-PRESSED

While organic is the safest choice because you're limiting your exposure to pesticides, at the very least, make sure your oil is expeller-pressed and not conventionally extracted with hexane, a toxic chemical, or deodorized with dangerously high temperatures that can damage the oil's fatty acids.

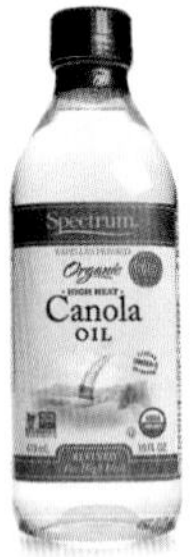

***

CLEANEST

ORGANIC EXPELLER-PRESSED

Olive oil, canola oil, coconut oil, sesame oil, and sunflower oil are all healthy options for clean eating. But while the type of oil you choose is important, so is the method that's used to make it. To keep the food you're cooking clean, buy organic expeller-pressed oils.

CHILE, GARLIC & GINGER–INFUSED SESAME OIL

1 **bottle (8 ounces) expeller-pressed sesame oil**

4 **cloves garlic, fresh or roasted, peeled, and smashed (see Note)**

2 **slices (¼-inch) jalapeño or other medium-heat chile**

1 **slice (¼-inch) fresh ginger, lightly crushed**

1. **COMBINE** the sesame oil, garlic, jalapeño, and ginger in a small saucepan. Heat over low heat until the mixture starts to lightly bubble, about 5 minutes. Remove from the heat and let cool thoroughly.

2. **DISCARD** the garlic and jalapeño. Transfer to an airtight container and store in the refrigerator for up to 1 month.

Note: If you prefer to use roasted garlic, here are the instructions for roasting: Preheat the oven to 425°F. Cut the top off a head of garlic so that the garlic cloves are exposed. Drizzle 1 teaspoon olive oil over the exposed garlic tops. Wrap in foil and bake until golden, about 30 minutes.

MAKES 1 CUP ||| Prep time: 5 minutes ||| **Total time: 5 minutes + cooling time**

Did You Know?

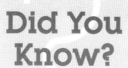

Canola oil has gotten a bad rap over the years, but it is actually one of the most heart-healthy oils out there. Canola oil is actually higher in anti-inflammatory omega-3s than most vegetable oils (including olive oil!), which may help reduce your risk of inflammatory illnesses like heart disease and cancer. The reason it's misunderstood is that much of it is produced from genetically modified plants, and extracted with the chemical solvent hexane. You can avoid these issues and reap canola's benefits by buying organic expeller-pressed oils.

ROSEMARY & SUNFLOWER SEED OAT CRACKERS

- **⅓ cup whole wheat flour**
- **⅓ cup rolled oats**
- **¼ teaspoon coarse sea salt**
- **½ teaspoon dried rosemary**
- **1 tablespoon sunflower oil**
- **½ teaspoon honey**
- **¼ cup plus 1 tablespoon sunflower seeds**

1. HEAT the oven to 425°F.

2. STIR together the flour, oats, salt, and ¼ teaspoon of the rosemary in a small bowl.

3. STIR in the oil, honey, and 3 tablespoons water. Mix with your hands until a sticky dough forms. Knead in the ¼ cup sunflower seeds and form the dough into a ball, adding more flour if needed to make the dough dry enough to handle.

4. ROLL the dough out on a floured surface as thin as you can get it without it tearing. Aim for the thickness of a tortilla.

5. BRUSH the surface lightly with water and sprinkle on the remaining 1 tablespoon sunflower seeds and ¼ teaspoon rosemary. Cut into 1-inch squares. Prick the center of each cracker with a skewer to make a single hole (or multiple holes, depending on your aesthetic preference).

6. BAKE on an ungreased baking sheet until crisp and golden, 8 to 10 minutes. Transfer to a wire rack and cool completely before serving.

MAKES 50 CRACKERS ||| Prep time: 5 minutes ||| **Total time: 15 minutes**

Protein Powder

Protein powder can instantly make a smoothie more satisfying and boost muscle-building potential after a workout. According to most experts, as long as you don't have an intolerance, your best bet is whey—a complete protein that enters your bloodstream quickly and contains a high amount of leucine, an amino acid that delivers energy to muscles. But still, choose your whey wisely.

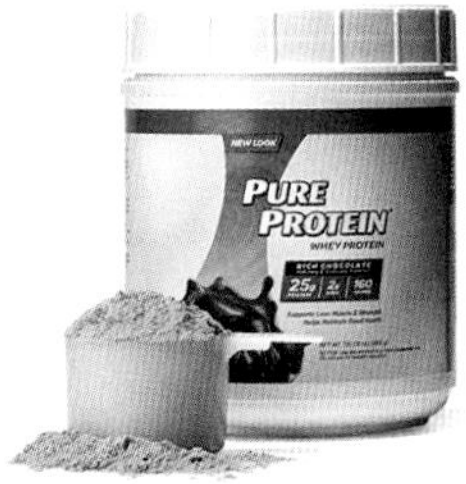

✷

NOT CLEAN

WHEY PROTEIN WITH ADDED SUGAR

Steer clear of whey proteins that have been flavored, or sweetened with sugar or artificial sweeteners to make them more palatable. These are often highly processed and contain corn- and soy-based ingredients.

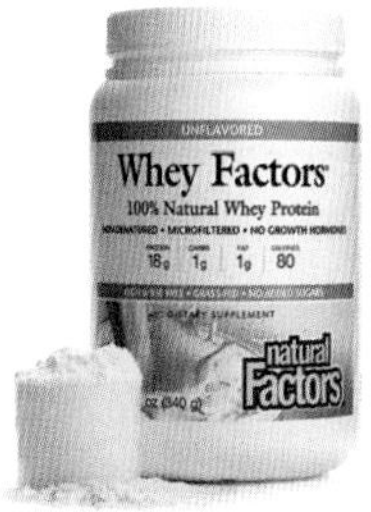

✷✷

CLEAN

WHEY PROTEIN ISOLATE OR HYDROLYSATE WITH SHORT INGREDIENT LIST

Whey protein isolate and hydrolysate are two other good options, delivering high amounts of protein, but you can't be guaranteed that they're made from high-quality, organic dairy. Plus, a recent study found that some whey protein isolates contained trace amount of harmful metals, so be sure to buy yours from a reputable source.

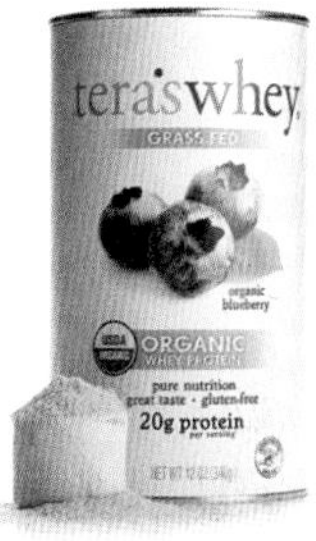

✷✷✷

CLEANEST

CONCENTRATED WHEY PROTEIN FROM ORGANIC GRASS-FED DAIRY

Your cleanest whey protein powder will be a whey concentrate (80% protein) that's organic and made with milk from grass-fed cows. This means your powder contains no hormones, pesticides, or additives. No other variations of whey protein (e.g., isolate and hydrolysate) meet these specifications.

BLUEBERRY PROTEIN PANCAKES

- **½ cup rolled oats**
- **1 tablespoon unflavored whey protein powder**
- **¼ teaspoon baking powder**
- **¼ teaspoon fine sea salt**
- **1 medium banana, mashed**
- **1 large egg**
- **½ teaspoon vanilla extract**
- **⅓ cup fresh or frozen blueberries**
- **1 teaspoon coconut oil**

1. **PULSE** the oats in a blender or food processor to a flour consistency. Transfer to a medium bowl.

2. **ADD** the protein powder, baking powder, and salt to the oats.

3. **WHISK** together the banana, egg, and vanilla in a separate bowl until smooth.

4. **FOLD** the oat mixture into the banana mixture until just smooth. Gently stir in the blueberries.

5. **HEAT** a skillet over medium heat. Add 1 teaspoon coconut oil. Pour about ¼ cup batter onto the skillet for each pancake. Cook until small bubbles begin to appear on the surface of the pancakes, then flip and cook until browned on the second side, about 3 minutes total.

MAKES 2 SERVINGS ||| Prep time: 5 minutes ||| **Total time: 15 minutes**

HEALTHY HACK

Don't just use protein powder for smoothies or shakes. Consider adding a scoop or two to your next batch of cookies, muffins, granola bars, or oatmeal to help thicken treats while infusing them with more stomach-filling, sugar-stabilizing protein.

PINEAPPLE & AVOCADO GREEN PROTEIN SMOOTHIE

- **2 cups 1% milk or unsweetened milk alternative such as almond milk**
- **1 banana, frozen**
- **1 cup chopped pineapple, frozen**
- **¼ avocado**
- **2 cups spinach**
- **¼ cup parsley sprigs**
- **2 tablespoons unflavored whey protein powder**
- **1 teaspoon chia seeds (optional)**

COMBINE all the ingredients (except the chia seeds) in a blender and process until smooth, 2 to 5 minutes depending on the power of your blender. If desired, stir in chia seeds before drinking.

MAKES 2 SERVINGS ||| Prep time: 3 minutes ||| **Total time: 5 minutes + freezing time (for the fruit)**

PROTEIN-PACKED CARROT-GINGER SOUP

- 1 tablespoon olive oil
- 1 rib celery, chopped
- 1 cup chopped onion
- 1½ tablespoons minced fresh ginger
- 2 teaspoons minced garlic
- 1 leek, white and light green parts, thinly sliced
- 4 cups vegetable stock
- 4 cups chopped carrots (about 1½ pounds)
- 1 can (15 ounces) white beans, rinsed and drained
- ½ teaspoon fine sea salt
- ½ teaspoon black pepper
- 2 ounces (about ¼ cup) unflavored whey protein powder
- 2 tablespoons plain 0% Greek yogurt
- 2 tablespoons chopped fresh chives

1. HEAT the olive oil in a Dutch oven or large saucepan over medium heat. Add the celery and onion and cook until soft, about 10 minutes.

2. ADD the ginger and garlic and cook until fragrant, about 2 minutes longer. Add the leek, vegetable stock, carrots, and beans and bring to a simmer. Cook until the carrots are soft, about 25 minutes. Remove from the heat.

3. STIR the protein powder into the soup, 2 tablespoons at a time, until incorporated. Add the salt and pepper. Blend the soup in the pot with an immersion blender until smooth (or puree in a stand blender).

4. TOP each serving with Greek yogurt and chives

MAKES 2 TO 4 SERVINGS ||| Prep time: 10 minutes ||| **Total time: 55 minutes**

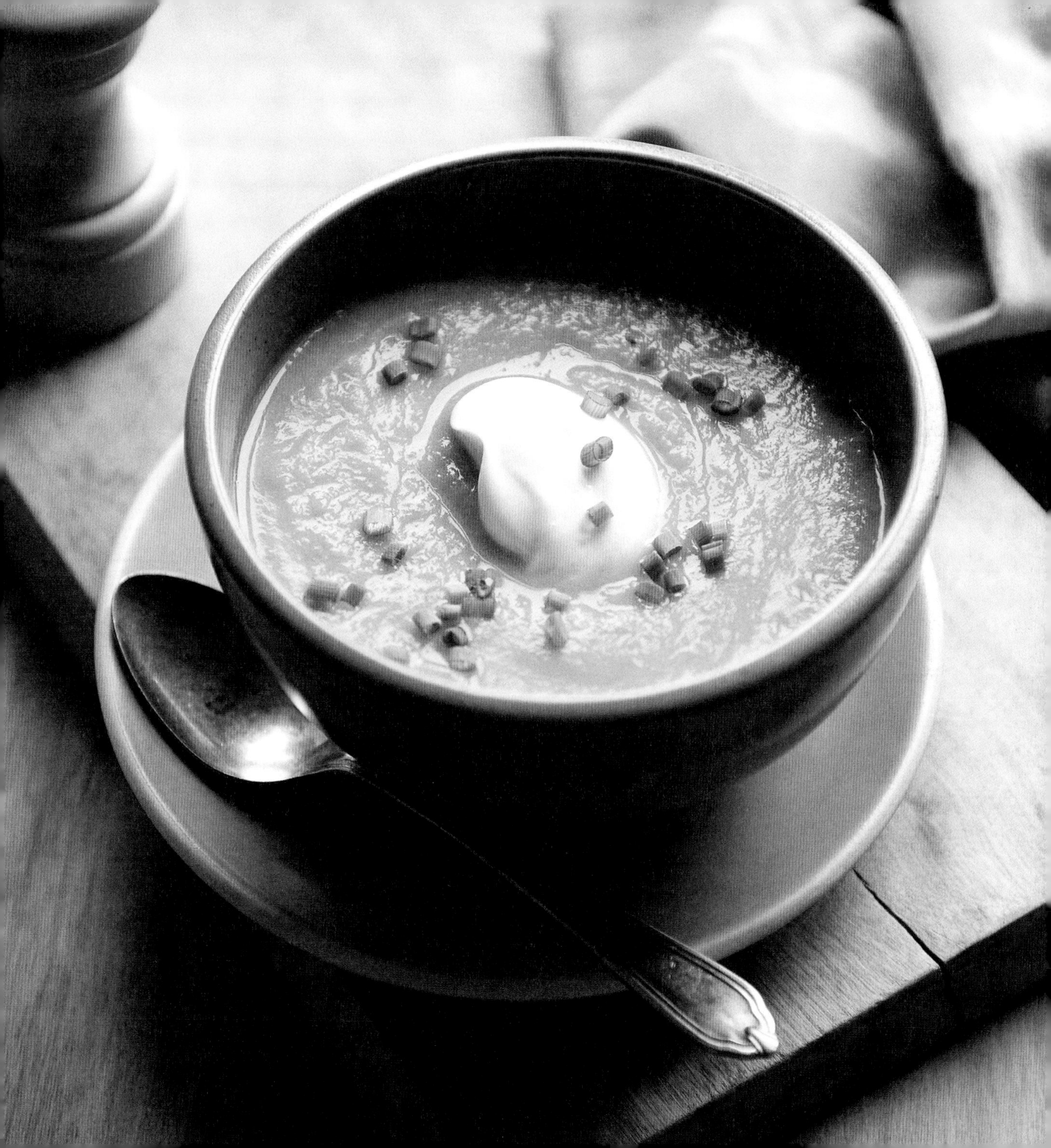

Umami Flavor

Umami is considered the fifth of our basic primary tastes:

sweet, sour, salty, bitter, umami. This literally translates from the Japanese as "savory" and can add an incredibly satisfying depth of flavor to meals. Just be sure you're getting it from safe, natural sources.

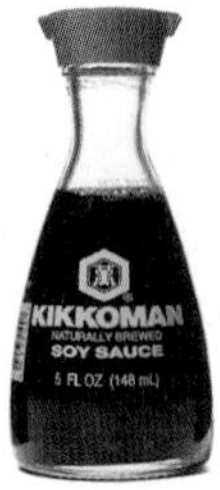

*

NOT CLEAN

SOY SAUCE

While soy sauce may be the most familiar form of umami flavor, it's the least clean. Like tamari, soy sauce is extremely high in sodium and often made from soybeans that are genetically modified. Surprisingly, it's also made with wheat.

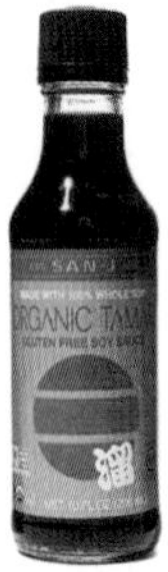

**

CLEAN

WHEAT-FREE TAMARI

Tamari is basically gluten-free soy sauce and a byproduct of fermented soybeans. While it's high in sodium and doesn't have all the benefits of mushrooms, it is believed to help in digestion. To ensure you're getting a product free of GMOs, go organic.

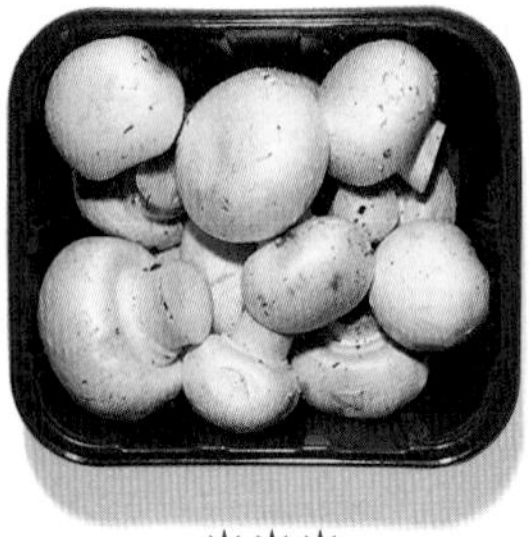

***

CLEANEST

ORGANIC MUSHROOMS

Consider incorporating more sautéed or roasted mushrooms into your dishes. In addition to their savory, almost-meaty flavor, mushrooms contain a type of fiber called beta-glucan, which helps lower cholesterol and improve cardiovascular health and helps protect against cold, flu, and other viruses.

CHANTERELLE MUSHROOM & ROOT VEGETABLE LATKES WITH SPICED PEACH BUTTER

- ½ **cup shredded parsnips**
- ½ **cup shredded sweet potato**
- ½ **cup shredded russet potato**
- ½ **cup finely chopped chanterelle mushrooms (about 2 ounces)**
- ¼ **cup finely chopped red or yellow onion**
- ½ **teaspoon minced garlic**
- ½ **teaspoon chopped thyme**
- 2 **teaspoons chopped dill**
- 2 **teaspoons chopped parsley**
- ⅛ **teaspoon fine sea salt**
- ¼ **teaspoon black pepper**
- ¼ **teaspoon ground cumin**
- ⅛ **teaspoon red-pepper flakes**
- 3 **tablespoons whole wheat flour**
- 1 **large egg, lightly beaten**
- ½ **teaspoon balsamic vinegar**
- 1 **tablespoon grapeseed oil**
- ¼ **cup Spiced Peach Butter (page 47)**

1. PLACE the shredded parsnips, sweet potato, and potato in a colander lined with paper towels. Set aside for 20 minutes. Squeeze the mixture over the sink to remove excess moisture.

2. TRANSFER the potato mixture to a medium bowl. Stir in the mushrooms, onion, garlic, thyme, dill, and parsley.

3. COMBINE the salt, pepper, cumin, pepper flakes, and flour in a small bowl. Add the flour mixture and egg to the potato mixture. Drizzle with the vinegar and stir well to combine.

4. HEAT ½ tablespoon of the oil in a large skillet over medium-high heat. Divide and form the batter into 4 patties. Place 2 of the latkes in the pan and cook until browned, 3 to 4 minutes on each side. Set aside on a plate lined with paper towel or a cutting board. Repeat with the remaining oil and batter.

5. SERVE with the peach butter.

MAKES 2 SERVINGS (2 LATKES EACH) ||| Prep time: 25 minutes ||| **Total time: 35 minutes + 20 minutes standing time**

PORCINI MUSHROOM MANICOTTI WITH HOMEMADE RICOTTA CHEESE

MANICOTTI SHELLS

- **1 large egg**
- **¼ cup plus 2 tablespoons 2% milk or unsweetened milk alternative**
- **1½ tablespoons plus 1 teaspoon unsalted butter, melted**
- **½ cup whole wheat flour**
- **Fine sea salt**

SAUCE

- **½ tablespoon unsalted butter**
- **1½ cups chopped fresh porcini mushrooms (6 ounces)**
- **¼ cup chopped red or yellow onion**
- **2 teaspoons minced garlic**
- **2 tablespoons dry white wine**
- **½ cup 2% milk or unsweetened milk alternative**
- **2 tablespoons whole wheat flour**
- **1 cup low-sodium vegetable broth**
- **½ cup chopped fresh basil**

1. MAKE the manicotti shells: Combine the egg, ¼ cup water, milk, 1½ tablespoons of the melted butter, the flour, and a dash of salt in a blender. Pulse for about 30 seconds, or until blended and smooth.

2. PLACE a medium nonstick skillet over medium-high heat and add ¼ teaspoon of the melted butter to the pan. Pour ⅓ cup of batter in the pan and swirl to spread evenly. Cook for 30 seconds on one side, and 10 seconds on the other side. Set aside on a plate or cutting board. Repeat, adding another ¼ teaspoon melted butter each time, until all of the batter has been used. You should end up with 4 crepes.

3. MAKE the sauce: Melt the butter in a medium skillet over medium-low heat. Add the mushrooms and onion. Cook until the mushrooms are softened and the onion is translucent, about 10 minutes, stirring every few minutes to ensure that it does not burn. Add the garlic and cook until browned, about 2 minutes. Add the wine and cook for 5 minutes longer. Use a wooden spoon or wire whisk to slowly stir in the milk and flour. Let cook, stirring frequently, until slightly thickened, about 1 minute. Pour the vegetable broth slowly into the sauce, whisking or stirring the mixture thoroughly to prevent lumps. Cook until thickened to the consistency of cake batter, about 10 minutes. Stir in the basil.

4. HEAT the oven to 375°F.

5. PREPARE the filling: Combine the ricotta, egg, Parmesan, mozzarella, basil, parsley, and rosemary in a medium bowl.

FILLING

- 1 cup Homemade Ricotta Cheese (page 212)
- 1 large egg
- ¼ cup grated Parmesan
- ¼ cup shredded part-skim mozzarella
- 2 tablespoons chopped fresh basil
- 2 tablespoons chopped fresh curly parsley
- 1 tablespoon finely chopped fresh rosemary

- ¼ cup grated Parmesan

6. SPREAD half of the sauce in the bottom of an ungreased 8 x 8-inch glass baking dish. Scoop and spread one-fourth of the filling down the middle of a manicotti shell. Roll up and place in the baking dish. Repeat with the remaining manicotti shells and filling. Pour the rest of the sauce on top of the shells and spread to cover. Sprinkle the ¼ cup Parmesan on top.

7. COVER with foil and bake for 10 minutes. Remove the foil and bake until the sauce is bubbling, about 10 minutes longer. Let stand for a few minutes before serving.

MAKES 2 SERVINGS ||| Prep time: 25 minutes ||| **Total time: 1 hour 10 minutes**

SMART SWAP

Want to get max nutrition out of your next cheesey meal? Skip the low-fat stuff. Two recent studies in the *American Journal of Clinical Nutrition* suggest that whole-fat dairy—what nutritionists have been telling us to shun for years—might actually be healthier in two major ways. In one study, researchers found that people who consumed more low-fat and nonfat dairy like milk and cheese also ate significantly more carbs, while those who consumed mostly whole-fat dairy ate fewer carbs. In the second study, whole-fat dairy like yogurt and cheese was associated with a 23% reduced risk of developing type 2 diabetes while eating low-fat and nonfat dairy had no benefit.

STUFFED PORTOBELLO MUSHROOMS

- **1 tablespoon grapeseed oil or unsalted butter**
- **1¾ cups chopped yellow or red onions**
- **½ teaspoon balsamic vinegar**
- **1¼ cups vegetable broth**
- **½ cup semi-pearled farro**
- **1 large egg, lightly beaten**
- **3 tablespoons low-fat plain yogurt**
- **Fine sea salt and black pepper**
- **2 portobello mushroom caps, stemmed**
- **½ cup crumbled feta cheese (2 ounces)**

1. HEAT the oil or butter in a cast-iron skillet over low heat. Add the onions and stir to coat evenly. Let cook until caramelized, about 45 minutes, stirring every 5 to 10 minutes. Stir in the balsamic vinegar.

2. MEANWHILE, bring the broth and farro to a boil in a medium saucepan. Reduce the heat to medium-low, cover, and simmer until the farro is tender, about 30 minutes. Transfer to a medium bowl and set aside.

3. HEAT the oven to 350°F. Line a baking sheet with heavy-duty foil and lightly oil the foil.

4. STIR the egg, yogurt, a dash of salt and pepper, and sautéed onions into the bowl of farro.

5. SET the mushroom caps on the prepared baking sheet and scoop the farro stuffing into each of the mushroom caps. Bake for 35 minutes, or until the farro stuffing is set.

6. SPRINKLE the mushrooms with feta cheese before serving.

MAKES 2 SERVINGS ||| Prep time: 20 minutes ||| **Total time: 2 hours 15 minutes**

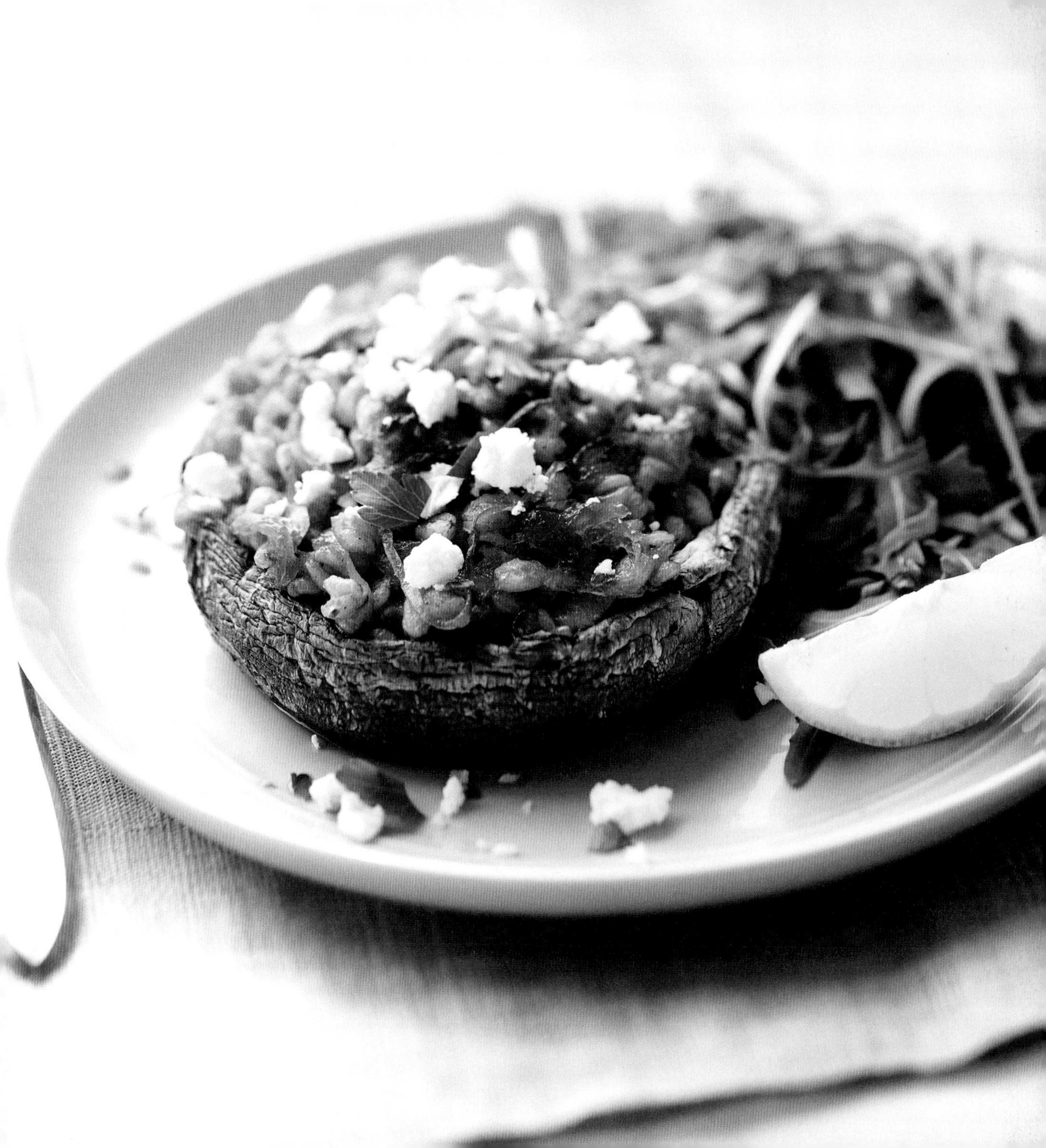

Packaged Soups/Broths

Soup is one of those comforting, soothing meals that never gets old. But unfortunately, most store-bought soup is loaded with preservatives or packed in cans that contain toxic chemicals. Consider making your own to get only the perks.

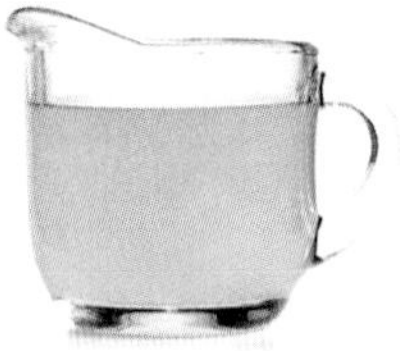

*

NOT CLEAN

SOUP AND BROTH IN CANS

Unless specified on the label, the epoxy lining of cans generally contains BPS and BPA, two chemicals that have been associated with hormone disruption, prostate cancer, diabetes, obesity, and aggressive behavior in children. A few brands such as Eden Organics, offer canned soups free of BPA and BPS. Canned soup also often contains excessive levels of sodium, sugar, artificial colors, and preservatives.

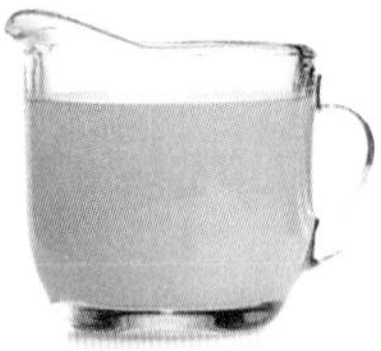

**

CLEAN

SOUP AND BROTH IN TETRA PAK

If you're buying soup or broth, know that it's safer to buy them in a Tetra Pak rather than a can.

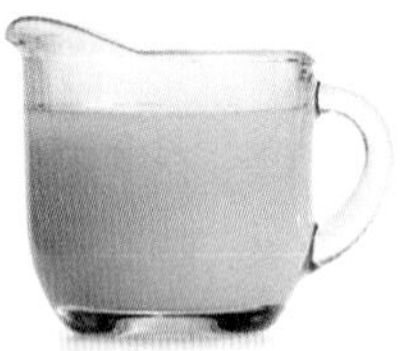

***

CLEANEST

HOMEMADE SOUPS AND BROTHS

After you've roasted a chicken, don't ditch that carcass—make a soup that's loaded with organic veggies, whole grains such as brown rice or whole wheat pasta, and beans. Start with our Homemade Bone Broth (opposite page). Not a meat eater? Try our hearty Homemade Veggie Broth (page 276) as a base for your favorite soups.

HOMEMADE BONE BROTH

Bones from 1 whole roasted chicken
2 carrots, roughly chopped
½ large onion, roughly chopped
2 cloves garlic, peeled and crushed
¾ teaspoon fine sea salt
¼ teaspoon dried rosemary
¼ teaspoon dried thyme
1 bay leaf
2 teaspoons apple cider vinegar

COMBINE all the ingredients plus 10 cups water in a large Dutch oven and bring to a boil. Reduce to a simmer, cover, and cook for 6 hours. Strain and discard the solids.

MAKES 6 CUPS ||| Prep time: 5 minutes ||| **Total time: 6 hours**

HEALTHY HACK

You'll get a boost of antioxidants from the veggies and a dose of collagen from the chicken broth, which can help heal a damaged gut and promote skin health.

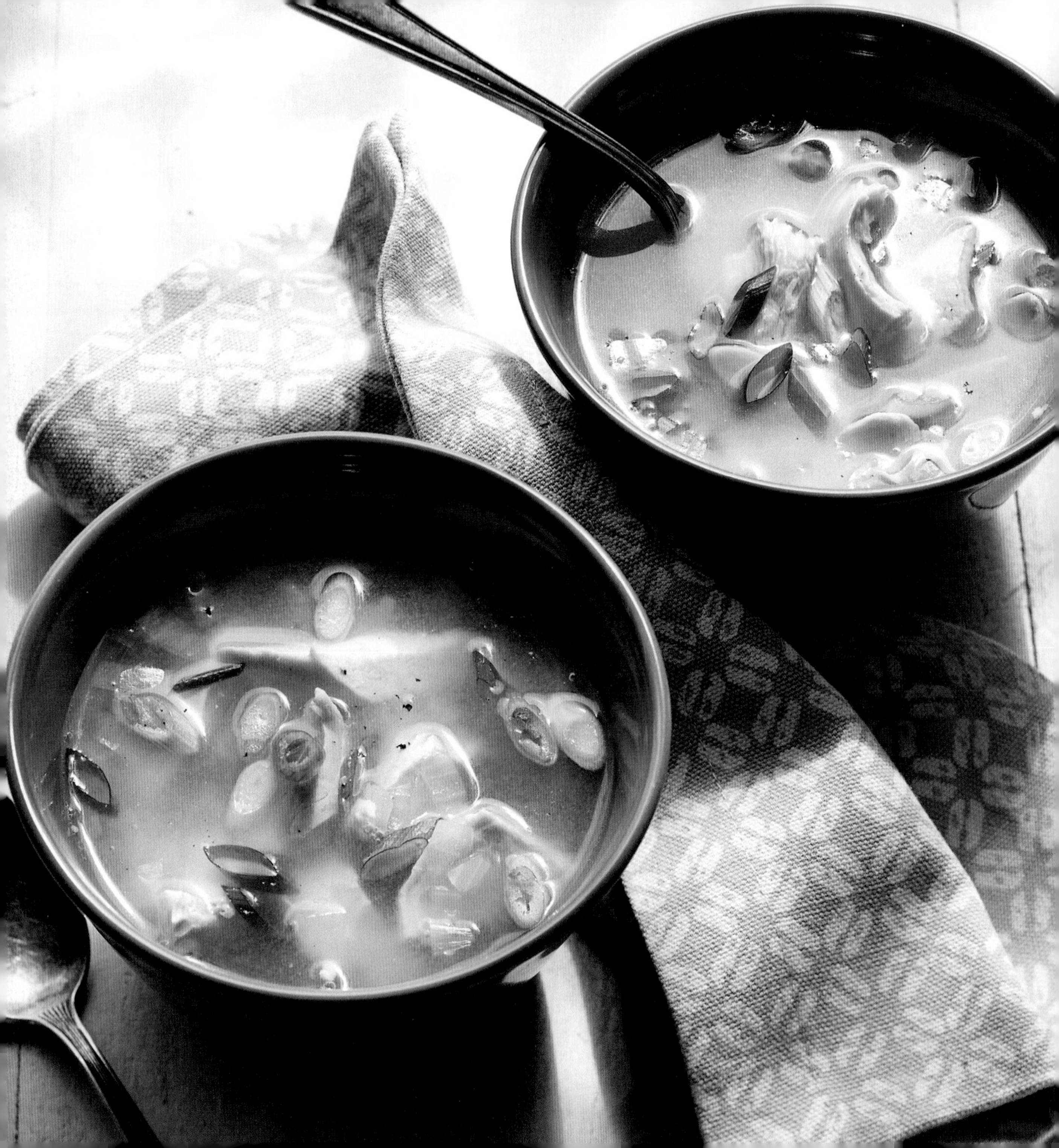

QUICK MISO-SCALLION CHICKEN SOUP

- **4 cups Homemade Bone Broth (page 273)**
- **4 teaspoons white miso paste**
- **¼ medium yellow onion, chopped**
- **½ teaspoon paprika**
- **1 clove garlic, chopped**
- **Pinch of black pepper**
- **½ pound boneless, skinless chicken breast, chopped**
- **2 scallions, sliced**

1. PLACE all the ingredients except the scallions in a saucepan over medium-high heat and bring to a boil. Reduce to a simmer and cook until the chicken is cooked through, about 15 minutes. Stir to ensure that the miso is fully incorporated.

2. LADLE the soup into 2 bowls and sprinkle with the scallions.

MAKES 2 SERVINGS ||| Prep time: 5 minutes ||| **Cook time: 20 minutes**

Did You Know?

It's not just an old wives' tale: There's something to that age-old comfort food remedy of chicken soup. Researchers have found that chicken soup prepared with lots of veggies mitigates some of the inflammation responsible for cold symptoms, like a runny nose and congestion.

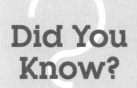

HOMEMADE VEGGIE BROTH

1 large carrot, roughly chopped
2 ribs celery, roughly chopped
1 medium onion, roughly chopped
1 medium turnip, roughly chopped
1 small sweet potato, roughly chopped
5 cremini mushrooms, halved
¾ teaspoon fine sea salt
¼ teaspoon black pepper
¼ teaspoon ground cumin
¼ teaspoon turmeric
¼ teaspoon dried oregano

COMBINE all the ingredients plus 10 cups water in a large Dutch oven and bring to a boil. Reduce to a simmer, cover, and cook for 4 hours. Strain and discard the solids.

MAKES 6 CUPS ||| Prep time: 5 minutes ||| **Total time: 4 hours**

Flavoring

Take organic vegetables, whole grains, and lean proteins to another level of flavor with the right herbs and spices. Just don't fall victim to the convenience of packaged spice blends and most conventional condiments.

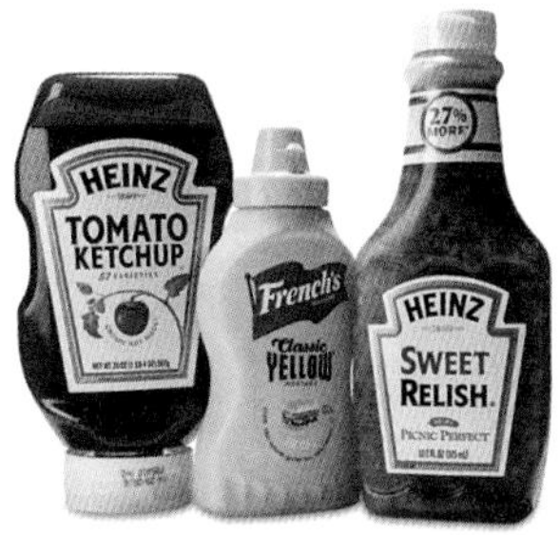

✱

NOT CLEAN

STORE-BOUGHT CONDIMENTS OR SAUCE PACKETS WITH SYNTHETIC INGREDIENTS AND ADDED SUGAR

Store-bought sauce packets and condiments generally contain synthetic ingredients as well as added sugar and salt—and bring nothing to the table as far as health benefits go.

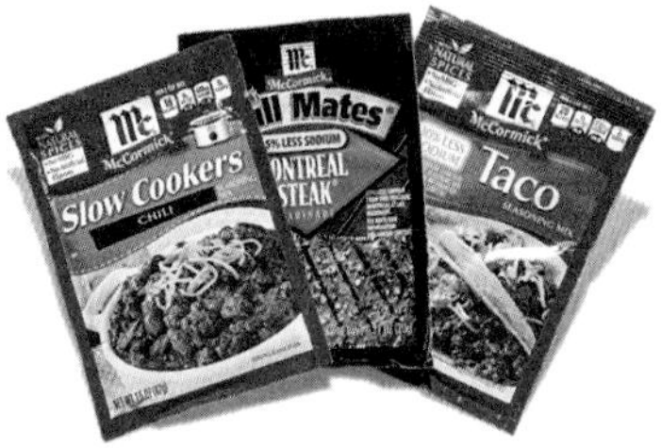

✱✱

CLEAN

STORE-BOUGHT SPICE PACKETS

These typically contain a mix of herbs, spices, and salt. They're unlikely to be organic, but they're generally not loaded with loads of funky additives and preservatives either.

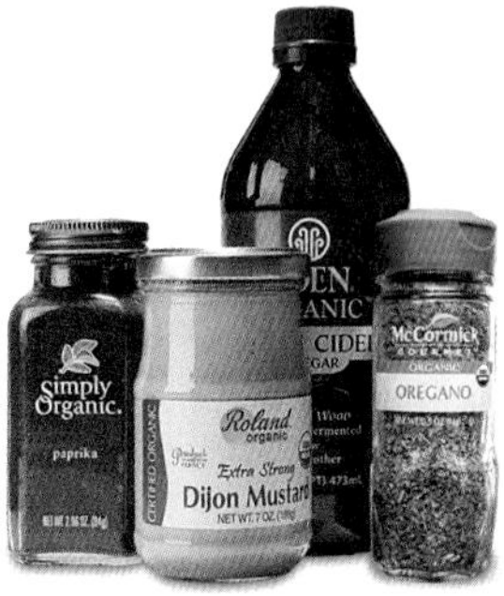

✱✱✱

CLEANEST

FRESH HERBS, ORGANIC JARRED HERBS AND SPICES, VINEGARS, SALT, MUSTARD AND OTHER LOW- OR NO-SUGAR CONDIMENTS

Use organic spices and herbs, vinegars, salt, and mustard to enhance the flavors of the meals you're preparing. All are very minimally processed and even pack health benefits of their own—herbs and spices contain a variety of antioxidants and phytonutrients, and vinegars contain acids that help curb cravings.

ITALIAN SEASONING BLEND

- **2 tablespoons dried oregano**
- **2 tablespoons dried basil**
- **2 tablespoons dried Italian parsley**
- **1 tablespoon garlic powder**
- **1 teaspoon dried thyme**
- **1 teaspoon dried rosemary**
- **1 teaspoon dried sage**

PULSE all the ingredients in a spice grinder until just mixed. Store in an airtight container.

MAKES 6 TABLESPOONS ||| Prep time: 5 minutes ||| **Total time: 5 minutes**

Keep it Fresh!

Many home cooks buy bottled herbs and spices and keep them forever and ever—or until the bottle runs dry. And while we applaud that thriftiness, the habit usually results in some less-than-stellar dinners: Herbs and spices can lose their potent flavor over time. To avoid this, purchase them in small quantities and always check that the expiration date is at least 6 months away. Store them in glass jars with tight lids (not plastic bags) and never near your oven, as heat will age them more quickly. If you have herbs that are slightly stale but still good, rub them vigorously with your hands to reactivate their flavor before adding to dishes.

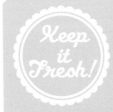

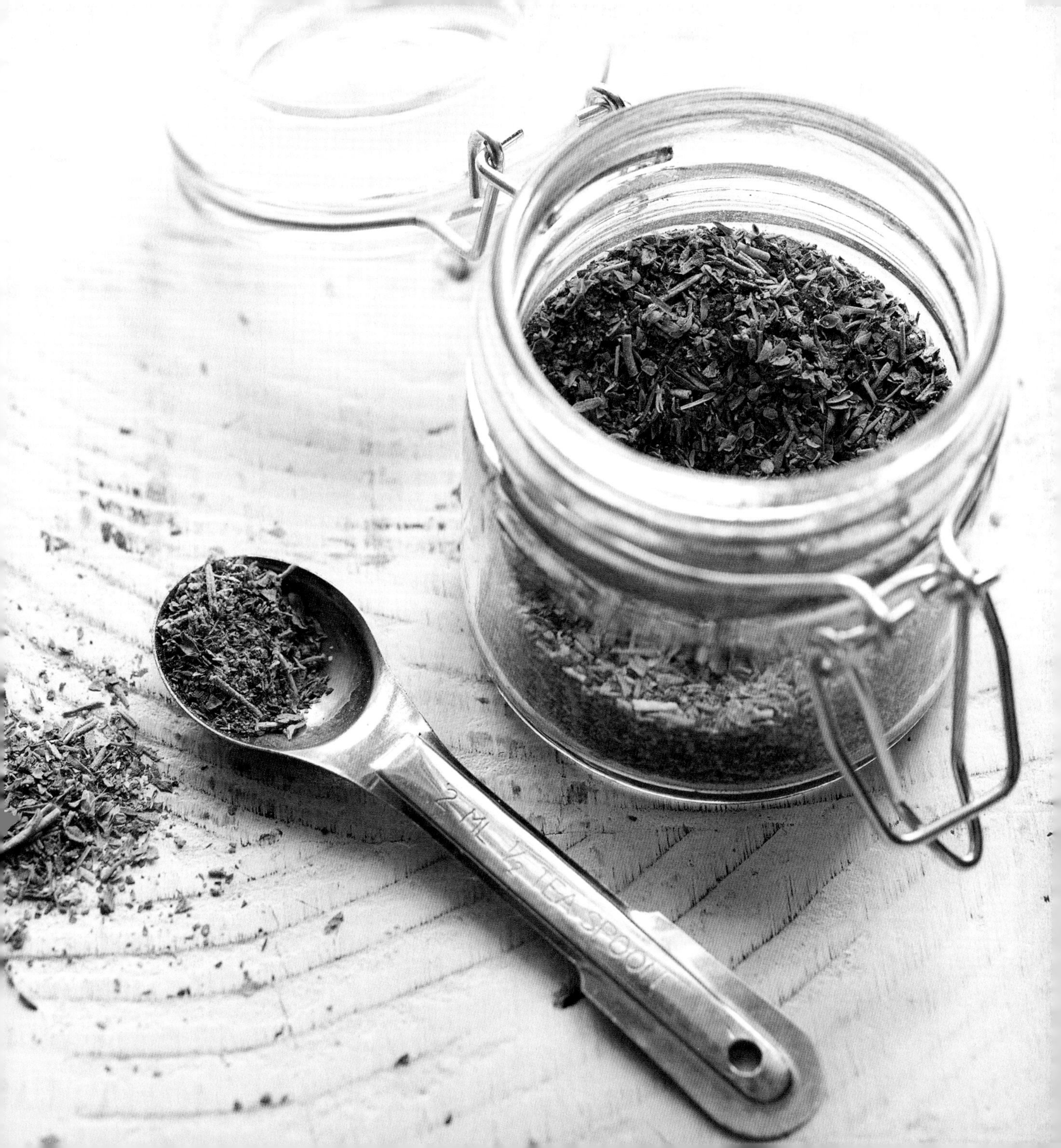
2 ML ½ TEA SPOON

CUMIN-LEMON SEA SALT

- ¼ cup sea salt
- 1 teaspoon grated lemon zest
- ¼ teaspoon ground cumin

COMBINE all the ingredients in a jar and shake vigorously for at least 10 seconds to really meld the flavors. Store in an airtight container.

MAKES ¼ CUP ||| Prep time: 5 minutes ||| **Total time: 5 minutes**

HONEY-ROSEMARY MUSTARD

- ½ cup apple cider vinegar
- ½ cup brown mustard seeds
- ½ cup yellow mustard seeds
- 1½ teaspoons kosher salt
- ½ teaspoon dried rosemary
- ¼ teaspoon black pepper
- ¼ teaspoon turmeric
- ¼ teaspoon garlic powder
- Pinch of ground cloves
- ¼ cup honey

1. **COMBINE** 1 cup water, the vinegar, mustard seeds, salt, rosemary, pepper, turmeric, garlic powder, and cloves in a bowl. Cover and let sit for 2 days.
2. **POUR** all the ingredients from the bowl into a blender or food processor. Add the honey and blend until the mustard seeds break open and the mixture looks creamy, about 5 minutes.
3. **STORE** in a sealed jar in the refrigerator.

MAKES 1¼ CUPS ||| Prep time: 10 minutes ||| **Total time: 10 minutes + 2 days soaking time**

Cooking Methods

You've filled your pantry with clean foods, so what's next?

How you cook matters, so pick a method that preserves your food's health perks and doesn't diminish them.

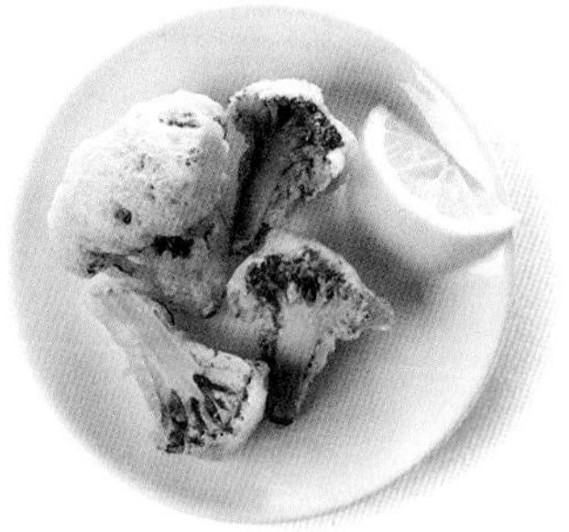

✷

NOT CLEAN

DEEP-FRY

Deep-frying is best avoided. In addition to an unhealthy amount of added fats, cooking foods at this high temperature causes cancer-causing and inflammatory compounds such as heterocyclic amines (HCAs), advanced glycation end products (AGEs), and polycyclic aromatic hydrocarbons (PAHs) to form on your food.

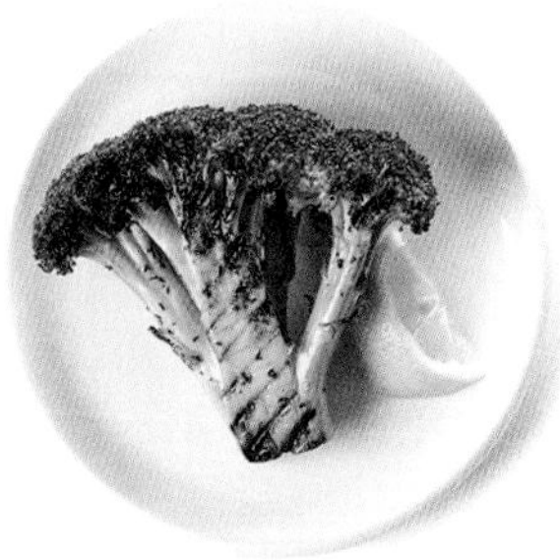

✷✷

CLEAN

GRILL WITH A MARINADE THAT'S LOW IN SUGAR

Because grilling exposes meat to such high heat, the same cancer-causing compounds (HCAs, AGEs, and PAHs) can form on your foods as deep-frying. This can be greatly diminished, however, if you use a marinade, provided it's not loaded with sugar.

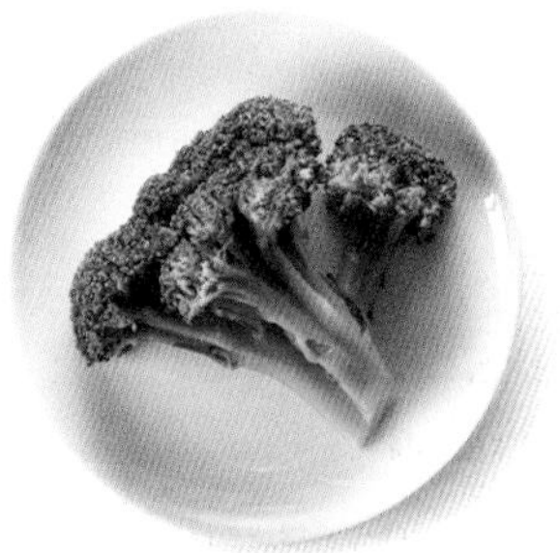

✷✷✷

CLEANEST

STEAM, BROIL, ROAST, OR PAN-FRY

To ensure maximum nutrition, steam, broil, roast, and pan-fry foods. Steaming is a great option if you want to cook without adding fat; broiling can produce the same results as grilling, but you have more control over the heat; pan-frying is a good choice for vegetables and proteins as long as you're cooking them in a healthy oil; and roasting veggies can enhance their natural sweetness.

PAN-FRIED BLACK BEAN VEGGIE PATTIES WITH SPICY GINGER-ALMOND SAUCE

- **3 teaspoons grapeseed oil**
- **¼ cup finely chopped bell pepper (any color)**
- **1 tablespoon finely chopped onion**
- **2 tablespoons finely chopped carrot**
- **1 teaspoon minced garlic**
- **⅔ cup slightly mashed cooked black beans**
- **¼ cup cooked quinoa**
- **½ teaspoon Sriracha sauce (optional)**
- **1 egg white**
- **2 tablespoons whole wheat flour**
- **1 teaspoon chili powder**
- **1 teaspoon ground cumin**
- **Fine sea salt**
- **¼ cup Spicy Ginger-Almond Sauce (page 148)**

1. HEAT 1 teaspoon of oil in a medium skillet over medium-low heat. Add the bell pepper, onion, carrot, and garlic and cook until the onion is tender and translucent, about 10 minutes.

2. TRANSFER the sautéed vegetables to a medium bowl and add the mashed beans, quinoa, Sriracha (if using), and egg white. Stir together the flour, chili powder, cumin, and a dash of salt in a small bowl. Add to the bean mixture and stir until combined. Divide and shape the mixture into 2 patties.

3. HEAT the remaining 2 teaspoons of oil in the same skillet used to cook the vegetables over medium heat. Add the patties and cook for approximately 6 minutes per side, or until slightly browned and warmed throughout.

MAKES 2 SERVINGS ||| Prep time: 10 minutes ||| **Total time: 45 minutes**

ITALIAN-HERBED BROILED TURKEY BREAST

- **¼ cup dry white wine**
- **2 tablespoons fresh lemon juice**
- **4 teaspoons grapeseed oil**
- **2 teaspoons minced garlic**
- **¼ cup finely chopped fresh basil**
- **¼ cup finely chopped fresh parsley**
- **2 tablespoons finely chopped fresh oregano**
- **4 teaspoons finely chopped fresh thyme**
- **2 teaspoons finely chopped fresh rosemary**
- **Fine sea salt and black pepper**
- **½ pound turkey breast, cut into ½-inch thick slices**

1. COMBINE the wine, lemon juice, oil, garlic, basil, parsley, oregano, thyme, rosemary, and a dash of salt and pepper in a small bowl.

2. PLACE the turkey breast slices in a shallow glass dish. Pour the marinade over the turkey. Cover and marinate in the refrigerator for 3 hours.

3. POSITION a rack 5 inches from the heat source and heat the oven to broil.

4. DRAIN the marinade from the turkey and discard. Arrange the turkey on a broiler pan and broil until cooked through, about 8 minutes, flipping halfway through. Let stand for a few minutes before serving.

MAKES 2 SERVINGS ||| Prep time: 10 minutes ||| **Total time: 20 minutes + marinating time**

HEALTHY HACK

Beer marinades can reduce levels of carcinogenic compounds that form on grilled meat in a major way. In one recent study, researchers found that marinating pork chops in a dark beer like Guinness for 4 hours reduced the levels of dangerous polycyclic aromatic hydrocarbons (PAHs) by half. The extra antioxidants in dark beer might be responsible for the benefit, as PAHs form with the help of free radicals, and antioxidants can help counter free radicals. To make a healthy marinade at home, simply whisk the following together in a bowl: 1 cup dark beer, ½ cup olive oil, ¼ cup lemon juice, 4 cloves smashed garlic, salt, pepper, and spices of your choice.

ROASTED BUTTERNUT SQUASH & MILLET BOWL WITH CRUMBLED PISTACHIOS

- **1 pound butternut squash, peeled and cut into ½-inch cubes (about 2 cups)**
- **1 tablespoon grapeseed oil**
- **Fine sea salt and black pepper**
- **½ cup minced red onion**
- **1 tablespoon finely chopped fresh rosemary**
- **1 tablespoon finely chopped fresh sage**
- **½ cup millet**
- **1¼ cups low-sodium vegetable broth**
- **½ cup finely chopped unsalted dry-roasted pistachios**

1. HEAT the oven to 400°F.

2. TOSS the butternut squash with the grapeseed oil and a dash of salt and pepper in a large bowl. Spread out in a nonstick baking sheet. Roast for 15 minutes. Remove the pan from the oven and flip the butternut squash with a metal spatula. (Leave the oven on.)

3. FOLD the red onion, rosemary, and sage into the butternut squash. Return to the oven and roast until tender and slightly browned, 10 to 15 minutes.

4. COOK the millet in a medium saucepan over medium-low heat until it turns golden brown and fragrant, about 4 minutes. Adjust to a lower heat if necessary to avoid burning the millet. Carefully add the broth to the pan and stir. Increase the heat to high and bring to a boil. Reduce to a simmer and cook until the grains have absorbed most of the broth, 10 to 15 minutes. Remove from the heat and let sit for 10 minutes.

5. COMBINE the roasted squash mixture and millet. Serve topped with the pistachios.

MAKES 2 SERVINGS ||| Prep time: 20 minutes ||| **Total time: 1 hour 15 minutes**

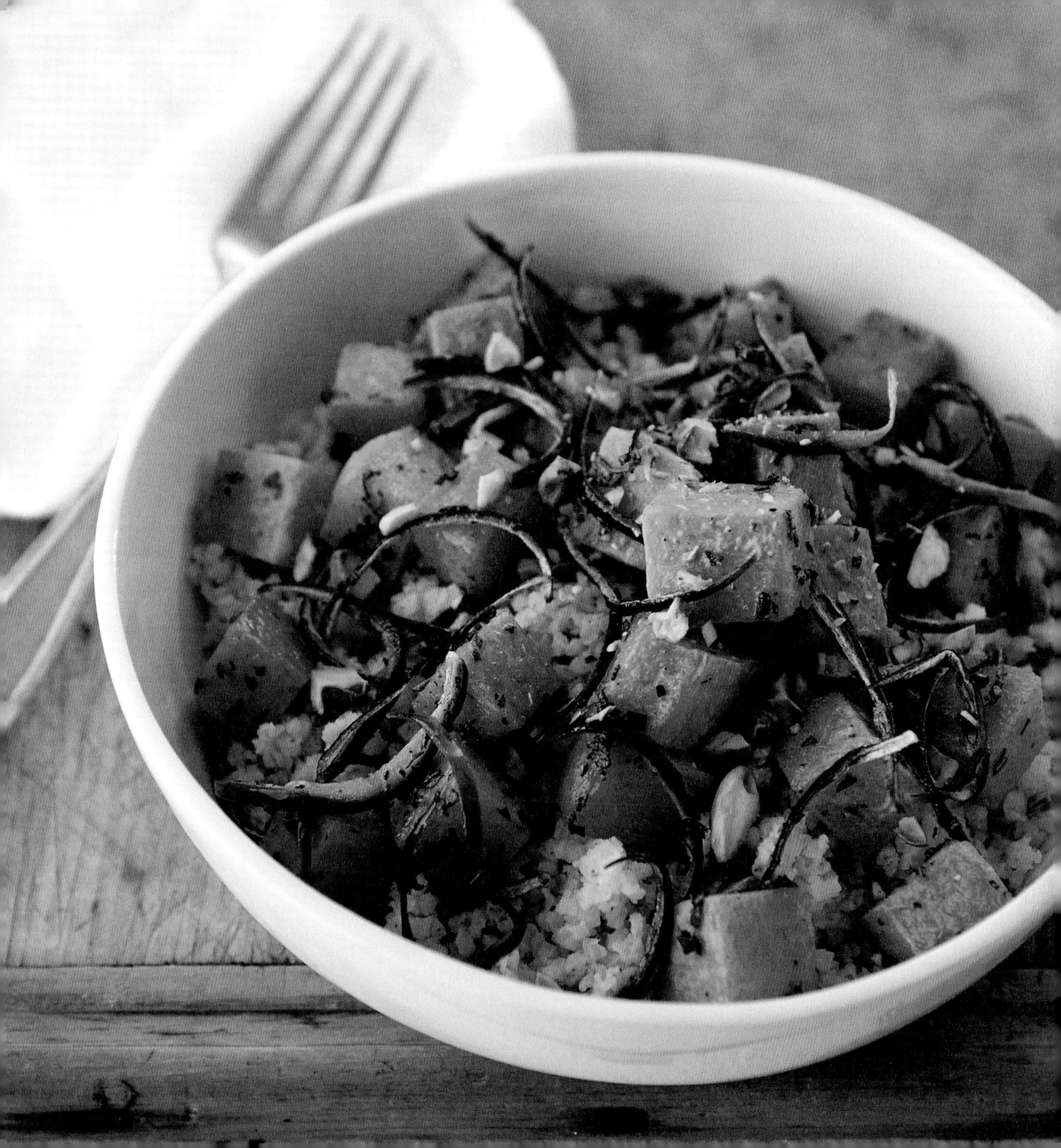

Thanks to the *Prevention* editors who helped write and create this book, mainly Stephanie Eckelkamp and Sarah Toland, along with Caroline Praderio and our leading editorial visionaries, Anne Alexander and Bruce Kelley.

We're also extremely grateful to Dr. Wendy Bazilian for immediately resonating with the concept and bringing her extensive experience in nutrition science and counseling to the *Eat Clean* team.

A special thanks to Amy King for the beautiful design and Mitch Mandel for the lovely photography throughout; to Stephanie Clarke and Willow Jarosh of C&J Nutrition for creating the mouthwatering clean meals inside these pages; to food stylist Khalil Hymore and prop stylist Kira Corbin for turning each dish into a work of art; and to food stylist Chris Barsh for making the cover really pop. Chelsea Zimmer spent a frenetic 48 hours shopping for all the delicious food featured here and even found time to bake a delicious—and clean!—apple pie.

Of course, the book would not have been possible without the tireless dedication of the Rodale book team, including senior editor Marisa Vigilante, who championed *Eat Clean, Stay Lean* from conception to finished book, and assistant editor Jess Fromm, whose dedication to every crucial detail helped turn an idea into an actual book, as well as invaluable support from senior project editor Nancy Bailey, editorial director Jennifer Levesque, and publisher Mary Ann Naples.

Underscored page references indicate boxed text. **Boldface** references indicate photographs.